Encyclopedia of Parkinson's Dis
Novel Treatments

Volume VII

Encyclopedia of Parkinson's Disease: Novel Treatments

Volume VII

Edited by **Kate White**

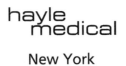

hayle
medical

New York

Published by Hayle Medical,
30 West, 37th Street, Suite 612,
New York, NY 10018, USA
www.haylemedical.com

Encyclopedia of Parkinson's Disease: Novel Treatments
Volume VII
Edited by Kate White

International Standard Book Number: 978-1-63241-195-2 (Hardback)

Printed in the United States of America.

Contents

Preface

The world is advancing at a fast pace like never before. Therefore, the need is to keep up with the latest developments. This book was an idea that came to fruition when the specialists in the area realized the need to coordinate together and document essential themes in the subject. That's when I was requested to be the editor. Editing this book has been an honour as it brings together diverse authors researching on different streams of the field. The book collates essential materials contributed by veterans in the area which can be utilized by students and researchers alike.

The novel treatments in the field of Parkinson's disease (PD) are discussed in this book. Recent Parkinson's disease medications treat symptoms; though none decrease the rate of dopaminergic neuron degeneration. Parkinson's disease is caused mainly due to the death of dopaminergic neurons in the substantia nigra. The primary problem in development of neuroprotective therapies is a restricted comprehension of the crucial molecular mechanisms that incite neurodegeneration. The discovery of PD genes has led to the hypothesis that dysfunction of the ubiquitin-proteasome pathway and misfolding of proteins are both critical to pathogenesis of the disease and earlier labeled as responsible in the neurodegeneration of this disease, oxidative stress, and mitochondrial dysfunction may also act in part by causing the collection of misfolded proteins, along with the production of other harmful events in dopaminergic neurons. Models based on neurotoxin have been crucial in explaining the molecular cascade of cell death in dopaminergic neurons. PD models based on the manipulation of PD genes should prove crucial in explaining significant characteristics of the disease, like selective vulnerability of substantia nigra dopaminergic neurons to the degenerative process. This book includes important topics in the novel treatments of PD such as distribution & regulation of G-protein, inflammation in PD, embryonic stem cells in PD and the role of neuropeptide substance.

Each chapter is a sole-standing publication that reflects each author's interpretation. Thus, the book displays a multi-facetted picture of our current understanding of application, resources and aspects of the field. I would like to thank the contributors of this book and my family for their endless support.

Editor

Distribution and Regulation of the G Protein-Coupled Receptor Gpr88 in the Striatum: Relevance to Parkinson's Disease

Renaud Massart[1], Pierre Sokoloff[3] and Jorge Diaz[1,2]
[1] INSERM UMR-894, Psychiatry and Neurosciences Center, Paris,
[2]Paris Descartes University, Faculty of Pharmacy / Laboratory
of Neurobiology and Molecular Pharmacology
(UMRs894 INSERM), Paris,
[3]Pierre Fabre Research Institute, Neurology and Psychiatry Department, Castres,
France

1. Introduction

The human basal ganglia constitutes a functional neural network located at the base of the forebrain. It receives most of its afferent inputs through the striatum, the major nucleus of the basal ganglia accomplishing fast neurotransmitter-mediated operations through somatotopically organized projections to the principal neuron cell type, the striatal GABAergic spiny projection neurons. This spiny projection neurons, which make up 95 % of the neuron population of striatum (Kemp & Powell 1971), receive excitatory glutamatergic inputs from all areas of the cortex and specific thalamic nuclei (Gerfen & Wilson 1996; Bolam et al., 2000; Voorn et al., 2004; Doig et al., 2010), and also modulatory dopaminergic inputs from the substantia nigra pars compacta (Smith & Kieval 2000; Utter. & Basso 2008). Spiny Projection Neurons include two major subpopulations giving rise to the direct striato-nigral pathway, and the indirect striato-pallidal pathway which communicates information to the basal ganglia output structures; the internal segment of the globus pallidus and the substantia nigra pars reticulata (Smith, Y. & Kieval 2000; Gerfen & Wilson 1996). Although the two neuron subpopulations are GABAergic, they differ in a number of properties including the expression of different complements of dopamine, Adenosine, NMDA and acetylcholine receptor subtypes as well as of peptide content; the direct striato-nigral pathway neurons coexpress substance P and dynorphin, whereas the indirect striato-pallidal pathway neurons express enkephalin (Gerfen et al., 1990, 1991; Reiner & Anderson 1990; Gerfen & Wilson 1996; Le Moine & Bloch, 1995).

Based on the fact that striatal medium-spiny neurons are the major input targets and the major projection neurons of striatum, it is thought that integration of neurotransmission in these neurons is an important determinant of the functional organization of the striatum. Thus, changes in neurotransmission on striatal spiny projection neurons have been involved in the regulation of voluntary movement, behavioral control, cognitive function and reward mechanisms. For instance, massive spiny projection neuron loss and major dopamine deficits in striatum lead to severe motor disorders, such as the excess of involuntary movements encountered in Huntington's disease and the rigidity and poverty of movements that typifies Parkinson's disease, respectively (Ross et al., 1997; Wolfgang & Stanley, 2003). Therefore, investigations addressed to characterize new receptor proteins displaying high densities and potential involvement in neurotransmission mechanisms within the striatum can provide new insight into the basal ganglia physiology and pathophysiology and also new clues for therapy of severe motor disorders.

A previous study reported a novel striatum-specific transcript, the strg/Gpr88, encoding an orphan G protein-coupled receptor of human and rodents (Mizushima et al., 2000). It display highest sequence homology with 5HT1D and β3 receptors. Since the original description, little data have been documented on the biological function (s) and the the cellular and subcellular distribution of the Gpr88 protein. Hence, the Gpr88 endogenous putative ligand, the detailed Gpr88 protein distribution and GPR88 functional roles are unknown. One approach to gain functional insights into this novel gene coding for an orphan receptor is the precise analysis of its spatial and temporal expression to provide information about the neural morphological substrates supporting Gpr88 functions in the striatal complex.

Hence, the present findings provide *in situ* hybridization and light-level immunohistochemical evidence for Gpr88 localization in the rat and monkey striatum and its subcellular distribution in striatal neurons by using a validated polyclonal antibody specifically recognizing Gpr88, (Massart et al 2009). We also describe morphological data on the spatiotemporal Gpr88 expression in the developing rat striatum, suggesting that both nigrostriatal and corticostriatal pathways control its normal striatal pattern of expression. Using treatments with l-DOPA and dopamine antagonists, in unilateral 6-hydroxydopamine- and cortical ibotenate-lesioned rats, we further demonstrated that striatal Gpr88 expression is modulated by dopamine- and glutamate-regulated mechanisms involving trans-synaptic influences of the corticostriatal pathway input activity.

2. Widespread Gpr88 expression within the striatal complex

Using *in situ* hybridization and immunohistochemistry approaches, we demonstrated that Gpr88 mRNA and protein expression are specially abundant within restricted basal telencephalic structures including the dorsal striatum, nucleus accumbens, and olfactory tubercle and also in the inferior olivary complex (Fig. 1).

2.1 All striatal GABAergic spiny projection neurons express Gpr88

Gpr88 is expressed throughout the two anatomical and functional patch/striosome-matrix compartments in the rat and monkey striatal complex (Figures 1F, 2A) with higher receptor expression in patch/striosome than in the surrounding matrix compartment. The prevalence of Gpr88 in the patch/striosome compartment and also within the dorsolateral striatal sector, indicates that Gpr88 may play a central role in the modulation of both limbic and motor cortical-basal ganglia circuits (Ragsdale & Graybiel; 1988; Graybiel A.M., 1995; Gerfen & Wilson, 1996). Immunofluorescent stainings and double labelling *in situ* hybridization experiments demonstrated that Gpr88 is present in all the spiny projection neurons of both the direct striato-nigral pathway and the indirect striato-pallidal pathway (Figure 2 C,D).

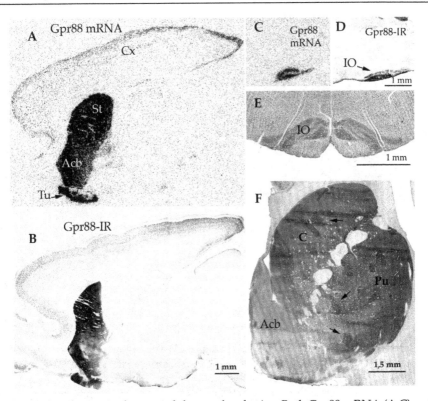

Fig. 1. Gpr88 distribution in the rat and the monkey brains. Both Gpr88 mRNA (A,C) and Gpr88 protein (B,D,E,F) are particularly concentrated throughout the striatum (St), nucleus accumbens (Acb), olfactory tubercle (Tu) and the inferior olive complex (IO) of the rat (A-E). Similar levels and distribution-pattern of Gpr88 immunorreactivity is detected in nucleus caudatus (C), putamen (Pu) and nucleus accumbens (Acb) of the monkey brain (F). Significant levels of Gpr88 are also present with a laminar distribution throughout the neocortex. Arrows in (F), point out small and intense Gpr88 stained areas corresponding to striosome striatal subcompartments. RT-QPCR data from rodents suggest that Gpr88 displays the highest expression levels compared to other known GPCRs of the striatum (Massart et al., 2007, 2008). The pattern of Gpr88 throughout the striatum of adult rats and monkeys is characterized by widespread distribution and regional differences (Figure 1), suggesting a central role of this orphan receptor in the modulation of sensorimotor related informations (Flaherty & Graybiel1994; Voorn et al., 2004). Although Gpr88 is prevalent in the striatal complex, we also detected moderate levels of both Gpr88 transcripts and protein throughout the cerebral neocortex (Figure 1A,B). Both signals display a similar non-homogeneous laminar distribution characterized by higher expression in the upper neocortical layers II-IV than in the lower layers V-VI. No Gpr88 expression was detected in the cortical layer I. Moreover, cortical Gpr88 expression represents about 20% of the GPR88 striatal expression, as assessed by different quantitive approaches including Western blot, immunohistochemistry and *in situ* hybridization. Double immuno-fluorescent labellings for Gpr88 and different neural cell-type specific markers have demonstrated that Gpr88 is an exclusive neuronal receptor of the brain, being absent from glial cells (Massart et al., 2009).

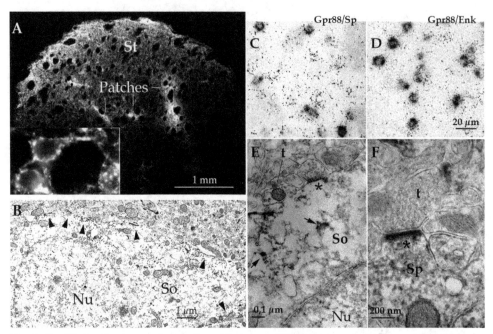

Fig. 2. Gpr88 distribution in the rat dorsal striatum. (A) The immunofluorescent Gpr88 signal is heterogeneously distributed within the dorsal striatum and characterized by its marked concentration in the striatal dorsolateral region and the patches compartments. The inset illustrates putative medium spiny neurons displaying intense Gpr88 labelling on the cell surface along the soma and dendrites. (C, D) double-labelling *in situ* hybridization indicates that all Substance P (dark-stained cells in C) and enkephalin (dark-stained cells in D) neurons, also express Gpr88 transcripts (detected by silver grain labellings). The distribution of the electron-dense immunoreactive reaction product, reflects the subcellular GPR88 presence in submembranous sites around the perikaryon (arrow-heads in B asterisk and arrows in E). The receptor is concentrated in symmetrical synapses in the cell body (asterisk in E) but also in asymmetrical synapses (asterisk in F) in dendritic spines (Sp). Note the absence of immunolabelling in synaptic contacts of two adjacent nerve terminals (t) in E. (Enk) Enkephalin, (Nu) Cell nucleus, (So) neuronal cell body, (Sp) Substance P in C, (Sp) dendritic spine in F.

Electron microscopic analysis of the Gpr88 immunolabelling in the rat dorsal striatum demonstrated a high proportion of electron dense Gpr88 positive dendritic spines, dendrite shafts and cell bodies (Figure 2 B,E,F) that are characteristic features of GABAergic spiny projection neurons (Somogyi et al., 1982; Bolam et al., 1983). However, no axonal or terminal Gpr88 immunolabeled profiles were observed. Likewise, globus pallidus and substantia nigra pars reticulata, two basal ganglia regions receiving the striato-pallidal and striato-nigral terminals respectively (Surmeier et al., 2007), lack Gpr88 immunoreactivity. All these morphological findings highlight a potential functional role for Gpr88 in synaptic events occurring on somatodendritic compartments and their integration in striato-nigral and striato-pallidal medium spiny neurons. Gpr88 immunoreactivity was often concentrated on discrete postsynaptic sub-membranous sites in a large proportion of asymmetrical (excitatory) synapses that generally receive glutamate as neurotransmitter (Bouyer et al., 1984; Bolam et al., 2000) and also on symmetrical (inhibitory) synapses which could be supplied by terminals originating from GABAergic aspiny or cholinergic interneurons or even by intrastriatal GABAergic axon-collaterals from medium-spiny projection neurons. Double immunofluorescent labellings in the same section demonstrated no association between Gpr88 immunoreactivity and tyrosine hydroxylase immunolabelled axon-terminals. In contrast, the Gpr88 immunoreactive signal was often juxtaposed to most vesicular glutamate transporter1 immunoreactive terminals, indicating that Gpr88 is preferentially located on synapses supplied by cortical inputs, rather than by vesicular glutamate transporter2 immunoreactive thalamic inputs contacting medium spiny neurons (Herzog et al., 2001; Kaneko & Fujiyama, 2002; Fremeau et al., 2004). Moreover, electron microscopy analysis demonstrates that Gpr88 immunoreactive signal is often present on the head of spines, where corticostriatal inputs mainly contact the dendritic tree of striatal spiny projection neurons (Bouyer et al., 1984; Dube et al., 1988; Ribak & Roberts 1990; Smith et al., 1994).

The preferential subcellular distribution of Gpr88 in striatal asymmetrical synapses of virtually all GABAergic projection neurons suggests a role for Gpr88 in the modulation of medium spiny neurons activity to cortical glutamatergic inputs and a potential role in the regulation of the flow of cortical information through the basal ganglia. Several lines of evidence indicate that cortical excitatory signals are modulated by dopaminergic synaptic contacts located on the neck of spines (Arbuthnott et al., 2000). Gpr88 location at specific synaptic sites, where corticostriatal and nigrostriatal afferents converge, further suggests involvement of Gpr88 in the modulation of both glutamatergic and dopaminergic signals received by the striatal medium spiny neurons.

3. Spatial and temporal Gpr88 expression in the developing rat striatum

To gain functional insights into striatal Gpr88 we have determined the profile of GPR88 expression in the prenatal and postnatal developing striatum of the rat by *in situ* hybridization and immunohistochemistry. Morphological data indicate that Gpr88 expression emerges with a homogeneous distribution, in the ventrolateral portion of the developing striatum at the embryonic day 16 (E16) of rat development (Figure 3A,B,C), a time when striatal neurons are both morphologically and functionally immature (van der Kooy & Fishell, 1987) and also when the patch-matrix striatal compartments, are not yet differentiated. The homogeneous Gpr88 mRNA distribution becomes heterogeneous when clusters of developing neurons displaying dense Gpr88 expression are seen throughout the dorsal and ventral striatal regions by the fetal stage E19-E20 (Figures 3D,E). Using double immunohistochemistry stained brain sections for Gpr88 and tyrosine hydroxylase, we confirmed that rich Gpr88 small areas strictly match the densely dopamine innervated striatal patch/striosome compartments (Gerfen et al., 1987). Levels of Gpr88 expression in patches compartments increase until the end of the first postnatal week and then decline in the second postnatal week with the ongoing development to eventually reach adult expression levels. Such developmental profile of Gpr88 expression in the prenatal and postnatal rat striatum suggests that the pattern of Gpr88 expression may be under the influence of afferent inputs reaching to the striatal primordia. This idea is based on the fact that the patchy-pattern profile of intense GPR88 expression in developing rat striatum closely matches the reported spatial and temporal development of the nigrostriatal dopamine afferents (Voorn et al., 1988), suggesting that the nigral dopamine inputs influence the patterning of striatal GPR88 expression. Such type of influence by the dopamine inputs has been demonstrated for the establishment of the pattern of opiate receptors expression in the embryonic patch compartment (van der Kooy & Fishell, 1992). The cortical projections are the second major afferent input to the striatum that may act in concert with nigral dopamine inputs to guide development of striatal subcompartment phenotypes. For instance, studies in the monkey have shown the patchy distribution of corticostriatal afferents before the day of birth (Goldman-Rakic, 1981). Moreover, organotypic assays involving co-cultures of the striatum with substantia nigra or cortex indicate that afferents from these structures have a prominent influence on the development of striatal patch/matrix compartments (Snyder-Keller & Costantini 1996; Snyder-Keller et al., 2001; Snyder-Keller, 2004). The mutual influence of dopaminergic and glutamatergic pathways within the developing striatum is probably important for the setting up of striatal neurotransmission circuits, as previously shown by dopamine manipulations that influence corticostriatal synaptic configurations (Meshul & Tan, 1994; Meshul et al., 1999; Meshul & Allen, 2000; Avila-Costa et al., 2005). These observations support the idea that cortical glutamatergic inputs and/or dopamine glutamate interactions may exert a control on Gpr88 expression in the developing medium spiny neurons.

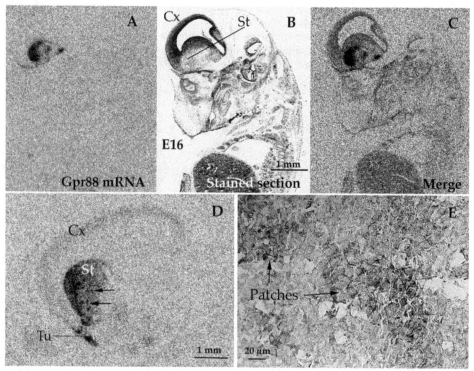

Fig. 3. Developmental profile of Gpr88 expression in the rat striatum. Gpr88 mRNA (A, D) and Gpr88-protein (E) expression in the developing striatum. (A) Homogeneous distribution of Gpr88 transcripts in the dorsolateral sector of differentiating striatum at E16. (D) Heterogeneous distribution of Gpr88-mRNA at E19. (F) Clusters of striatal developing neurons displaying dense Gpr88 immunoreactive signal (Gpr88-rich patches) at E20. (Cx) cortex, (St) striatum, (Tu) olfactory tubercle.

Although dopamine and glutamate afferents are the most likely candidates to modulate Gpr88 expression in developing medium-spiny projection neurons, other factors associated with nigral and cortical inputs may also play an important role in controlling Gpr88 expression within the striatal primordium. For instance, the nigrostriatal and corticostriatal pathways supply the striatum with brain-derived neurotrophic factor (BDNF) (Altar et al., 1997; Seroogy et al., 1994) which has been shown to influence survival, sprouting, and synaptogenesis in different neural systems (Hammond et al., 1999; Alsina et al., 2001; Mamounas et al., 2000). Moreover, studies in mature animals have shown that BDNF has profound effects on neurotransmission, activity-dependent synaptic remodeling, neurogenesis and receptors expression (Altar et al., 1997; Lessmann, 1998; Guillin et al., 2001; Tanaka et al., 2008; Taliaz, 2010). Rather than exclusive effects of either dopamine or glutamate on striatal Gpr88, continuous interplay among afferent signaling systems, including dopamine, glutamate and BDNF, is likely to refine the pattern expression of Gpr88 throughout the period of striatal development. Based on the spatiotemporal profile of GPR88 expression during striatal differentiation, we propose that the early receptor expression is modulated at least in part through a nigrostriatal and corticostriatal pathway dependent mechanisms. In support to the hypothesis of BDNF regulating Gpr88 expression during development, heterozygote BDNF-knockout mice have diminished Gpr88 mRNA levels in both the caude putamen and the shell of the nucleus accumbens (Massart et al., 2005).

4. Modulation of striatal Gpr88 expression by nigrostriatal and corticostriatal pathways in the rat in a model of Parkinson's disease

The demonstration of the regulation of striatal Gpr88 expression by nigrostriatal dopamine and cortical glutamate inputs was carried out in a rat model of Parkinson's disease (Schwarting & Huston 1996; Massart et al., 2009). Unilateral lesion of dopamine nigrostriatal pathway, caused by infusion of 6-OHDA in the medial forebrain bundle, produced a decrease in Gpr88 protein and mRNA expressions (Table 1). However, *in situ* hybridization analysis with double labelling showed that the effects of dopamine depletion were different in the two subpopulations of striatal medium spiny neurons. At the cellular level, 6-OHDA lesion induced a decrease in mRNA expression in striato-pallidal pathway neurons and inversely, a rise in striato-nigral projection neurons, in the dopamine depleted striatum (Table 1). Recently reported data (Heiman et al., 2008; Massart et al., 2009) showed that striatal Gpr88 mRNA expression is twice as high in striato-pallidal output neurons as in striato-nigral output neurons of rodents, the overall lesion-induced Gpr88 downregulation is consistent with the strong decrease in Gpr88 expression occurring in striato-pallidal pathway neurons, not compensated by the limited increase occurring in striato-nigral pathway neurons. These opposed variations are nearly completely reversed by a typical antiparkinsonian treatment with l-DOPA (Table 1).

Our finding revealed that D1 receptors, but not D2 receptors, activation exerts a positive influence on Gpr88 expression in the indirect striato-pallidal pathway of the dopamine-depleted hemisphere. On the contrary, D2 receptors stimulation controls Gpr88 expression in the direct striato-nigral pathway. This is rather surprising since D1 and D2 receptors are largely segregated to striatal neurons of the striato-nigral and striato-pallidal pathways, respectively (Gerfen et al., 1990; Le Moine & Bloch, 1995). In fact, in striato-pallidal medium spiny neurons harboring D2 receptors/Enk, in contrast to striato-nigral medium spiny

	Treatment	Gpr88 protein – immunohistochemistry		Gpr88 mRNA - *In situ* hybridization					
				Total mRNA		mRNA / SP+ cells		mRNA / ENK+ cells	
		Intact	Lesioned	Intact	Lesioned	Intact	Lesioned	Intact	Lesioned
6-OHDA lesion	Vehicle	107 ± 3.8	91 ± 2.9 *	69 ± 3.2	56 ± 1.4 *	22 ± 1.4	29 ± 1.9 ***	42 ± 2.1	31 ± 1.8 ***
	L- DOPA	99 ± 5.1	90 ± 4.6	73 ± 4.2	70 ± 3.7	22 ± 1.4	26 ± 1.7	40 ± 0.8	38 ± 1.3
	L-DOPA + SCH23390	108 ± 5.9	92 ± 5.6	76 ± 6.8	62 ± 3.2	23 ± 2.7	21 ± 1.6	43 ± 3.3	26 ± 4.3 ***
	L-DOPA + Haloperidol	100 ± 5.5	92 ± 6.1	74 ± 4.4	75 ± 3.0	37 ± 1.9 ***	26 ± 0.9	40 ± 1.4	39 ± 1.1
Ibotenate lesion	Vehicle	107 ± 3	83 ± 3 ***	89 ± 3.8	78 ± 1.9 ***	19 ± 0.5	17 ± 0.5	32 ± 0.9	23 ± 1.2 ***

Table 1. Effects on Gpr88 expression of dopamine depletion, induced by unilateral 6-OHDA infusion into the medial forebrain bundle, or of a bilateral lesion of the cortex induced by multiple infusions of ibotenate. All data are expressed as group mean ±SEM. The raw data for 6-OHDA (nigro-striatal) lesion were analysed by two-way ANOVA with lesion and treatment as independent variable and the Bonferroni test for multiple comparisons was applied in post hoc analysis to determine which values were significantly different. For data from ibotenate-induced lesion, the Student's unpaired two-tailed t-test was used to compare Ibotenate-injected vs. vehicle-injected rats. Alpha level level was set at 0.05. GraphPad 5 software (La Jolla, California, USA) was used to perform statistical analysis . * $P < 0.05$; **$P < 0.01$; ***$P < 0.001$ vs. intact side (6-OHDA lesion) or intact, vehicle-infused animals (ibotenate lesion). See Massart et al. 2009 for details.

neurons containing D1 receptors/Sp, Gpr88 expression was downregulated by the 6-OHDA lesion and the reversion of this effect by l-DOPA was dependent on D1 receptor stimulation, as indicated by its blockade by the D1 receptor-selective antagonist SCH23390, but not by haloperidol, a D2 receptor-selective antagonist (Table 1). In parallel, in D1 receptor/Sp-expressing striato-nigral neurons, Gpr88 expression was upregulated by the lesion, in contrast to D2 receptor/Enk striato-pallidal output neurons. The reversion of this effect by l-DOPA was dependent of D2 receptors stimulation, as indicated by the absence of effects of SCH23390 (Table 1). Moreover, co-administration of l-DOPA and D2-receptor antagonist haloperidol raised Gpr88 expression in striato-nigral medium spiny neurons of the contralateral hemisphere (See Massart et al 2009; Taymans., 2005).

These results suggest that l-DOPA effects on Gpr88, in each of the two medium spiny neuron subsets, are not directly mediated by the respective dopamine receptor subtypes they express, but indirectly by dopamine receptor transmission through a different neurotransmitter afferent input to the medium spiny neurons. In particular l-DOPA and intrastriatal dopamine transmission can act as a neuromodulator of glutamate release in the dopamine depleted striatum (Jonkers et al., 2002; David et al., 2005; Stephens 2005). l-DOPA effects on Gpr88 expression in striato-pallidal pathway neurons are likely regulated through D1 receptor present on the soma and dendrites of excitatory corticostriatal projection neurons, leading to activation of the corticostriatal inputs. In contrast, l-DOPA/D2 receptors stimulation-induced Gpr88 decrease in striato-nigral neurons was probably mediated by reduced glutamate release from corticostriatal inputs by stimulation of presynaptic D2 receptors (Cepeda et al., 2001). Thus, l-DOPA-induced differential changes in Gpr88 levels on both striato-nigral and striato-pallidal medium spiny neurons, may be mediated through dopamine-induced influences in corticostriatal glutamatergic neurotransmission mechanisms, as previously suggested for the modulation of other striatal markers expressed in these neurons (Uhl et al., 1988; Salin et al., 1997; Zeng et al., 2000; Blandini et al., 2003; Robelet et al 2004; Carta et al., 2005).

In support to the above hypothesis, corticostriatal deafferentation, elicited by ibotenate infusions, induced a marked Gpr88 mRNA and protein down-regulation in striato-pallidal neurons without significantly affecting Gpr88 in striato-nigral neurons (Table 1). These data agree with the involvement of corticostriatal glutamatergic input in the effects of dopamine depletion induced Gpr88 changes in the striatal medium spiny projections neurons, and with a greater influence of cortical inputs on Gpr88 expression in the striato-pallidal pathway neurons.

5. Conclusions

Gpr88 is an important constituent of the basal ganglia, being one of the most abundant GPCR in this brain region. Although its function is unknown, detailed analysis of its gene expression in striatal spiny projection neurons suggests that Gpr88 has typical features of a GPCR in charge of transducing extracellular signals. First, it is expressed at the plasma membrane of striatal medium-spiny projection neurons, and probably exposed to the extracellular signals. Second, establishment of Gpr88 expression during development is concomitant with major dopaminergic and glutamatergic afferences reaching the embryonic striatum. Third, Gpr88 expression is enriched in the patch/striosome compartment, which suggests its involvement in the modulation of both limbic and motor cortical-basal ganglia circuits. Fourth, Gpr88 expression is influenced by modifications of cortical and nigral inputs to medium spiny neurons occurring in a situation modeling the pronounced loss of dopamine-producing neurons, occurring in Parkinson's disease.

Striato-nigral and striato-pallidal pathways neurons play an important role in integrating circuits of the basal ganglia/basal forebrain and finding on new proteins in these two major striatal output pathways, may contribute to a better understanding of certain pathophysiologic states (e.g., movement and psychiatric disorders). Hence, the rich and selective expression of GPR88 in the two striatal subpopulations medium-spiny projection neurons, directly receiving dopaminergic and glutamatergic inputs provides an anatomical basis for potential therapeutic applications, particularly in the striatum where modulation of glutamatergic and dopaminergic functions have important consequences for Parkinson's disease and its treatment.

6. References

Altar, C. A.; Cai, N.; Bliven, T.; Juhasz, M.; Conner, J. M.; Acheson, A. L.; Lindsay, R. M. & Wiegand, S. J. (1997) Anterograde transport of brain-derived neurotrophic factor and its role in the brain. *Nature*, Vol. 389, No. 6653, (February 1998), pp. 856-860, ISSN 0028-0836

Alsina, B.; Vu, T. & Cohen-Cory S. 2001. Visualizing synapse formation in arborizing optic axons in vivo: dynamics and modulation by BDNF. *Nat Neurosci.*, Vol. 4, No. 11, (October 2001), pp. 1093-1101, ISSN 1097-6256

Arbuthnott, G. W.; Ingham, C. A. & Wickens, J. R. (2000). Dopamine and synaptic plasticity in the neostriatum. *J Anat.*, Vol. 196, No.4 , (August 2000), pp. 587-596 ISSN 0021-8782

Avila-Costa, M. R.; Colın-Barenque, L.; Aley-Medina, P.; Valdez, A. L.; Librado, J. L.; Martinez, E. F. & Fortoul, T. I. (2005). Bilateral increase of perforated synapses after unilateral dopamine depletion. *Int. J. Neurosci.*, Vol. 115, No. 1, (March 2005), pp. 79–86, ISSN 0020-7454

Blandini, F.; Fancellu, R.; Orzi, F.; Conti, G.; Greco, R.; Tassorelli, C. & Nappi G. (2003). Selective stimulation of striatal dopamine receptors of the D1 or D2-class causes opposite changes of fos expression in the rat cerebral cortex. Eur. *J. Neurosci.*, Vol. 17, No. 4, (February 2003), pp. 763-70, ISSN 0953-816X

Bolam, J. P.; Somogyi, P.; Takagi, H.; Fodor, I. & Smith, A. D. (1983). Localisation of substance P-like immunoreactivity in neurons and nerve terminals in the neostriatum of the rat: a correlated light and electron microscopic study. *J. Neurocytol.*, Vol. 12, No. 2, (April 1983), pp. 325-344, ISSN 0300-4864

Bolam, J. P.; Hanley, J. J.; Booth, P. A. C. & Bevan, M. D. (2000). Synaptic organisation of the basal ganglia. *J. Anat.*, Vol. 196, No. 4, (August 2000), pp. 527-542, ISSN 0021-8782

Bouyer, J. J.; Park D. H.; Joh, T. H. & Pickel V. M. (1984). Chemical and structural analysis of the relation between cortical inputs and tyrosine hydroxylase-containing terminals in rat neostriatum. *Brain Research*, Vol. 302, No. 2, (June 1984), pp. 267-275, ISSN 0006-8993

Carta, A. R.; Tronci, E.; Pinna, A. & Morelli M. (2005). Different responsiveness of striatonigral and striatopallidal neurons to L-DOPA after a subchronic intermittent L-DOPA treatment. *Eur. J. Neurosci.*, Vol. 21, No. 5, (April 2005), pp. 1196-204, ISSN 0953-816X

Cepeda, C.; Hurst, R. S.; Altemus, K. L.; Flores-Hernandez, J.; Calvert. C. R.; Jokel, E. S.; Grandy, D. K.; Low, M. J.; Rubinstein, M.; Ariano, M. A. & Levine, M. S. (2001). Facilitated glutamatergic transmission in the striatum of D2 dopamine receptor-deficient mice. *J. Neurophysiol.*, Vol. 85, No. 2, (February 2001), pp. 659–670, ISSN 0022-3077

David, H. N.; Ansseau, M. & Abraini, J. H. (2005). Dopamine–glutamate reciprocal modulation of release and motor responses in the rat caudate–putamen and nucleus accumbens of "intact" animals, *Brain Res. Rev.*, Vol. 50, No. 2, (November 2005), pp. 336–360, ISBN/ISSN (*no mentioned*)

Doig, N. M.; Moss, J. & Bolam, J. P. (2010). Cortical and Thalamic Innervation of Direct and Indirect Pathway Medium-Sized Spiny Neurons in Mouse. *J. Neurosci.*, Vol. 30, No. 44, (November 2010), pp.14610 –14618, ISSN 1529-2401 (Electronic), ISSN 0270-6474 (Linking)

Dube, L.; Smith, A. D. & Bolam, J. P. (1988) Identification of synaptic terminals of thalamic or cortical origin in contact with distinct medium-size spiny neurons in the rat neostriatum. *J. Comp. Neurol.*, Vol. 267, No. 4, (January 1988), pp. 455-471, ISSN 0021-9967

Flaherty, A. W. & Graybiel, A. M. (1994). Input-output organization of the sensorimotor striatum in the squirrel monkey. *J. Neurosci.*, Vol. 14, No. 2, (February 1994), pp. 599-610, ISSN 0270-6474

Fremeau, R. T.; Kam, K.; Qureshi, T.; Johnson, J.; Copenhagen, D. R.; Storm-Mathisen, J.; Chaudhry, F. A.; Nicoll, R. A. & Edwards, R. H. (2004). Vesicular glutamate transporters 1 and 2 target to functionally distinct synaptic release sites. *Science*, Vol. 304, No. 5678, (May 2004), pp. 1815-1819, ISSN 1095-9203 (Electronic), ISSN 0036-8075 (Linking)

Fujiyama, F.; Unzai, T.; Nakamura, K.; Nomura, S. & Kaneko, T. (2006). Difference in organization of corticostriatal and thalamostriatal synapses between patch and matrix compartments of rat neostriatum. *Eur. J. Neurosci.*, Vol. 24, No. 10, (December 2006), pp. 2813–2824, ISSN 0953-816X

Gerfen, C. R.; Herkenham, M. & Thibault J. (1987). The neostriatal mosaic: II. Patch- and matrix-directed mesostriatal dopaminergic and non-dopaminergic systems. *J Neurosci.*, Vol. 7, No. 12, (December 1987), pp. 3915-3934, ISSN 0270-6474

Gerfen, C. R.; Engber, T. M.; Mahan, L. C.; Susel, Z.; Chase, T. N.; Monsma, F. J. & Sibley, D. R. (1990). D1 and D2 dopamine receptor-regulated gene expression of striatonigral and striatopallidal neurons. *Science*, Vol. 250, No. 4986, (December 1990), pp. 1429-1432, ISSN 0036-8075

Gerfen, C. R.; McGinty, J. F. & Young, W. S. (1991). Dopamine differentially regulates dynorphin, substance P, and enkephalin expression in striatal neurons: in situ hybridisation histochemical analysis. *J. Neurosci.*, Vol. 11, No. 4, (April 1991), pp. 1016-1031, ISSN 0270-6474

Gerfen, C. R. & Wilson, C. (1996). The basal ganglia. In: *Handbook of chemical neuroanatomy. Integrated systems of the CNS, part III. Vol. 12*, Swanson, L. W., Björklund, A. & Hökfelt, T. (eds), pp. 371-468, Elsevier, ISBN 0-444-82451-0, Amsterdam, Netherlands

Gerfen, C. R. (2000). Molecular effects of dopamine on striatal-projection pathways. *Trends Neurosci.*, Vol. 23, No. 10 Suppl, (October 2000), pp. 64-70, ISSN 0166-2236

Goldman-Rakic P. S. (1981). Prenatal formation of cortical input and development of cytoarchitectonic compartments in the neostriatum of the rhesus monkey. *J Neurosci.*, Vol. 1, No. 7, (September 1981), pp. 721-735, ISSN 0270-6474

Graybiel, A. M. (1995). The basal ganglia. *Trends Neurosci.*, Vol. 18, No. 2, (February 1995), pp. 60-62, ISSN 0166-2236

Guillin, O.; Diaz, J.; Carroll, P.; Griffon, N.; Schwartz, J.-C. & Sokoloff, P. (2001). BDNF controls dopamine D3 receptor expression and triggers behavioral sensitisation. *Nature*, Vol. 411, No. 6833, (May 2001), pp. 86-89, ISSN 0028-0836

Hammond, E. N.; Tetzlaff, W.; Mestres, P. & Giehl, K. M. (1999). BDNF, but not NT-3, promotes long-term survival of axotomized adult rat corticospinal neurons in vivo. *Neuroreport*, Vol. 10, No. 12, (November 1999), pp. 2671-2675, ISSN 0959-4965

Heiman, M.; Schaefer, A.; Gong, S.; Peterson, J. D.; Day, M.; Ramsey, K. E.; Suarez-Farinas, M.; Schwarz, C.; Stephan, D. A.; Surmeier, D. J.; Greengard, P. & Heintz, N. (2008). A Translational Profiling Approach for the Molecular Characterization of CNS Cell Types. *Cell*, Vol. 135, No. 4, (November 2008), pp. 738–748, ISSN 1097-4172 (Electronic), ISSN 0092-8674 (Linking)

Herzog, E.; Bellenchi, G. C.; Gras, C.; Bernard, V.; Ravassard, P.; Bedet, C.; Gasnier, B.; Giros, B. & El Mestikawy, S. (2001). The existence of a second vesicular glutamate transporter specifies subpopulations of glutamatergic neurons. *J. Neurosci.*, Vol. 21, No. 22, (November 2001), pp. RC181, ISSN 1529-2401 (Electronic), ISSN 0270-6474 (Linking)

Jonkers, N.; Sarre, S.; Ebinger, G. & Michotte, Y. (2002). MK801 suppresses the L-DOPA-induced increase of glutamate in striatum of hemi-Parkinson rats. *Brain Res.*, Vol. 926, No. 1-2, (January 2002), pp. 149–155, ISSN 0006-8993

Kaneko, T. & Fujiyama, F. (2002). Complementary distribution of vesicular glutamate transporters in the central nervous system. *Neurosci. Res.*, Vol. 42, No. 4, (May 2002), pp. 243-250, ISSN 0168-0102

Kemp, J. M. & Powell, T.P. (1971). The structure of the caudate nucleus of the cat: light and electron microscopy. *Philos. Trans. R. Soc. Lond. B. Biol. Sci.*, Vol. 262, No. 845, (September 1971), pp. 383-401, ISSN 0962-8436

Le Moine, C. & Bloch, B. (1995). D1 and D2 dopamine receptor gene expression in the rat striatum: sensitive cRNA probes demonstrate prominent segregation of D1 and D2 mRNAs in distinct neuronal populations of the dorsal and ventral striatum. *J. Comp. Neurol.*, Vol. 355, No. 3, (May 1995), pp. 418-426, ISSN 0021-9967

Lessmann, V. (1998). Neurotrophin-dependent modulation of glutamatergic synaptic transmission in the mammalian CNS. *Gen Pharmacol.*, Vol. 31, No. 5, (November 1998), pp. 667-74, ISSN 0306-3623

Mamounas, L. A.; Altar, C. A.; Blue, M. E.; Kaplan, D. R.; Tessarollo, L. & Lyons, W. E. (2000). BDNF promotes the regenerative sprouting, but not survival, of injured serotonergic axons in the adult rat brain. *J Neurosci.*, Vol. 20, No. 2, (January 2000), pp. 771-782, ISSN 1529-2401 (Electronic), ISSN 0270-6474 (Linking)

Massart, R.; Diaz, J.; Griffon, N.; Vernier, P. & Sokoloff, P. (1995). Regional and cellular expression pattern of the striatum-specific orphan G protein-coupled receptor Gpr88. 7e Colloque de la Société des Neurosciences, France, May 2005

Massart, R.; Guilloux, J. P; Mignon, V.; Lauressergues, E.; Cussac, D.; Sokoloff, P. & Diaz, J. (2007). Complex regulation of the orphan G protein-coupled receptor GPR88 in the unilaterally 6-OHDA lesioned rat model of Parkinson's disease. 37th Annual Meeting of Neuroscience, San-Diego, USA, November 2007

Massart, R.; Guilloux, J. P.; Mignon, V.; Lauressergues, E.; Cussac, D.; Sokoloff, P. & Diaz, J. (2008) Striatal synaptic and cortical nuclear GPR88, a promising target for psychiatric and movement disorders. ECNP Workshop, Nice, France, Mars 2008

Massart, R.; Guilloux, J. P.; Mignon, V.; Sokoloff, P. & Diaz, J. (2009). Striatal Gpr88 expression is confined to the whole projection neuron population and is regulated by dopaminergic and glutamatergic afferents. *Eur J Neurosci.*, Vol. 30, No. 3, (August 2009), pp. 397-414, ISSN 1460-9568 (Electronic), ISSN 0953-816X (Linking)

Meshul, C. K. & Tan, S. E. (1994). Haloperidol-induced morphological alterations are associated with changes in calcium/calmodulin kinase II activity and glutamate immunoreactivity. *Synapse.*, Vol. 18, No. 3, (November 1994), pp. 205-217, ISSN 0887-4476

Meshul, C. K.; Emre, N.; Nakamura, C. M.; Allen, C.; Donohue, M. K. & Buckman, J. F. (1999). Time-dependent changes in striatal glutamate synapses following a 6-hydroxydopamine lesion. *Neuroscience.*, Vol. 88, No. 1, (March 1999), pp. 1–16, ISSN 0306-4522

Meshul, C. K. & Allen, C. (2000). Haloperidol reverses the changes in striatal glutamatergic immunolabeling following a 6-OHDA lesion. *Synapse*, Vol. 36, No. 2, (May 2000), pp. 129-142, ISSN 0887-4476

Mizushima, K.; Miyamoto, Y.; Tsukahara, F.; Hirai, M.; Sakaki, Y. & Ito, T. (2000). A novel G-protein-coupled receptor gene expressed in striatum. *Genomics*, Vol. 69, No. 3, (November 2000), pp. 314-321, ISSN 0888-7543

Ragsdale, C. W. & Graybiel, A. M. (1988). Fibers from the basolateral nucleus of the amygdala selectively innervate striosomes in the caudate nucleus of the cat. *J. Comp. Neurol.*, Vol. 269, No. 4, (March 1988), pp. 506-522, ISSN 0021-9967

Reiner, A. & Anderson, K. D. (1990). The patterns of neurotransmitter and neuropeptide co-occurrence among striatal projection neurons: conclusions based on recent findings. *Brain Res Rev.*, Vol. 15, No. 3, (September 1990), pp. 251-65, ISBN/ISSN (*no mentioned*)

Ribak, C. E. & Roberts, R. C. (1990). GABAergic synapses in the brain identified with antisera to GABA and its synthesizing enzyme, glutamate decarboxylase. *Journal of Electron Microscopy Technique*, Vol. 15, No. 1, (May 1990), pp. 34-48, ISSN 0741-0581

Robelet, S.; Melon, C.; Guillet, B.; Salin, P. & Kerkerian-Le Goff, L. (2004). Chronic l-DOPA treatment increases Extracellular glutamate levels and GLT1 expression in the basal ganglia in a rat model of Parkinson's disease. *Eur. J. Neurosci.*, Vol. 20, No. 5, (September 2004), pp. 1255-1266, ISSN 0953-816X

Ross, C. A.; Becher, M. W.; Colomer, V.; Engelender, S.; Wood J. D. & Sharp A. H. (1997). Huntington's disease and dentatorubral- allidoluysian atrophy: proteins, pathogenesis and pathology. *Brain Pathol.*, Vol. 7, No. 3, (July 1997), pp. 1003-1016, ISSN 1015-6305

Salin, P.; Dziewczapolski, G.; Gershanik, O. S.; Nieoullon, A. & Raisman-Vozari, R. (1997). Differential regional effects of long-term L-DOPA treatment on preproenkephalin and preprotachykinin gene expression in the striatum of 6-hydroxydopamine-lesioned rat. *Brain Res.Mol. Brain Res.*, Vol. 47, No. 1-2, (July 1997), pp. 311-321, ISSN 0169-328X

Schwarting, R. K. W. & Huston, J. P. (1996). Unilateral 6-hydroxydopamine lesions of meso-striatal dopamine neurons and their physiological sequelae. *Prog. Neurobiol.*, Vol. 49, No. 3, (June 1996), pp. 215-266, ISSN 0301-0082

Seroogy, K. B.; Lundgren, K. H.; Tran, T. M.; Guthrie, K. M.; Isackson, P. J. & Gall, C. M. (1994). Dopaminergic neurons in rat ventral midbrain express brain-derived neurotrophic factor and neurotrophin-3 mRNAs. *J Comp Neurol.*, Vol. 342, No. 3, (April 1994), pp. 321-334, ISSN 0021-9967

Smith, Y.; Bennett, B. D.; Bolam, J. P.; Parent, A. & Sadikot, A. F. (1994). Synaptic relationships between dopaminergic ,fferents and cortical or thalamic input in the sensorimotor territory of the striatum in monkey. *J. Comp. Neurol.*, Vol. 344, No. 1, (June 1994), pp. 1-19, ISSN 0021-9967

Smith, Y. & Kieval, J. Z. (2000) Anatomy of the dopamine system in the basal ganglia. *Trends Neurosci.*, 23, No. 10 Suppl, (October 2000), pp. 28-33, ISSN 0166-2236

Snyder-Keller, A. & Costantini, L. C. (1996). Glutamate receptor subtypes localize to patches in the developing striatum. *Brain Res Dev Brain Res.*, Vol. 94, No. 2, (July 1996), pp. 246-250, ISSN 0165-3806

Snyder-Keller, A.; Costantini, L. C. & Graber, D. J. (2001). Development of striatal patch/matrix organization in organotypic co-cultures of perinatal striatum, cortex and substantia nigra. *Neuroscience*, Vol. 103, No. 1, (April 2001), pp. 97-109, ISSN 0306-4522

Snyder-Keller, A. (2004). Pattern of corticostriatal innervation in organotypic cocultures is dependent on the age of the cortical tissue. *Exp Neurol.*, Vol. 185, No. 2, (January 2004), pp. 262-271, ISSN 0014-4886

Somogyi, P.; Priestley, J. V.; Cuello, A. C.; Smith, A. D. & Takagi, H. (1982). Synaptic connections of enkephalin-immunoreactive nerve terminals in the neostriatum: a correlated light and electron microscopic study. *J. Neurocytol.*, Vol. 11, No. 5, (October 1982), pp. 779-807, ISSN 0300-4864

Stephens, B.; Mueller, A. J.; Shering, A. F.; Hood, S. H.; Taggart, P.; Arbuthnott, G. W.; Bell, J. E.; Kilford, L.; Kingsbury, A. E.; Daniel, S. E. & Ingham, C.A. (2005). Evidence of a breakdown of corticostriatal connections in Parkinson's disease. *Neuroscience*, Vol. 132, No. 3, (April 2005), pp. 741-754, ISSN 0306-4522

Surmeier, D. J.; Ding, J.; Day, M.; Wang, Z. & Shen, W. (2007). D1 and D2 dopamine-receptor modulation of striatal glutamatergic signaling in striatal medium spiny neurons. *Trends Neurosci.*, Vol. 30, No.5 , (May 2007), pp. 228-235, ISSN 0166-2236

Taliaz, D .; Stall, N .; Dar, D. E. & Zangen. A. (2010). Knockdown of brain-derived neurotrophic factor in specific brain sites precipitates behaviors associated with depression and reduces neurogenesis. *Mol Psychiatry.*, Vol. 15, No. 1, (July 2009), pp. 80-92, ISSN 1476-5578 (Electronic), ISSN 1359-4184 (Linking)

Tanaka J.; Horiike Y.; Matsuzaki M.; Miyazaki, T.; Ellis-Davies G. C. & Kasai H. (2008). Protein synthesis and neurotrophin-dependent structural plasticity of single dendritic spines. *Science*, Vol. 319, No. 5870, (March 2008), pp. 1683-87, ISSN 1095-9203 (Electronic), 0036-8075 (Linking)

Taymans, J. M.; Kia, H. K.; Groenewegen, H. J.; Leysen, J.E. & Langlois, X. (2005). Bilateral control of brain activity by dopamine D1 receptors : evidence from induction patterns of regulator of G protein signalling 2 and c-fos mRNA in D1-challenged hemiparkinsonian rats. *Neuroscience*, Vol. 134, No. 2, (June 2005), pp. 643-56, ISSN 0306-4522

Uhl, G. R.; Navia, B. & Douglas, J. (1988). Differential expression of preproenkephalin and preprodynorphin mRNAs in striatal neurons: high levels of preproenkephalin expression depend on cerebral cortical afferents. *J. Neurosci.*, Vol. 8, No. 12, (December 1988), pp. 4755–4764, ISSN 0270-6474

Utter, A. A. & Basso, M. A. (2008). The basal ganglia: An overview of circuits and function. *Neuroscience and Biobehavioral Reviews.* Vol. 32, No. 3, (January 2008), pp. 333–342, ISSN 0149-7634

van der Kooy, D. & Fishell, G. (1987). Neuronal birthdate underlies the development of striatal compartments. *Brain Res.*, Vol. 401, No. 1, (January 1987), pp. 155-161, ISSN 0006-8993

van der Kooy, D. & Fishell, G. (1992). Embryonic lesions of the substantia nigra prevent the patchy expression of opiate receptors, but not the segregation of patch and matrix compartment neurons, in the developing rat striatum. *Brain Res Dev Brain Res.*, Vol. 66, No. 1, (March 1992), pp. 614-623, ISSN 0165-3806

Voorn, P.; Kalsbeek, A.; Jorritsma-Byham, B. & Groenewegen, H. J. (1988). The pre- and postnatal development of the dopaminergic cell groups in the ventral mesencephalon and the dopaminergic innervation of the striatum of the rat. *Neuroscience.*, Vol. 25, No. 3, (June 1988), pp. 857-887, ISSN 0306-4522

Voorn, P.; Vanderschuren, L. J.; Groenewegen, H. J.; Robbins, T.W. & Pennartz, C. M. A. (2004). Putting a spin on the dorsal-ventral divide of the striatum. *Trends Neurosci.*, Vol.27, No. 8, (August 2004), pp. 468-474, ISSN 0166-2236

Wolfgang, H. O. & Stanley, F. (2003) . Parkinsonism. In: *Movement Disorders. Neurological Disorders: Course and Treatment*, Second Edition, pp. 1021-1079, Elsevier Science, ISBN 978-0-12-125831-3, USA

Zeng, B. Y.; Pearce, R. K.; MacKenzie, G. M. & Jenner P. (2000). Alterations in preproenkephalin and adenosine-2a receptor mRNA, but not preprotachikinin mRNA correlate with occurrence of dyskinesia in normal monkeys chronically treated with L-DOPA. *Eur. J. Neurosci.*, Vol. 12, No. 3, (April 2000), pp. 1096-1104, ISSN 0953-816X

2

Inflammation in Parkinson's Disease: Causes and Consequences

Louise M. Collins, André Toulouse and Yvonne M. Nolan
Department of Anatomy and Neuroscience, University College Cork
Ireland

1. Introduction

Parkinson's disease (PD) is the second most common progressive neurodegenerative disorder after Alzheimer's disease (AD) with a prevalence of 0.5-1% among persons older than 65 years of age (Toulouse & Sullivan, 2008). The incidence increases to 2.6% in persons aged 85 and older, and has a mean age of onset of 55 years. Statistics released in 1990 from a unique global study carried out by the World Health Organisation, suggest that there are approximately 4 million PD patients worldwide. However, despite intensive research, the aetiology of this neurodegenerative disease still remains unclear and despite substantial efforts, a cure remains elusive. This, coupled with the increasing aging demographics, makes the importance of research into PD imperative, and the development of novel drug treatments a primary aim, both for economic and humanitarian purposes. The disease is a chronic, progressive neurodegenerative motor disorder, resulting in the selective loss of dopaminergic (DA) neurons within the substantia nigra (SN) pars compacta (pc) of the midbrain. As the disease progresses there is gradual circuitry degeneration within the nigrostriatal pathway, producing motor, cognitive and psychiatric symptoms (Braak et al., 2003). Lewy bodies are classified as the focal pathological hallmark of PD and their presence is necessary for the *post-mortem* diagnosis of the disease. They are not unique to PD however and are also found in other diseases such as dementia with Lewy Bodies and diffuse Lewy Body disease (Braak et al., 2003). PD can be further characterised by the presence of an accumulation of activated microglia within the SNpc (McGeer et al., 1988).

PD exists in many forms and can be classified into both familial and idiopathic (also referred to as sporadic) forms, with epidemiological studies indicating approximately 5-10% of cases as being familial, and 90-95% as idiopathic (Tomiyama et al., 2008). Familial PD can be transmitted in an autosomal dominant (AD-PD) or recessive fashion (AR-PD). The study of genetic forms of PD has led to a better understanding of the underlying molecular mechanisms occurring during the disease progression. To date, six genes (SNCA, LRRK2, PRKN, DJ-1, PINK1 and ATP13A2) have been implicated in familial forms of PD (Bekris et al., 2010). In contrast to idiopathic PD, the genetic forms of this disease display a significantly younger age of onset and a shorter disease duration (Pankratz & Foroud, 2007). Despite this, patients with the autosomal dominant form of the disease have similar clinical and pathological features to those with idiopathic PD. In idiopathic PD, environmental factors such as toxins, free radicals and inflammation have been considered the most likely candidates as causative agents. For example, pesticides can induce oxidative stress (an increased production of activated oxygen species such as superoxide anions and hydroxyl radicals) which leads to lipid peroxidation, DNA damage and mitochondrial dysfunction (Dick, 2006; Jenner, 2003). Moreover, there is evidence to suggest that the oxidative stress that occurs at a basal level in the SNpc is increased during PD (Jenner, 2003). The involvement of inflammation in the progression of PD has been well documented and is generally typified by an accumulation of activated microglia in damaged regions of the brain (Gao & Hong, 2008; Long-Smith et al., 2009). Initial evidence stems from a *post-mortem* study over twenty years ago, which demonstrated the presence of activated microglia and T-lymphocytes in the SNpc of a PD patient (McGeer et al., 1988). Since then, an abundance of studies have supported a role for neuroinflammation and activated microglia in the pathology of PD (Banati et al., 1998; Hirsch & Hunot, 2009; Imamura et al., 2003; McGeer & McGeer, 2004; Orr et al., 2002). Activated microglia are predominantly found in the SNpc in the vicinity of degenerating DA neurons in *post-mortem* PD brains, but have also been detected in the hippocampus, transentorhinal cortex, cingulate cortex and temporal cortex, where neuronal loss is also prevalent (Banati et al., 1998; Imamura et al., 2003; McGeer et al., 1988; Sawada et al., 2006). The presence of activated microglia in rat brains lesioned with 6-hydroxydopamine (6-OHDA), a neurotoxin used to model PD, has been reported by numerous groups (Akiyama & McGeer, 1989; Crotty et al., 2008; Depino et al., 2003; He et al., 2001). Further evidence implicating inflammation in PD comes from studies that report an increase in the expression of the pro-inflammatory cytokines, interleukin (IL)-1β, tumour necrosis factor-α (TNF-α) and IL-6 in PD patients compared with healthy subjects (Boka et al., 1994; Dobbs et al., 1999; Mogi et al., 1994a; Mogi et al., 1994b). Enzymes associated with inflammation, such as inducible nitric oxide synthase (iNOS) and cyclooxygenase-2 (COX-2), have also been identified *post-mortem* in PD brains (Hunot et al., 1996; Knott et al., 2000).

2. Neuroinflammation in Parkinson's disease

2.1 Microglia

Microglia are the resident immune-competent cells of the central nervous system (CNS). They monitor the brain for invading pathogens and immune insults and are capable of stimulating an adaptive immune response (Garden & Moller, 2006). Pio del Rio-Hortega first ignited interest in microglia in the early 20th century when he identified them as a separate glial entity (del Rio Hortega, 1932), providing a complete and comprehensive framework of their involvement in brain pathology (Raivich et al., 1999). There are currently two proposed subsets of microglia residing within the CNS. There are the *"resting"* microglia found ramified throughout the brain parenchyma and mostly a permanent population, and the perivascular microglia, which are periodically replaced by bone-marrow derived elements and are strategically located in the basal lamina of brain capillaries and the choroid plexus (Santambrogio et al., 2001). These two subsets differ in their expression of leucocyte common antigen, CD45, which is high (CD45^{high}) in perivascular and low (CD45^{low}) in parenchymal microglia (Sedgwick et al., 1991). The production of microglia is complex. There is an initial production of microglia during development, a constant turnover of microglia during adulthood and throughout senescence, and an up-regulated production of microglia in response to pathological conditions. Furthermore, each of these stages is likely to be governed by diverse mechanisms. The origin of microglia remains contentious, but the majority of the neuroscience community support the premise that they are derived from mesodermal precursor cells of hematopoietic lineage (Barron, 1995; Cuadros & Navascues, 1998) due to their expression of macrophage antigens, such as F4/80, Fc receptor (FcR) and macrophage-1 antigen (MAC-1) (Carson et al., 1998). Mesodermal precursor cells infiltrate the brain during embryonic and early postnatal phases of development and have the potential to differentiate into macrophages, dendritic cells (DCs) and granulocytes (Santambrogio et al., 2001). Factors which govern and propel this invasion are not widely understood but are believed to involve cell surface bound molecules and components of the extracellular matrix (Cuadros & Navascues, 1998). As with the origin of microglia, the mechanism of microglial renewal *in situ* remains controversial. This prolonged controversy to unequivocally differentiate activated endogenous microglia from those of infiltrating blood monocytes is due to a lack of distinguishable cell surface or enzymatic markers (Ransohoff & Cardona, 2010). In addition, the prevailing technique of lethally irradiated chimeras to examine this appears to be fraught with confounding factors. Ajami et al., (2007) utilised chimeric animals obtained through parabiosis, which does not require experimental manipulation, and found that microglial homeostasis is maintained independently of bone-marrow derived precursors. They also reported that mature resident microglia are capable of focal self-renewal and microgliosis in response to insult or injury (Ajami et al., 2007).

Within the healthy adult brain microglia reside as a ubiquitously distributed quiescent cell population, representing 10-20% of non-neuronal cells within the CNS parenchyma. They are functionally related to peripheral tissue macrophages and other cells of the monocyte lineage, but differ in their down-regulated expression of a number of cytoplasmic molecules (Perry, 1998). Historically referred to as *"resting"* microglia, which discriminates them morphologically from their active amoeboid form found during insult to the CNS, they are characterised by a small rod-shaped somata and numerous elongated, highly ramified processes. Through their protrusions, they are in direct contact with astrocytes, neuronal cell bodies and blood vessels, suggesting that they dynamically interact with a variety of neural elements (Nimmerjahn et al., 2005). As immune effector cells of the CNS, they are extremely receptive to subtle change in their microenvironment, rapidly undergoing morphological as well as functional transformations (Ladeby et al., 2005). Although research in recent years has greatly advanced our knowledge of activated microglia, little has been established concerning the function of the microglia residing in the unperturbed CNS. This is due in part to the exceedingly complex predicament many have faced while trying to culture *"resting"* microglia *in vitro*. The removal and dissociation of cells from CNS tissue, either by mechanical or proteolytic means inevitably leads to some level of activation (Garden & Moller, 2006). Many have observed microglial cells *in vitro* exhibiting an amoeboid morphology in a non-pathogenic environment. Eder and co-workers exposed murine microglia to astrocyte-conditioned medium and noted a dramatic transformation in morphology from a *"resting"* ramified appearance to *"active"* amoeboid microglia. within a few hours of treatment. As well as this, they observed a down-regulation in macrophage surface molecules such as major-histocompatibility complex (MHC) class-II, and the adhesion molecules leucocyte function-associated antigen-1 (LFA-1) and intercellular adhesion molecule-1 (ICAM-1) (Eder et al., 1999). Well-established histological approaches have allowed *"resting"* microglia to be examined *in situ*, capturing them in a "freeze-frame picture" at the time of being placed in fixative but this approach also has limitations and thus may obscure potentially important dynamic processes (Davalos et al., 2005). Advances in multi-photon *in vivo* microscopy however, have shed some light on the function of *"resting"* microglia *in situ*. By examining the behaviours of eGFP-expressing parenchymal microglia in heterozygous CX_3CR1-mice, it was revealed that microglial processes are incessantly palpating their microenvironment. The protrusions extend and retract rapidly and dynamically, reaching up to several micrometres in length over intervals of seconds to minutes (Davalos et al., 2005; Nimmerjahn et al., 2005). It was postulated that their high motility serves as a "housekeeping" function allowing them to effectively manage the brain milieu and to clear the parenchyma of accumulated metabolic products and deteriorated tissue components (Nimmerjahn et al., 2005). Indeed it has been estimated that they are capable of probing the entire volume of the brain every 4-5 hours. The highly ramified form of microglia covers 30-40µm in diameter and though their processes are in close proximity, they are not in direct contact, suggesting that each cell occupies its own exclusive patrol territory (McGeer & McGeer, 2007; Raivich et al., 1999). As such, they are now more appropriately termed *"surveillant"* microglia to properly describe their rapid and continuous monitoring of the surrounding vicinity (Ransohoff & Cardona, 2010).

"Surveillant" ramified microglia respond to activating stimuli with a rapid morphological transformation into *"active"* amoeboid microglia (Nakajima & Kohsaka, 2001). Activated microglia are found in the brain under almost all pathological conditions and are involved in tissue repair, amplification of inflammatory effects, neuronal degeneration and the phagocytosis of dead cells and cellular debris (Davalos et al., 2005). Microglia express a perplexing array of cell surface receptors such as complement receptor 3 and MHC class I and II, whose up-regulation is concomitant with activation of microglia (Nakajima & Kohsaka, 2001). These receptors play a pivotal role in enabling microglia to detect subtle changes in their microenvironment, triggering them to extend their processes to the surrounding area of insult, and to engulf damaged cells via phagocytosis (Davalos et al., 2005). In addition, microglia are considered the main antigen presenting cell (APC) population within the CNS, as both *in vivo* and *in vitro* studies have demonstrated their capacity for antigen presentation in response to a variety of CNS pathological conditions (Graeber & Streit, 2010). Activation of microglia and the consequent up-regulation of MHC class II, CD40 and ICAM-1 stimulate T cell proliferation and the production of IL-2, IFNγ and IL-4. However, the ability of endogenous microglia to act as APCs has been brought into question, with many postulating that it may be the role of perivascular macrophages or invading DCs (Perry, 1998). Today, growing evidence suggests that DCs do in fact participate in the regulation of T-cell responses (Teo & Wong, 2010). Microglia in common with other cells of the myeloid lineage also have the ability to secrete immunomodulatory molecules such as cytokines, chemokines, neurotrophins, reactive oxygen and nitrogen species, which communicate signals to surrounding cells to regulate the innate immune response (Garden & Moller, 2006). Cytokines, such as ILs, IFNs and TNFα/β are low-molecular weight proteins that are usually classified as pro- or anti-inflammatory, and microglia express receptors for these cytokines in an autocrine feedback loop that is critical for down-regulating inflammation and restoration of homeostasis. In the brain, it has been reported that cytokines function in growth promotion, inhibition and proliferation of astrocytes and oligodendrocytes (Hanisch, 2002), modulation of neurotransmitter release (Zalcman et al., 1994) long-term potentiation (Nolan et al., 2005) behavioural impairments such as memory impairment (Yirmiya et al., 2002) anhedonia (Konsman et al., 2002) and anxiety (Anisman & Merali, 1999).

2.2 Activated microglia in Parkinson's disease

The first evidence for a role of inflammation in PD came from McGeer and colleagues who observed activated microglia and T cells in the *post-mortem* SNpc of a PD patient (McGeer et al., 1988). We now know from a multitude of studies that microglial activation and consequent neuroinflammatory processes play a role in PD (Hirsch & Hunot, 2009). Whereas mild activation of microglia has apparent beneficial effects, chronic microglial activation in response to neuronal damage, as is evident in PD, results in the death of otherwise viable cells. Activation of microglia either directly via a toxin, pathogen or endogenous protein or indirectly from dying neurons may be both long-lived and self-propelling due to positive feedback from degenerating neurons even after the initial insult has ceased (Gao & Hong, 2008). This repetitive cycle of neurotoxic activation of microglia in response to neuronal damage is referred to as *reactive microgliosis* (Block et al., 2007) and is a feature of several brain pathologies (Carson et al., 1998). DA neurons in the SNpc are particularly susceptible to microglial-mediated neurotoxicity due to the high densities of microglia present (Kim et al., 2000). Thus, microglial activation and hence neuroinflammation, may be propagated and potentially amplify the destruction of neurons in PD (Gao & Hong, 2008). Substances which are produced by dying DA neurons and can activate microglia include α-synuclein-aggregates (Zhang et al., 2005), neuromelanin (Wilms et al., 2003), adenosine triphosphate (ATP) (Davalos et al., 2005) and matrix metalloproteinase-3 (MMP-3) (Kim et al., 2007; Kim et al., 2005).

Aggregated α-synuclein, the major constituent of Lewy bodies in PD, has been reported to be surrounded by activated microglia or inflammatory mediators (McGeer et al., 1988; Yamada et al., 1992). It has also been shown to activate microglia in primary mesencephalic cultures, which in turn amplify α-synuclein-mediated neurotoxicity (Zhang et al., 2005). The phagocytosis of extracellular aggregated α-synuclein and activation of NADPH-oxidase is essential to further activate microglia and propel DA neurodegeneration (Zhang et al., 2005). Neuromelanin, a neuro-pigment released from stressed DA neurons has been shown to induce microglial activation (Wilms et al., 2003) through proteasomal inhibition (Kim et al., 2006). Its accumulation in human SNpc correlates with age progression, and extra neural melanin has been found in close proximity to activated microglial cells in patients suffering from juvenile idiopathic and methyl-4-phenyl-2,3-dihydropyridine (MPTP)-induced Parkinsonism (Wilms et al., 2007). Supplementation of microglial cultures with human neuromelanin *in vitro* has been shown to induce chemotactic effects and stimulate the release of TNFα, IL-6 and NO (Wilms et al., 2003). Thus, the release of neuromelanin can augment microglial activation and contribute to a self-perpetuating cycle of neuronal degeneration and chronic inflammation (Kim et al., 2006). Extracellular ATP, a purinergic neurotransmitter, was initially described as an activator of microglial cells in 1993 (Kettenmann et al., 1993). The effects of ATP released from damaged neurons are mediated through its signalling with purinergic receptors, namely the metabotropic G-protein coupled P2Y receptors and the ligand gated ionotropic P2X receptors, both of which are expressed on microglia (Butt, 2011). Upon stimulation, activated microglia migrate along a chemotactic gradient to the site of injury or inflammation, facilitated by the release of pro-migratory factors such as extracellular ATP, UTP and members of the chemokine family from damaged cells. ATP then interacts with P2 receptors on microglia to stimulate the release of TNFα, IL-1β, iNOS and NO. Experiments by Kim *et al* have identified a pivotal role for the protease MMP-3 in DA neuronal activity (Kim et al., 2005). MPP+-stressed primary mesencephalic DA neurons induce and release active MMP-3, which is toxic to DA neurons. It has been reported that primary microglial cultures treated with catalytically active recombinant MMP-3 stimulated microglial activation, superoxide generation and enhanced DA neuronal cell death while MPTP-treated MMP-3-/- mice attenuated microglial activation, superoxide generation and DA degeneration (Kim et al., 2007).

Stimulation with the glycolipid endotoxin lipopolysaccharide (LPS) is currently one of the most common methods for activating microglia *in vitro*. LPS interacts with Toll-like receptor (TLR) 4, one of a family of pathogen recognition receptors (PPRs) responsive to microbial signals. Microglia have been reported to express 9 of the 12 TLRs (Jack et al., 2005). LPS-stimulated microglia release inflammatory cytokines (IL-1β, IL-1 receptor antagonist (IL-1RA), IL-6, IL-8, IL-10, IL-12, IL-18, macrophage colony stimulating factor), chemokines (macrophage inflammatory protein (MIP)-1α, MIP-1β, TNF-α, TNF-β, monocyte chemoattractant protein-1 (MCP-1), RANTES), and prostaglandins (Kim & de Vellis, 2005; Nakamura, 2002), as well as stimulating an increase in myristoylated alanine-rich C kinase substrate (MARCKS), MARCKS-related protein, protein kinase-C, iNOS and NO production (Garden & Moller, 2006). Cytokines produced by LPS-stimulated microglia can potentiate microglial activation through autocrine signalling to create a self-propagating cycle of expression. Pro-inflammatory cytokines IL-1β, TNFα, IL-2 and IL-6 are constitutively expressed at basal levels in PD patients as evidenced in *post-mortem,* serum and cerebrospinal fluid *in vivo* (Boka et al., 1994; Dobbs et al., 1999; Mogi et al., 1994a; Mogi et al., 1994b; Stypula et al., 1996). Moreover, the death signalling receptor TNF receptor type-1 (TNFR-1) is expressed on DA neurons in human SNpc (Boka et al., 1994; Mogi et al., 2000). Animal studies support an involvement of pro-inflammatory cytokines in the DA neuronal degeneration evident in PD. For example, induction of chronic expression of IL-1β in adult rat SNpc using a recombinant adenovirus resulted in DA neuronal cell death after three weeks (Ferrari et al., 2006). Another study using neutralising antibodies to IL-1β and TNF-α showed that approximately 50% of LPS-induced DA neuronal cell death in primary cultures of rat midbrain was mediated by the production of these two cytokines (Gayle et al., 2002).

It has been postulated that microglia are maintained in a quiescent state by numerous micro-environmental inhibitory influences, many of which are produced by neurons. Hence, microglial activation during pathological insult may be due to a *"switching-off"* of these inhibitory neuronal signals (Ransohoff & Cardona, 2010). One such neuron-cell inhibitory signalling mechanism is the direct cell-to-cell interactions between neuronal-CD200 (OX2) and its receptor CD200R, expressed on microglia. The CD200-CD200R interaction is essential for maintaining microglial homeostasis in the unperturbed CNS. A down-regulation of CD200 expression has been observed in neurons exposed to inflammatory conditions, and inhibition of CD200 causes microglial activation (Lyons et al., 2007). Therefore, there is a direct neuronal mechanism for regulating microglial activity, and loss of this interaction during neuronal cell degeneration may stimulate up-regulation of CD200, facilitating microglial activation. Recent evidence has implicated an impairment of CD200-CD200R interaction as a contributing factor in PD neurodegeneration (Wang et al., 2011). Blockade of CD200R selectively and significantly enhanced DA neuronal cell susceptibility to rotenone and iron-induced neurotoxicity in mesencephalic neuron-glia co-cultures. This was coupled with elevated microglial activation and superoxide generation and a decrease in CD200 expression on DA neurons. Microglia have also been shown to receive inhibitory inputs from a neuronal membrane-tethered chemokine CX3CL1, through its receptor CX3CR1. Removal of this inhibition also unleashed microglial activity (Shan et al., 2011). Other inhibitory signals exist between CD22-CD45, CD172A-CD47 and ICAM5-LFA-1 (Ransohoff & Perry, 2009).

3. Systemic inflammation and Parkinson's disease

It has been proposed that in chronic neurodegenerative diseases like PD, systemic infections and inflammation can exacerbate symptoms and promote neurodegeneration (Perry et al., 2007). A systemic response includes the liver acute phase response and the behavioural and metabolic components that induce sickness behaviour (Ferrari & Tarelli, 2011; Perry et al., 2007). Specifically, peripheral monocytes, macrophages and Kupffer cells express TLRs and PPRs, which innately recognise specific pathogen-associated molecular patterns (PAMPs) associated with invading pathogens (Dantzer, 2009). A prototypical PAMP, LPS, is specifically recognised by TLR4, which results in the production of pro-inflammatory cytokines IL-1α, IL-1β. Through autocrine signalling these cytokines induce self-synthesis and the synthesis of further cytokines (Dantzer, 2009) inducing general inflammation. Compromise of the blood-brain barrier (BBB) which is observed in neurological disorders, stimulates peripheral leucocytes and systemic inflammatory mediators such as cytokines, to migrate into the brain parenchyma where they induce the activation of microglia and the subsequent release of more cytokines (Ferrari & Tarelli, 2011). For example, peripheral TNFα can stimulate microglia to secrete chronically elevated pro-inflammatory mediators, which in turn can induce chronic self-perpetuating neuroinflammation, resulting in a slow and progressive loss of DA neurons in the SNpc (Qin et al., 2007). The brain recognises cytokines as molecular signals of sickness and induces symptoms of malaise, lassitude, fatigue, anhedonia, apathy, numbness, coldness, and reduced appetite and body temperature (Dantzer, 2009; Perry et al., 2007). To reinforce this theory, it has been demonstrated that a systemic inflammatory challenge in an animal with chronic neurodegeneration exhibits exaggerated brain inflammation, sickness behaviour and an increase in acute neurodegeneration (Perry et al., 2007). This emerging *"two-hit hypothesis"* in the aetiology of neurodegenerative diseases such as PD, suggests that the disease is multifactorial and a consequence of *"multiple-hits"* involving diverse inflammatory stimuli (Di Monte, 2003). Infectious agents may comprise the first *"hit"*, therefore sensitising the brain to subsequent *"hits"*, which may not have been pathogenic in the absence of an already *"primed"* system (Jang et al., 2009a). In this instance, microglia in the aged or diseased brain are said to be *"primed"* and can evoke an exaggerated response contributing to disease progression (Perry et al., 2007).

Clinical and epidemiological reports suggest a correlation between systemic inflammatory events, chronic neuroinflammation and the aetiology and progressive nature of PD (Ferrari & Tarelli, 2011; Long-Smith et al., 2009; Perry, 2010). Postulated risk factors implicated in idiopathic PD include age, genetic predisposition, bacterial or viral infections, neuronal injury such as traumatic brain injury or stroke, and environmental toxins (Koprich et al., 2008; Tansey & Goldberg, 2010). Associations were first established towards the end of the first world war (1924-1918) when the H1N1 influenza-A pandemic was coupled with a dramatic increase in post-encephalitic Parkinsonism (PEP) (also referred to as *"sleeping sickness"* or von Economo encephalitis) (Jang et al., 2009a; Rail et al., 1981; Tansey et al., 2007). People born during this time were at a 2-3 fold increased risk of developing PD, with PEP implicated in 50% of all Parkinsonism cases (Jang et al., 2009a; Tansey et al., 2007). PEP shares cardinal symptomatology with idiopathic PD including rigidity and bradykinesia but a lack of Lewy body formation (Jang et al., 2009a). Moreover, Takahashi et al., 1995 demonstrated that the H1N1 virus preferentially targets the SNpc, the primary site of pathology in PD (Takahashi et al., 1995). It has also been shown that exposure to the highly pathogenic neurotropic H5N1 influenza virus increases susceptibility to developing PD with an observed onset of post-influenzal encephalopathies (Jang et al., 2009b). Other viruses associated with secondary Parkinsonism include coxsackie virus (Poser et al., 1969; Walters, 1960), Japanese encephalitis B (Ogata et al., 1997), St. Louis virus (Pranzatelli et al., 1994), west Nile virus (Robinson et al., 2003) and HIV (Tse et al., 2004). Infection with Japanese-encephalitis virus (JEV), which occurs predominantly in India, China and Southeast Asia, for a prolonged period is likely to induce PEP (Ogata et al., 2000; Shoji et al., 1993; Tansey et al., 2007). People with JEV have similar neuropathological and locomotor symptoms to patients with idiopathic PD (Tansey et al., 2007), and the virus has previously been used to create a pre-clinical model of PD in rats (Ogata et al., 1997). This group demonstrated that in Fisher rats infected with JEV, there was marked gliosis and DA neuronal loss in the SNpc similar to that seen in PD, and bradykinesia which could be reversed with L-DOPA and monoamine oxidase (MAO) inhibitors. More recently, in a cohort of 60 JEV patients, transient-type Parkinsonian features were observed in 16 patients, with 19 displaying Parkinsonism with additional dystonia (Misra & Kalita, 2010).

Oxidative stress, through the generation of reactive oxygen species (ROS) is a key regulator of the neuroinflammatory process, with the underlying purpose of removing the cause of inflammation. Progressive neurodegenerative diseases like PD however, are associated with an overproduction of ROS causing neuronal oxidative damage as well as microglial activation, which subsequently leads to the generation of more ROS (Block & Hong, 2005). Moreover, oxidative stress preferentially affects DA neurons in the SNpc, which are particularly vulnerable as they operate under high oxidant conditions due to reduced levels of the anti-oxidant glutathione (Misra & Kalita, 2010; Sian et al., 1994). Accordingly, it has been postulated that pre-exposure to environmental toxins such as heavy metals, organophosphate compounds, neurotoxins, and pesticides like paraquat and rotenone which can induce oxidative stress and the generation of free radicals, increases the susceptibility to the development of PD in later life (Calne & Langston, 1983; Jang et al., 2009a). Pathological and clinical evidence has also identified the involvement of the gastrointestinal tract in enhancing susceptibility to idiopathic Parkinsonism, with *Helicobacter pylori* infection proposed as a potential trigger in disease progression (Tansey & Goldberg, 2010; Weller et al., 2005). Indeed, polymorphisms in the nucleotide-binding oligiomerisation domain 2 (NOD2) gene associated with Crohn's disease, a chronic inflammatory bowel disease, have been shown to be over-represented in patients with idiopathic PD (Bialecka et al., 2007).

Evidence now suggests that a disruption in neurovascular homeostasis with increased BBB permeability due to factors secreted by activated glia is associated with neuroinflammation in age-related neurodegenerative diseases. Activated glia have an up-regulated expression of cellular adhesion molecules and the subsequent induction of chemokine gradients direct peripheral leucocytes to the site of inflammation (Chung et al., 2010; Stone et al., 2009). Indeed, positron emission tomography (PET) and histological studies of PD patients as well as MPTP and LPS-induced models of PD reveal a pathogenic link between neuroinflammation, increased BBB permeability and the consequent infiltration of systemic inflammatory molecules, and DA neuronal death (Chung et al., 2010). PD patients have a reported dysfunction in the BBB transporter system (Kortekaas et al., 2005) and blood vessels in the midbrain (Faucheux et al., 1999). Increased levels of vascular endothelial growth factor (VEGF) and pigment epithelium-derived factor have been demonstrated in PD patients and in the MPTP model (Yasuda et al., 2007). A report from a study using animals provides evidence that nigral injection of VEGF to mice disrupted the BBB permeability and induced DA neuronal death in the ventral mesencephalon (VM) (X. Chen et al., 2008). In another study, systemic injection of high concentrations of LPS to rats caused functional breakdown of the BBB resulting in granulocyte infiltration and activation of parenchymal microglia. The subsequent infiltration of immune cells contributed to the degeneration of DA neurons in the SNpc (Brochard et al., 2009).

Assessment of serum obtained from PD subjects corroborates the involvement of systemic inflammation in PD (Hirsch & Hunot, 2009). Increased levels of CD4+ have been reported in the serum of patients with PD, suggesting peripheral activation of lymphocytes (Bas et al., 2001; Fiszer et al., 1994; Hirsch & Hunot, 2009). Infiltrating cytotoxic CD4+ and CD8+ T cells, but not B cells, have been observed in the inflamed SNpc of *post-mortem* PD human specimens and in the MPTP-induced mouse model of PD during the course of neurodegeneration (Brochard et al., 2009; Ferrari & Tarelli, 2011; Stone et al., 2009). In support of a role for systemic immune cells in the degeneration of nigral DA neurons, CD4-/- mice have been shown to be resistant to MPTP-induced neurotoxicity in the SN (Brochard et al., 2009). Amplified TNFα, IL-2, IL-6 and RANTES (Brodacki et al., 2008; Dobbs et al., 1999; Rentzos et al., 2007; Stypula et al., 1996) levels have also been detected in serum obtained from PD patients. Increases in serum cytokines may serve as a therapeutic marker for PD as a blood sample study of men with high plasma concentrations of IL-6 revealed an increased risk of developing PD (H. Chen et al., 2008). In a cohort of 46 PD patients, increased serum levels of soluble TNFR-1, which modulates TNFα activity were detected, which is in agreement with studies showing elevated TNFR-1 in the SNpc of PD brains (Mogi et al., 2000), although this was not associated with clinical parameters. Another group however, has demonstrated that LPS-induced increase of MCP-1, RANTES, MIP-1α, IL-8, IL-6 and IFNγ levels secreted by peripheral blood mononuclear cells significantly correlated with the severity of PD symptoms (Reale et al., 2009). Systemic low level of inflammation induced by a non-toxic dose of LPS has been shown to increase the severity of nigral DA neuronal cell loss in response to a subsequent low-dose of 6-OHDA in the rat model of PD (Koprich et al., 2008), while chronic systemic IL-1β also exacerbated neurodegeneration and microglial activation in the SN of 6-OHDA-treated rats (Pott Godoy et al., 2008). These data support the role of primed microglia, in the *"two-hit hypothesis"*.

Evidence now suggests that prenatal infections may be a risk factor for the development of PD in later life. Brains from postnatal day (P) 21 rat pups born to dams that were intraperitoneally injected with LPS at the gestation window of vulnerability (embryonic day (E) 10.5), displayed reduced numbers of tyrosine hydroxylase (TH) immunoreactive cells in the SN and ventral tegmental area. This apparent DA neuronal loss was associated with reduced striatal dopamine and an increase in TNFα in the striatum and mesencephalon. The loss of TH+ cells was still observed 33 days post- injection (Ling et al., 2002). It has thus been suggested that prenatal infections such as bacterial vaginosis (BV) in humans may be potential risk factors for PD. Indeed, during pregnancy, levels of LPS and TNFα are elevated in the chorioamniotic environment of women with BV, which may hinder typical DA neuron development (Ling et al., 2002). One group has reported loss of DA neurons up to 16 months post prenatal exposure of rats to LPS, which corresponds to the mean age in humans at which PD symptoms are first observed. Thus, prenatal exposure of rats to LPS has been suggested as a potential model of PD as it induces a slow, protracted loss of nigral DA neurons (Carvey et al., 2003). Further validation for this model was demonstrated by significant dopamine and serotonin reductions observed in the frontal cortex, nucleus accumbens, striatum, amygdala, hippocampus and hypothalamus, comparable to the neurochemical alterations evident in PD subjects (Wang et al., 2009). In a study to examine the effect of systemic inflammation on the progression of PD, prenatally LPS-exposed rats were subjected to a moderate dose of 6-OHDA at four-months. The data revealed that both prenatal LPS exposure and postnatal 6-OHDA-treatment produced significant DA neuron loss. However, the combined effect was additive and not synergistic. This may have been due to the young age of the animal or the toxin used (Ling et al., 2004). This model was subsequently investigated but with prenatally LPS-exposed rats treated with rotenone rather than 6-OHDA postnatally. The combined effects of LPS and rotenone produced a synergistic TH+ cell loss in the SN relative to controls, which was associated with increased striatal-dopamine activity, TNFα and increased reactive microglia (Ling et al., 2004).

4. Inflammation in animal models of Parkinson's disease

4.1 MPTP model

The MPTP model of PD has been extensively used to elucidate the basal ganglia response to nigrostriatal deficits as well as to examine the validity of novel drug treatments for PD. The MPTP neurotoxin was initially discovered during the 1980s in humans intoxicated with a by-product of an illicit drug synthesis scheme who presented with symptoms manifesting as severe Parkinsonism (Langston et al., 1983; Langston & Ballard, 1983). *Post-mortem* analysis, ranging between 3-16 years post-MPTP administration, revealed selective DA neurodegeneration and gliosis, with microglial clustering occurring around nerve cells (Langston et al., 1999). It was subsequently postulated that activated microglia might perpetuate DA neuronal degeneration after a primary insult of environmental or genetic origin (Hirsch et al., 2003). Currently, MPTP administration is the most universally used agent for reproducing PD pathologies. It is primarily used in murine and non-human primate models of PD but less frequently in rats, as rat DA neurons are elusively resistant to MPTP-toxicity and are incapable of recapitulating analogous symptoms (Przedborski & Vila, 2003). Motor-impairment symptoms of PD such as bradykinesia, tremor at rest, gait disturbances, postural instability and rigidity have all been observed in MPTP-treated primate models (Bove et al., 2005). While MPTP can mimic a wide range of PD-like symptoms it does not manifest one of the pathological hallmarks of PD, namely the formation of Lewy body-like inclusions, nor can it induce sustained motor impairments. MPTP is highly lipophilic and can easily infiltrate the BBB where it is spontaneously oxidised to an active form, 1-methyl-4-phenyl-2,3-dihydropyridium (1-MPP+) by MAO-B in glial cells. 1-MPP+ is released into the extracellular space where it is taken up by DA neurons via the DA transporter (DAT) (Przedborski & Vila, 2003). Here, it accumulates in the mitochondrial complex and is involved in potently inhibiting mitochondrial complex-1 of the electron transfer chain, leading to an increased production of ROS such as O_2^- and a decrease in ATP. In addition, 1-MPP+ can bind to vesicular monoamine transporter-2, enabling its translocation into the synaptic vesicles where it stimulates the extrusion of synaptic DA. This excess DA is auto-metabolised resulting in a burst of ROS such as hydrogen peroxide (H_2O_2) and superoxide radicals (O_2^-). Accumulation of ROS subsequently causes oxidative degradation of DNA, lipids and proteins resulting in the demise of nigral neurons. This MPTP-induced burst of ROS is generated by microglial

NADPH, therefore, activated microglia have been shown to play an essential role in MPTP-induce neurotoxicity (Gao et al., 2003; Wu et al., 2003). Moreover, cytosolic DA oxidation can be catalysed by COX-2, which has been shown to be up-regulated in nigral DA neurons in both MPTP-treated mice, rats and in human *post-mortem* samples (Teismann & Ferger, 2001; Teismann et al., 2003).

In an effort to examine a potential role for glia in DA neuronal degeneration, focus was initially placed on deciphering the temporal relationship between DA neurodegeneration and glial activation in MPTP-induced PD murine models. Significant depletion of DA fibres and activated astroglia in the striatum was observed 24-48 hours and 48 hours post-MPTP-administration, respectively (O'Callaghan et al., 1990). The duration of astroglia activation was directly dependent on the extent of DA neuronal damage, and was sustained for the duration of MPTP-administration. It was subsequently reported that microglial activation was observed in the striatum 48 hours post-MPTP administration (Francis et al., 1995), while further studies elucidated that activated microglia were present in the SNpc 24 hours post MPTP and that activation was sustained for 14 days (Czlonkowska et al., 1996; Kohutnicka et al., 1998). Other groups pinpoint microglial activation in the SN of mice as early as 12 hours and peaking at 24 hours post-MPTP-administration (Dehmer et al., 2000; Liberatore et al., 1999). It has since been reported that activated amoeboid microglia have been observed in the SN of monkeys years after systemic MPTP-injection (McGeer et al., 2003). A further study has implicated a role for cytokines and chemokines in the acute MPTP mouse model of PD by demonstrating that real-time PCR detected elevated mRNA expression of TNFα, MCP-1 and IL-1α in the mouse striatum 2-4 hours post MPTP-administration (Sriram et al., 2006). However, ablation of TNFα or TNFR-1 did not affect chronic MPTP-induced nigral DA neuronal cell degeneration in mice (Ferger et al., 2004; Leng et al., 2005).

4.2 6-OHDA model

6-OHDA is a hydroxylated analogue of DA, which is actively taken up into DA neurons via DAT expressed on the nerve terminals. It is directly toxic to DA neurons and is used to model PD in rodents. However, since it is unable to cross the BBB, it must be stereotaxically injected into the SN, which results in a widespread and almost immediate destruction of DA neurons (Stanic et al., 2003). The standard delivery method of 6-OHDA is unilateral injection into either the VM, the medial forebrain bundle or the striatum, avoiding areas containing noradrenergic neurons as 6-OHDA can be taken up via the noradrenaline transporter (Deumens et al., 2002). Striatal lesions result in destruction of the nigral DA neuronal terminals leading to a dying back mechanism whereby the cell bodies in the SN are affected secondarily and progressively (Kirik et al., 1998; Sauer & Oertel, 1994). This creates a therapeutic window of opportunity whereby potential neuroprotective strategies can be evaluated. Loss of TH+-immunoreactive cells are detectable as early as 24 hours post-6-OHDA lesion in the striatum, peaking in the third week post-lesion. However, loss of TH+ cells in the SN does not appear until the second week post-lesion (Blandini et al., 2007). Behavioural testing such as drug-induced rotations can then be performed to assess the anti-Parkinsonian abilities of potential therapies. While the 6-OHDA-lesion model remains one of the most popular animal models of PD to date, like the MPTP model, it fails to encapsulate all the hallmarks of PD pathology, particularly a lack of Lewy body formation. Secondly, PD is a chronic disorder potentially lasting 1-2 decades, so the 6-OHDA-model is in fact regarded as an acute model of PD. As in the MPTP-induced animal model of PD, activated microglia have been observed in the SN and nigrostriatal tract of 6-OHDA-lesioned rats (Akiyama & McGeer, 1989; Depino et al., 2003; He et al., 2001). Microglial activation was initially observed 1-day post 6-OHDA-lesion but appeared transient in nature (Akiyama & McGeer, 1989). We have observed a significant increase in the number of activated microglia, indicated by MHC class II in the SNpc of 6-OHDA-lesioned rats at 10-28 days post lesion (Crotty et al., 2008). Pro-inflammatory cytokines have also been implicated as neurotoxic mediators of 6-OHDA-induced DA neuronal death; blockade of the soluble form of the TNF-α receptor but not the transmembrane form was found to attenuate the death of DA neurons in 6-OHDA-lesioned rats (McCoy et al., 2006). We have previously demonstrated that conditioned-medium (CM) obtained from LPS-stimulated rat glial-enriched cortical cultures can induce loss of DA neurons in primary VM cultures and that this effect can be exacerbated by 6-OHDA treatment. IL-1β released from activated microglia in the CM mediated this effect as blockade of IL-1R1 with IL-1RA attenuated the CM-induced DA neuronal toxicity (Long-Smith et al., 2010).

4.3 LPS model

LPS is one of the main constitutes of gram-negative bacteria and is used as a tool to mimic general infection as it is a potent stimulator of immune cells. Intranigral injection of LPS in rats has been shown to manifest Parkinsonism-like symptoms, such as the selective loss of DA neurons in the SN (Arimoto et al., 2006; Castano et al., 1998; Herrera et al., 2000). Thus the LPS model has served as a valuable tool in deciphering the role of glial cells, especially microglia, in the DA neurodegeneration process and has been described by many as the neuroinflammatory model of PD. LPS binds to the serum LPS-binding protein (LBP), which facilitates binding to the CD14 receptor expressed on microglia. The LBP can then dissociate and allow the LPS-CD14 complex to bind to TLR4, resulting in a cascade of intracellular signalling. The adapter protein myeloid differentiation factor 88 (myD88) attaches to TLR4 and interacts with IL-1 receptor-associated kinase (IRAK), which phosphorylates, activating TNF-R-associated factor-6 (TRAF6). The mitogen-activated protein kinases (MAPK) p38 and c-Jun N-terminal kinase (JNK) are activated downstream of this, leading to the up-regulation of transcription factors such as nuclear-factor-κB (NF-κB). This up-regulation results in the production of pro-inflammatory cytokines (McGettrick & O'Neill, 2010).

Intranigral injection of LPS in rats has been shown to result in a significant decrease of DA levels in the striatum, microglial activation and a time and LPS-dose-dependent degeneration of DA neurons in the SN (Castano et al., 1998). In this study, microglial activation was observed at 6 hours and peaked at 1-2 days post LPS injection, while DA neuronal degeneration persisted up to at least 21 days after intranigral injection of LPS demonstrating that LPS-induced microglial activation can induce progressive degeneration of nigral DA neurons. Furthermore, it has been reported that prenatal exposure of LPS to rats results in sustained microglial activation and the development of fewer than normal nigral DA neurons (Ling et al., 2006). Systemic administration of LPS has also been found to induce progressive degeneration of nigral DA neurons in rats (Qin et al., 2007). It had previously been suggested that LPS-mediated DA neuronal toxicity required the presence of glia (Bronstein et al., 1995) and indeed a subsequent study reported that a single intranigral injection of LPS induced selective DA neuronal degeneration up to one year post injection (Herrera et al., 2000). Thus, unlike MPTP and 6-OHDA, LPS is not a direct toxin but rather causes indirect death of DA neurons by activating microglia, inducing an inflammatory reaction and subsequent DA neuronal death. Studies on rat mesencephalic cultures suggest that DA neurons are twice as sensitive to LPS as non-DA neurons and that the toxicity of LPS occurs via microglial activation (Bronstein et al., 1995; Gayle et al., 2002). Although many *in vitro* studies have supported an involvement of NO in microglial-mediated DA neuronal death after LPS-treatment (Chao et al., 1992; Gibbons & Dragunow, 2006), others have suggested that NO is not involved (Castano et al., 1998; Gayle et al., 2002). The pro-inflammatory cytokines IL-1β and TNF-α are thought to be involved in LPS-mediated toxicity (Gayle et al., 2002). In support of a role for LPS-induced pro-inflammatory cytokines in DA neurotoxicity, we have shown that IL-1β in CM released from LPS-stimulated microglia significantly reduces the percentage of DA neurons in embryonic rat neuronal-enriched cultures that IL-1R1 is expressed on these DA neurons, and that blockade of IL-1R1 prevented the CM-induced DA neuronal death (Long-Smith et al., 2010). Furthermore, blockade of the soluble form of the TNF-α receptor has been reported to reduce microglial activation in the *in vivo* LPS model of PD (McCoy et al., 2006). Also, Ling and co-workers found that the decreased numbers of nigral DA neurons in rats after prenatal exposure to LPS, was accompanied by elevated levels of TNF-α in the striatum (Ling et al., 2004).

5. Neuroinflammatory diagnostic tools for Parkinson's disease

Microglial responsiveness to injury and neurodegenerative disease suggests that it may serve as a marker for the diagnosis and progression of disease pathology in PD. There is a current drive to develop non-invasive imaging tools to assess and quantify the dynamics of activated microglia in neurodegenerative diseases like PD. Advances in this technology, especially for identification of microglial biomarkers at the early stages of disease, would have important implications for PD diagnosis, assessment of progression, and therapy. Currently, the best-studied imaging paradigm for microglial activation is the radiolabelled translocator protein (TSPO) ligand using PET (Dolle et al., 2009). This line of research initially started when a correlation was observed between increased binding of Ro5-4864 (a benzodiazepine) and PK11195 (an isoquinoline) to receptors on the surface of mitochondria primarily localised in glial cells (Arlicot et al., 2008; Chauveau et al., 2008). These receptors were originally referred to as peripheral type benzodiazepine receptors and were increased in activated microglia (Park et al., 1996; Stephenson et al., 1995). The nomenclature has since been changed to TSPO as further research elucidated that these receptors are expressed throughout the brain and body (Papadopoulos et al., 2006). Gene-expression analysis in brains of rodents, primates and humans have illustrated that TSPO expression is nearly absent in parenchyma-microglia (Winkeler et al., 2010) but is elevated in many neurodegenerative disorders including, stroke, AD, PD, multiple sclerosis, Huntington's disease and amyotrophic lateral sclerosis, (Arlicot et al., 2008) thus emphasising the involvement of microglial activation and neuroinflammation in these diseases. TSPOs are the prototypical biomarkers of neuroinflammatory changes in a variety of CNS disorders and have therefore been proposed as potential diagnostic targets for *in vivo* imaging (Arlicot et al., 2008; Chauveau et al., 2008).

Currently, functional PET and single photon emission tomography (SPECT), in conjunction with ligands for TSPO, can detect microglial activation *in vivo*. Examples of radiolabelled TSPO ligands include [¹¹C]Ro5-4864 and [¹¹C](R)-PK11195 (1-(2-chlorophenyl)-N-methyl-N-(1-methylpropyl)-3 isoquinoline carboxamide) (Chauveau et al., 2008). In PD subjects, PET imaging revealed microglial activation in the pons, basal ganglia, and frontal and temporal cortical areas. Longitudinal studies of these patients revealed stable [^{11}C](R)-PK11195 binding potential (BP; a parameter that mixes receptor density with ligand affinity), indicative of early activation of microglia in PD pathology (Gerhard et al., 2006; Winkeler et al., 2010). However, the [^{11}C](R)-PK11195 tracer is limited, as it is incapable of distinguishing between phenotypic differences, and thus possibly functional differences of microglia. To overcome this, a PET tracer for the dopamine-transporter, [^{11}C]CFT, has been used in conjunction with [^{11}C](R)-PK11195 to examine the viability of the presynaptic DA neurons (Ouchi et al., 2009). This study of 10 drug-naïve PD patients, demonstrated changes in microglial activity in conjunction with DAT density which were investigated using PET imaging with [^{11}C](R)-PK11195 and [^{11}C]CFT tracers. Subjects underwent magnetic resonance imaging (MRI) prior to PET measurement to define the regions of interest, which would allow for the evaluation of microglial activation in parallel with presynaptic neuronal degeneration *in vivo*. Elevated midbrain [^{11}C](R)-PK11195 BP levels were significantly inversely correlated with [^{11}C]CFT BP localised in the putamen. The elevated [^{11}C](R)-PK11195 BP also correlated with motor impairment. A follow-up 4-year scan revealed increased microglial activation spread over the extrastriatal region (Ouchi et al., 2009). PET imaging and *post-mortem* analysis of the brain of a rat lesioned with 6-OHDA revealed reduced [^{11}C]CFT BP in the striatum, indicative of DA degeneration, while [^{11}C](R)-PK11195 BP was markedly increased in the striatum and SNpc. *Post-mortem* immunohistochemical analysis corroborated this finding by showing activated microglia in the striatum and SNpc at 4 weeks post-lesion (Cicchetti et al., 2002). Alternative SPECT imaging biomarkers for TSPO such as [^{123}I]CLINDE (2-(4'iodophenyl)-3-(N,N-diethyl)-imidazo[1,2-a]pyridine-3-acetamide) have been examined *in vivo* and also pose as potential image-guided diagnostic tools for microglial activation in neurodegenerative diseases like PD (Arlicot et al., 2008).

6. Immunomodulatory therapies

As the wealth of evidence continues to accumulate regarding the role of microglial activation in the pathogenesis of PD, a large number of inhibitory drugs have been investigated. The use of broad spectrum steroidal and non-steroidal anti-inflammatory drugs, specific microglial inhibitors or anti-inflammatory cytokines have not only helped decipher the role of microglial activation in neuroinflammation in PD but also indicated that inhibiting the specific processes involved in microglial activation may be a therapeutic avenue for PD.

The glucocorticoids are well known for their broad range of anti-inflammatory effects and have long been used in clinical settings for the treatment of brain inflammation (Castano et al., 2002). Microglial cells express the glucocorticoid receptor which is involved in the regulation of the transcription factors NF-κB and activator protein-1 (AP-1) (Scheinman et al., 1995) which in turn are key regulators of pro-inflammatory cytokine expression (Nadeau & Rivest, 2003). Of particular interest, the synthetic steroid dexamethasone was shown to provide neuroprotection against LPS or MPTP-induced toxicity in rodent models. In both models, the delivery of dexamethasone prevented the activation of microglia usually associated with neurodegeneration (Castano et al., 2002; Kurkowska-Jastrzebska et al., 2004). However, the severe side-effects associated with glucocorticoid use prevent any long-term usage in neuroprotective therapies for PD. Large scale epidemiological studies have shown that the chronic use of non-steroidal anti-inflammatory drugs (NSAID) such as aspirin or ibuprofen could provide some level of protection against PD (Chen et al., 2005; Chen et al., 2003). Other studies suggest that the role of NSAIDs in decreasing the risk of PD is extremely limited (Hancock et al., 2007; Hernan et al., 2006). A recent meta-analysis of studies published between 1966 and 2008 showed that while NSAIDs as a class do not modify the risk of developing PD, the chronic intake of ibuprofen may have a beneficial effect (Gagne & Power, 2010; Gao et al., 2011; Samii et al., 2009). Ibuprofen possibly mediates this effect via its inhibition of COX activity to inhibit the production of pro-inflammatory lipid mediator prostaglandins (Mitchell et al., 1993). Some of the beneficial effects observed could also be mediated via other mechanisms associated with NSAIDs such as inactivation of the pro-inflammatory nuclear receptor NF-κB (Grilli et al., 1996; Kopp & Ghosh, 1994), activation of peroxisome proliferator-activated receptor gamma (PPARγ), a nuclear factor mediating anti-inflammatory effects in microglia (Bernardo et al., 2005) or activation of the Rho kinase pathway (Zhou et al., 2003). Results from animal models of PD demonstrate that aspirin and indomethacin have both been shown to prevent MPTP-induced loss of striatal dopamine in the mouse (Aubin et al., 1998; Kurkowska-Jastrzebska et al., 2002). The NSAID Celecoxib reversed striatal DA neuronal fibre and nigral DA neuronal cell loss in 6-OHDA-treated rats (Sanchez-Pernaute et al., 2004) while aspirin has been shown to prevent 6-OHDA-induced striatal dopamine depletion (Di Matteo et al., 2006).

Other neuroimmunomodulatory strategies include the use of the second generation tetracycline analogue, minocycline. It has been shown to inhibit microglial activation and prevent iNOS and NADPH oxidase generation as well as IL-1β up-regulation (Du et al., 2001). It is a lipophilic molecule which easily crosses the BBB and is reported to have anti-inflammatory and neuroprotective activities (Kim & Suh, 2009). Some studies in experimental models of PD have shown that it is neuroprotective against MPTP-, LPS, or 6-OHDA induced neurodegeneration (Du et al., 2001; He et al., 2001; Tomas-Camardiel et al., 2004; Wu et al., 2002) while others showed that it exacerbated the deleterious effects of MPTP in rodents and non-human primates (Diguet et al., 2004; Yang et al., 2003). While the reason for the discrepancies is unknown, differences between the various studies include doses and timing of intervention and may reflect the dual role of microglia in inflammation. Despite these contradictory results, a phase II randomized double-blind futility clinical trial was set-up. Results after 12 and 18 months suggest that minocycline is well tolerated and does not negatively impact on symptomatic treatment. It is therefore currently recommended for phase III clinical trials to assess its long-term effect on disease progression (NINDS-NET-PD-Investigators, 2006, 2008).

In addition to the role of glial-associated innate immunity, an adaptive immune response may also be involved in triggering cell death in DA neurons. Manipulating this adaptive response mediated by T cells could be a successful approach for neuroprotection. This immuno-intervention aims at redirecting the harmful T cell response towards an anti-inflammatory and protective immune response by means of an antigen-based immunisation. Preclinical results using glatiramer acetate (a random amino acid polymer composed of alanine, glutamine, lysine and tyrosine amino acids) as the immunisation agent showed that this approach could be successful. Glatiramer-acetate primed T cells transferred to MPTP-treated mice were shown to reach the brain where they suppressed microglial activation and provided neuroprotection to the nigrostriatal neurons by inducing the neurotrophic factor glial cell-derived neurotrophic factor (GDNF). Furthermore, specific depletion of the donor T cells abrogated this neuroprotective effect confirming that the effect is donor T cell dependent (Benner et al., 2004). Interestingly, the donor T cells were shown to secrete high levels of anti-inflammatory cytokines IL-4, IL-10 and TGFβ (Benner et al., 2004). As glatiramer acetate has already been shown to be safe and tolerable in clinical trial and has had significant reduction effects on disability in multiple sclerosis patients (Comi et al., 2011), it represents a very attractive possibility. Interestingly, another neuropeptide, vasoactive intestinal peptide, has been reported to prevent MPTP-induced loss of nigral DA neurons and striatal DA fibres in the mouse while also down-regulating IL-1β and TNF-α expression and iNOS generation (Delgado & Ganea, 2003).

Alternatively, the delivery of anti-inflammatory cytokines such as IL-10 could be considered as an anti-inflammatory therapeutic strategy for PD. Pre-treatment of mesencephalic neuroglial cultures with IL-10 inhibited LPS-stimulated microglial activation and degeneration of DA neurons (Qian et al., 2006). Similar neuroprotective effects were observed *in vivo* after chronic infusion of IL-10 into the SNpc of rats that were challenged with LPS (Arimoto et al., 2006). More recently, gene therapy approaches have been developed to deliver IL-10 into the rat SNpc, and have proved effective in attenuating the neuronal loss and behavioural deficits in the 6-OHDA rat model of PD (Johnston et al., 2008). Furthermore, the blockade of pro-inflammatory cytokines should be considered as a potential therapeutic avenue. Blocking the soluble TNF signalling by delivery of a dominant-negative form has been shown to promote neuronal survival and reduce the behavioural deficits in the hemi-Parkinsonian rat model of PD (McCoy et al., 2006; McCoy et al., 2008). While these pre-clinical results are interesting, the availability of a broad spectrum of compounds acting on TNF signalling makes this molecule a very attractive target. Etanercept and Infliximab are a new generation of engineered inhibitors of TNF that are broadly used for the treatment of rheumatoid arthritis and other peripheral inflammatory diseases. Their use in CNS diseases is however limited by their general inability to cross the BBB (Tweedie et al., 2007). While direct intrastriatal delivery or long-term gene transfer as illustrated above are possibilities, other inhibitors of TNF synthesis may prove useful such as the infamous antiemetic compound thalidomide. Thalidomide is a sedative, immunosuppressive and anti-inflammatory drug that has teratogenic effects (Smithells & Newman, 1992) and inhibits the synthesis of TNF-α (Sampaio et al., 1991). Thalidomide was shown to protect nigrostriatal neurons and prevent striatal DA depletion in the early stages of MPTP-induced neurodegeneration (Boireau et al., 1997; Ferger et al., 2004).

PPARγ has been shown to exert anti-inflammatory functions in both the periphery and the CNS where it is detected in glial and neuronal cells. Following activation by its naturally occurring ligands eicosanoids and prostaglandin J2, it regulates the expression of pro-inflammatory molecules such as iNOS, COX-2 and, indirectly, of broad array of cytokines through its interactions with the transcription factor NF-κB (Chaturvedi & Beal, 2008; Chung et al., 2008). Pioglitazone and rosiglitazone are two synthetic agonists of PPARγ that are approved for the treatment of type II diabetes. In the CNS they exhibit neuroprotective effects in models of neurodegenerative disorders, including PD, by preventing inflammation, oxidative damage and apoptosis (Chaturvedi & Beal, 2008). Specifically, pioglitazone prevents MPTP-induced activation of microglia and DA neuronal cell loss in murine SNpc *in vivo* (Dehmer et al., 2004). This has been shown to occur through inhibition of MAO-B, the enzyme responsible for conversion of MPTP to its toxic metabolite MPP+ (Quinn et al., 2008). When pioglitazone was administered to rats that were also injected intrastriatally with LPS, the resultant LPS-induced microglial activation and DA degeneration was attenuated (Hunter et al., 2007). Recently, the neuroprotective effects of rosiglitazone have been shown in the MPTP mouse model of PD; chronic administration of the drug prevented behavioural deficits, DA neuronal loss and microglial activation in the SNpc *in vivo* (Schintu et al., 2009).

As mentioned above, NF-κB plays an important role in the regulation of chronic diseases through the promotion of inflammation and of cell survival. Activation of NF-κB requires the activity of the IκB kinase (IKK) complex (Kim et al., 2006). Activated NF-κB has been detected in neurons and activated microglia in the SN of PD patients and MPTP-treated animals suggesting that some of the pro-inflammatory mechanisms regulated by the NF-κB pathways may play an important role in the pathogenesis of PD (Ghosh et al., 2007; Hunot et al., 1997). Recent studies have shown that blockade of NF-κB activity either directly or through IκB can inhibit components of the inflammatory pathways in microglia namely, the oxidative stress pathway and the production of pro-inflammatory cytokines (Anrather et al., 2006; Gauss et al., 2007). Selective inhibition of NF-κB activity by a peptide blocking the IKK complex prevented DA neuronal loss in MPTP-treated mice and suppressed microglial activation (Ghosh et al., 2007). Finally, a selective pharmacological IKKβ inhibitor has demonstrated neuroprotective properties in LPS- and MPTP-induced models of PD. Treatment with this compound prevented neuronal damage in a process dependant on the presence of microglia. Particularly, it prevented the activation of microglial oxidative pathways and the release of pro-inflammatory cytokines by specific blockade of the NF-κB signalling pathway (Zhang et al., 2010).

7. Conclusion

The death of dopaminergic neurons in the SNpc is the key pathology of PD. Therefore, it is imperative that research is undertaken, not only in areas which could provide protective strategies for the remaining neurons, or which involve dopaminergic neuronal cell replacement therapies, but also into understanding the fundamental mechanisms by which these cells die. Although the precise role of inflammation in the pathogenesis of PD remains unclear, an array of evidence from the clinic and from animal models now points to its substantial involvement in this debilitating disease.

8. Acknowledgment

The authors thank Declan Conroy and Aoife Nolan for technical assistance.

9. References

Ajami, B., Bennett, J.L., Krieger, C., Tetzlaff, W. & Rossi, F.M. (2007). Local self-renewal can sustain CNS microglia maintenance and function throughout adult life. *Nat Neurosci,* Vol.10, No.12, pp. 1538-1543

Akiyama, H. & McGeer, P.L. (1989). Microglial response to 6-hydroxydopamine-induced substantia nigra lesions. *Brain Res,* Vol.489, No.2, pp. 247-253

Anisman, H. & Merali, Z. (1999). Anhedonic and anxiogenic effects of cytokine exposure. *Adv Exp Med Biol,* Vol.461, No., pp. 199-233

Anrather, J., Racchumi, G. & Iadecola, C. (2006). NF-kappaB regulates phagocytic NADPH oxidase by inducing the expression of gp91phox. *J Biol Chem*, Vol.281, No.9, pp. 5657-5667

Arimoto, T., Choi, D.Y., Lu, X., Liu, M., Nguyen, X.V., Zheng, N., Stewart, C.A., Kim, H.C. & Bing, G. (2006). Interleukin-10 protects against inflammation-mediated degeneration of dopaminergic neurons in substantia nigra. *Neurobiol Aging*, Vol.28, No.6, pp. 894-906

Arlicot, N., Katsifis, A., Garreau, L., Mattner, F., Vergote, J., Duval, S., Kousignian, I., Bodard, S., Guilloteau, D. & Chalon, S. (2008). Evaluation of CLINDE as potent translocator protein (18 kDa) SPECT radiotracer reflecting the degree of neuroinflammation in a rat model of microglial activation. *Eur J Nucl Med Mol Imaging*, Vol.35, No.12, pp. 2203-2211

Aubin, N., Curet, O., Deffois, A. & Carter, C. (1998). Aspirin and salicylate protect against MPTP-induced dopamine depletion in mice. *J Neurochem*, Vol.71, No.4, pp. 1635-1642

Banati, R.B., Daniel, S.E. & Blunt, S.B. (1998). Glial pathology but absence of apoptotic nigral neurons in long-standing Parkinson's disease. *Mov Disord*, Vol.13, No.2, pp. 221-227

Barron, K.D. (1995). The microglial cell. A historical review. *J Neurol Sci*, Vol.134 Suppl, No., pp. 57-68

Bas, J., Calopa, M., Mestre, M., Mollevi, D.G., Cutillas, B., Ambrosio, S. & Buendia, E. (2001). Lymphocyte populations in Parkinson's disease and in rat models of parkinsonism. *J Neuroimmunol*, Vol.113, No.1, pp. 146-152

Bekris, L.M., Mata, I.F. & Zabetian, C.P. (2010). The genetics of Parkinson disease. *J Geriatr Psychiatry Neurol*, Vol.23, No.4, pp. 228-242

Benner, E.J., Mosley, R.L., Destache, C.J., Lewis, T.B., Jackson-Lewis, V., Gorantla, S., Nemachek, C., Green, S.R., Przedborski, S. & Gendelman, H.E. (2004). Therapeutic immunization protects dopaminergic neurons in a mouse model of Parkinson's disease. *Proc Natl Acad Sci U S A*, Vol.101, No.25, pp. 9435-9440

Bernardo, A., Ajmone-Cat, M.A., Gasparini, L., Ongini, E. & Minghetti, L. (2005). Nuclear receptor peroxisome proliferator-activated receptor-gamma is activated in rat microglial cells by the anti-inflammatory drug HCT1026, a derivative of flurbiprofen. *J Neurochem*, Vol.92, No.4, pp. 895-903

Bialecka, M., Kurzawski, M., Klodowska-Duda, G., Opala, G., Juzwiak, S., Kurzawski, G., Tan, E.K. & Drozdzik, M. (2007). CARD15 variants in patients with sporadic Parkinson's disease. *Neurosci Res*, Vol.57, No.3, pp. 473-476

Blandini, F., Levandis, G., Bazzini, E., Nappi, G. & Armentero, M.T. (2007). Time-course of nigrostriatal damage, basal ganglia metabolic changes and behavioural alterations following intrastriatal injection of 6-hydroxydopamine in the rat: new clues from an old model. *Eur J Neurosci*, Vol.25, No.2, pp. 397-405

Block, M.L. & Hong, J.S. (2005). Microglia and inflammation-mediated neurodegeneration: multiple triggers with a common mechanism. *Prog Neurobiol*, Vol.76, No.2, pp. 77-98

Block, M.L., Zecca, L. & Hong, J.S. (2007). Microglia-mediated neurotoxicity: uncovering the molecular mechanisms. *Nat Rev Neurosci*, Vol.8, No.1, pp. 57-69

Boireau, A., Bordier, F., Dubedat, P., Peny, C. & Imperato, A. (1997). Thalidomide reduces MPTP-induced decrease in striatal dopamine levels in mice. *Neurosci Lett*, Vol.234, No.2-3, pp. 123-126

Boka, G., Anglade, P., Wallach, D., Javoy-Agid, F., Agid, Y. & Hirsch, E.C. (1994). Immunocytochemical analysis of tumor necrosis factor and its receptors in Parkinson's disease. *Neurosci Lett*, Vol.172, No.1-2, pp. 151-154

Bove, J., Prou, D., Perier, C. & Przedborski, S. (2005). Toxin-induced models of Parkinson's disease. *NeuroRx*, Vol.2, No.3, pp. 484-494

Braak, H., Del Tredici, K., Rub, U., de Vos, R.A., Jansen Steur, E.N. & Braak, E. (2003). Staging of brain pathology related to sporadic Parkinson's disease. *Neurobiol Aging*, Vol.24, No.2, pp. 197-211

Brochard, V., Combadiere, B., Prigent, A., Laouar, Y., Perrin, A., Beray-Berthat, V., Bonduelle, O., Alvarez-Fischer, D., Callebert, J., Launay, J.M., Duyckaerts, C., Flavell, R.A., Hirsch, E.C. & Hunot, S. (2009). Infiltration of CD4+ lymphocytes into the brain contributes to neurodegeneration in a mouse model of Parkinson disease. *J Clin Invest*, Vol.119, No.1, pp. 182-192

Brodacki, B., Staszewski, J., Toczylowska, B., Kozlowska, E., Drela, N., Chalimoniuk, M. & Stepien, A. (2008). Serum interleukin (IL-2, IL-10, IL-6, IL-4), TNFalpha, and INFgamma concentrations are elevated in patients with atypical and idiopathic parkinsonism. *Neurosci Lett*, Vol.441, No.2, pp. 158-162

Bronstein, D.M., Perez-Otano, I., Sun, V., Mullis Sawin, S.B., Chan, J., Wu, G.C., Hudson, P.M., Kong, L.Y., Hong, J.S. & McMillian, M.K. (1995). Glia-dependent neurotoxicity and neuroprotection in mesencephalic cultures. *Brain Res*, Vol.704, No.1, pp. 112-116

Butt, A.M. (2011). ATP: A ubiquitous gliotransmitter integrating neuron-glial networks. *Semin Cell Dev Biol*, Vol.22, No.2, pp. 205-213

Calne, D.B. & Langston, J.W. (1983). Aetiology of Parkinson's disease. *Lancet*, Vol.2, No.8365-66, pp. 1457-1459

Carson, M.J., Reilly, C.R., Sutcliffe, J.G. & Lo, D. (1998). Mature microglia resemble immature antigen-presenting cells. *Glia*, Vol.22, No.1, pp. 72-85

Carvey, P.M., Chang, Q., Lipton, J.W. & Ling, Z. (2003). Prenatal exposure to the bacteriotoxin lipopolysaccharide leads to long-term losses of dopamine neurons in offspring: a potential, new model of Parkinson's disease. *Front Biosci*, Vol.8, No., pp. s826-837

Castano, A., Herrera, A.J., Cano, J. & Machado, A. (1998). Lipopolysaccharide intranigral injection induces inflammatory reaction and damage in nigrostriatal dopaminergic system. *J Neurochem*, Vol.70, No.4, pp. 1584-1592

Castano, A., Herrera, A.J., Cano, J. & Machado, A. (2002). The degenerative effect of a single intranigral injection of LPS on the dopaminergic system is prevented by dexamethasone, and not mimicked by rh-TNF-alpha, IL-1beta and IFN-gamma. *J Neurochem*, Vol.81, No.1, pp. 150-157

Chao, C.C., Hu, S., Molitor, T.W., Shaskan, E.G. & Peterson, P.K. (1992). Activated microglia mediate neuronal cell injury via a nitric oxide mechanism. *J Immunol*, Vol.149, No.8, pp. 2736-2741

Chaturvedi, R.K. & Beal, M.F. (2008). PPAR: a therapeutic target in Parkinson's disease. *J Neurochem*, Vol.106, No.2, pp. 506-518

Chauveau, F., Boutin, H., Van Camp, N., Dolle, F. & Tavitian, B. (2008). Nuclear imaging of neuroinflammation: a comprehensive review of [11C]PK11195 challengers. *Eur J Nucl Med Mol Imaging*, Vol.35, No.12, pp. 2304-2319

Chen, H., Jacobs, E., Schwarzschild, M.A., McCullough, M.L., Calle, E.E., Thun, M.J. & Ascherio, A. (2005). Nonsteroidal antiinflammatory drug use and the risk for Parkinson's disease. *Ann Neurol*, Vol.58, No.6, pp. 963-967

Chen, H., O'Reilly, E.J., Schwarzschild, M.A. & Ascherio, A. (2008). Peripheral inflammatory biomarkers and risk of Parkinson's disease. *Am J Epidemiol*, Vol.167, No.1, pp. 90-95

Chen, H., Zhang, S.M., Hernan, M.A., Schwarzschild, M.A., Willett, W.C., Colditz, G.A., Speizer, F.E. & Ascherio, A. (2003). Nonsteroidal anti-inflammatory drugs and the risk of Parkinson disease. *Arch Neurol*, Vol.60, No.8, pp. 1059-1064

Chen, X., Lan, X., Roche, I., Liu, R. & Geiger, J.D. (2008). Caffeine protects against MPTP-induced blood-brain barrier dysfunction in mouse striatum. *J Neurochem*, Vol.107, No.4, pp. 1147-1157

Chung, J.H., Seo, A.Y., Chung, S.W., Kim, M.K., Leeuwenburgh, C., Yu, B.P. & Chung, H.Y. (2008). Molecular mechanism of PPAR in the regulation of age-related inflammation. *Ageing Res Rev*, Vol.7, No.2, pp. 126-136

Chung, Y.C., Ko, H.W., Bok, E., Park, E.S., Huh, S.H., Nam, J.H. & Jin, B.K. (2010). The role of neuroinflammation on the pathogenesis of Parkinson's disease. *BMB Rep*, Vol.43, No.4, pp. 225-232

Cicchetti, F., Brownell, A.L., Williams, K., Chen, Y.I., Livni, E. & Isacson, O. (2002). Neuroinflammation of the nigrostriatal pathway during progressive 6-OHDA dopamine degeneration in rats monitored by immunohistochemistry and PET imaging. *Eur J Neurosci*, Vol.15, No.6, pp. 991-998

Comi, G., Cohen, J.A., Arnold, D.L., Wynn, D. & Filippi, M. (2011). Phase III dose-comparison study of glatiramer acetate for multiple sclerosis. *Ann Neurol*, Vol.69, No.1, pp. 75-82

Crotty, S., Fitzgerald, P., Tuohy, E., Harris, D.M., Fisher, A., Mandel, A., Bolton, A.E., Sullivan, A.M. & Nolan, Y. (2008). Neuroprotective effects of novel phosphatidylglycerol-based phospholipids in the 6-hydroxydopamine model of Parkinson's disease. *Eur J Neurosci*, Vol.27, No.2, pp. 294-300

Cuadros, M.A. & Navascues, J. (1998). The origin and differentiation of microglial cells during development. *Prog Neurobiol*, Vol.56, No.2, pp. 173-189

Czlonkowska, A., Kohutnicka, M., Kurkowska-Jastrzebska, I. & Czlonkowski, A. (1996). Microglial reaction in MPTP (1-methyl-4-phenyl-1,2,3,6-tetrahydropyridine) induced Parkinson's disease mice model. *Neurodegeneration*, Vol.5, No.2, pp. 137-143

Dantzer, R. (2009). Cytokine, sickness behavior, and depression. *Immunol Allergy Clin North Am*, Vol.29, No.2, pp. 247-264

Davalos, D., Grutzendler, J., Yang, G., Kim, J.V., Zuo, Y., Jung, S., Littman, D.R., Dustin, M.L. & Gan, W.B. (2005). ATP mediates rapid microglial response to local brain injury in vivo. *Nat Neurosci*, Vol.8, No.6, pp. 752-758

Dehmer, T., Heneka, M.T., Sastre, M., Dichgans, J. & Schulz, J.B. (2004). Protection by pioglitazone in the MPTP model of Parkinson's disease correlates with I kappa B alpha induction and block of NF kappa B and iNOS activation. *J Neurochem*, Vol.88, No.2, pp. 494-501

Dehmer, T., Lindenau, J., Haid, S., Dichgans, J. & Schulz, J.B. (2000). Deficiency of inducible nitric oxide synthase protects against MPTP toxicity in vivo. *J Neurochem,* Vol.74, No.5, pp. 2213-2216

del Rio Hortega, P. (1932). *Microglia.* In: Penfield, W. (Ed.), Cytology and cellular pathology of the nervous system. Hoeber, New York, pp. 481-534.

Delgado, M. & Ganea, D. (2003). Neuroprotective effect of vasoactive intestinal peptide (VIP) in a mouse model of Parkinson's disease by blocking microglial activation. *FASEB J,* Vol.17, No.8, pp. 944-946

Depino, A.M., Earl, C., Kaczmarczyk, E., Ferrari, C., Besedovsky, H., del Rey, A., Pitossi, F.J. & Oertel, W.H. (2003). Microglial activation with atypical proinflammatory cytokine expression in a rat model of Parkinson's disease. *Eur J Neurosci,* Vol.18, No.10, pp. 2731-2742

Deumens, R., Blokland, A. & Prickaerts, J. (2002). Modeling Parkinson's disease in rats: an evaluation of 6-OHDA lesions of the nigrostriatal pathway. *Exp Neurol,* Vol.175, No.2, pp. 303-317

Di Matteo, V., Pierucci, M., Di Giovanni, G., Di Santo, A., Poggi, A., Benigno, A. & Esposito, E. (2006). Aspirin protects striatal dopaminergic neurons from neurotoxin-induced degeneration: an in vivo microdialysis study. *Brain Res,* Vol.1095, No.1, pp. 167-177

Di Monte, D.A. (2003). The environment and Parkinson's disease: is the nigrostriatal system preferentially targeted by neurotoxins? *Lancet Neurol,* Vol.2, No.9, pp. 531-538

Dick, F.D. (2006). Parkinson's disease and pesticide exposures. *Br Med Bull,* Vol.79-80, No.1, pp. 219-231

Diguet, E., Fernagut, P.O., Wei, X., Du, Y., Rouland, R., Gross, C., Bezard, E. & Tison, F. (2004). Deleterious effects of minocycline in animal models of Parkinson's disease and Huntington's disease. *Eur J Neurosci,* Vol.19, No.12, pp. 3266-3276

Dobbs, R.J., Charlett, A., Purkiss, A.G., Dobbs, S.M., Weller, C. & Peterson, D.W. (1999). Association of circulating TNF-alpha and IL-6 with ageing and parkinsonism. *Acta Neurol Scand,* Vol.100, No.1, pp. 34-41

Dolle, F., Luus, C., Reynolds, A. & Kassiou, M. (2009). Radiolabelled molecules for imaging the translocator protein (18 kDa) using positron emission tomography. *Curr Med Chem,* Vol.16, No.22, pp. 2899-2923

Du, Y., Ma, Z., Lin, S., Dodel, R.C., Gao, F., Bales, K.R., Triarhou, L.C., Chernet, E., Perry, K.W., Nelson, D.L., Luecke, S., Phebus, L.A., Bymaster, F.P. & Paul, S.M. (2001). Minocycline prevents nigrostriatal dopaminergic neurodegeneration in the MPTP model of Parkinson's disease. *Proc Natl Acad Sci U S A,* Vol.98, No.25, pp. 14669-14674

Eder, C., Schilling, T., Heinemann, U., Haas, D., Hailer, N. & Nitsch, R. (1999). Morphological, immunophenotypical and electrophysiological properties of resting microglia in vitro. *Eur J Neurosci,* Vol.11, No.12, pp. 4251-4261

Faucheux, B.A., Bonnet, A.M., Agid, Y. & Hirsch, E.C. (1999). Blood vessels change in the mesencephalon of patients with Parkinson's disease. *Lancet,* Vol.353, No.9157, pp. 981-982

Ferger, B., Leng, A., Mura, A., Hengerer, B. & Feldon, J. (2004). Genetic ablation of tumor necrosis factor-alpha (TNF-alpha) and pharmacological inhibition of TNF-synthesis attenuates MPTP toxicity in mouse striatum. *J Neurochem,* Vol.89, No.4, pp. 822-833

Ferrari, C.C., Pott Godoy, M.C., Tarelli, R., Chertoff, M., Depino, A.M. & Pitossi, F.J. (2006). Progressive neurodegeneration and motor disabilities induced by chronic expression of IL-1beta in the substantia nigra. *Neurobiol Dis,* Vol.24, No.1, pp. 183-193

Ferrari, C.C. & Tarelli, R. (2011). Parkinson's disease and systemic inflammation. *Parkinsons Dis,* Vol.2011, No., pp. 436813

Fiszer, U., Mix, E., Fredrikson, S., Kostulas, V., Olsson, T. & Link, H. (1994). gamma delta+ T cells are increased in patients with Parkinson's disease. *J Neurol Sci,* Vol.121, No.1, pp. 39-45

Francis, J.W., Von Visger, J., Markelonis, G.J. & Oh, T.H. (1995). Neuroglial responses to the dopaminergic neurotoxicant 1-methyl-4-phenyl-1,2,3,6-tetrahydropyridine in mouse striatum. *Neurotoxicol Teratol,* Vol.17, No.1, pp. 7-12

Gagne, J.J. & Power, M.C. (2010). Anti-inflammatory drugs and risk of Parkinson disease: a meta-analysis. *Neurology,* Vol.74, No.12, pp. 995-1002

Gao, H.M. & Hong, J.S. (2008). Why neurodegenerative diseases are progressive: uncontrolled inflammation drives disease progression. *Trends Immunol,* Vol.29, No.8, pp. 357-365

Gao, H.M., Liu, B., Zhang, W. & Hong, J.S. (2003). Critical role of microglial NADPH oxidase-derived free radicals in the in vitro MPTP model of Parkinson's disease. *FASEB J,* Vol.17, No.13, pp. 1954-1956

Gao, X., Chen, H., Schwarzschild, M.A. & Ascherio, A. (2011). Use of ibuprofen and risk of Parkinson disease. *Neurology,* Vol.76, No.10, pp. 863-869

Garden, G.A. & Moller, T. (2006). Microglia biology in health and disease. *J Neuroimmune Pharmacol,* Vol.1, No.2, pp. 127-137

Gauss, K.A., Nelson-Overton, L.K., Siemsen, D.W., Gao, Y., DeLeo, F.R. & Quinn, M.T. (2007). Role of NF-kappaB in transcriptional regulation of the phagocyte NADPH oxidase by tumor necrosis factor-alpha. *J Leukoc Biol,* Vol.82, No.3, pp. 729-741

Gayle, D.A., Ling, Z., Tong, C., Landers, T., Lipton, J.W. & Carvey, P.M. (2002). Lipopolysaccharide (LPS)-induced dopamine cell loss in culture: roles of tumor necrosis factor-alpha, interleukin-1beta, and nitric oxide. *Brain Res Dev Brain Res,* Vol.133, No.1, pp. 27-35

Gerhard, A., Pavese, N., Hotton, G., Turkheimer, F., Es, M., Hammers, A., Eggert, K., Oertel, W., Banati, R.B. & Brooks, D.J. (2006). In vivo imaging of microglial activation with [11C](R)-PK11195 PET in idiopathic Parkinson's disease. *Neurobiol Dis,* Vol.21, No.2, pp. 404-412

Ghosh, A., Roy, A., Liu, X., Kordower, J.H., Mufson, E.J., Hartley, D.M., Ghosh, S., Mosley, R.L., Gendelman, H.E. & Pahan, K. (2007). Selective inhibition of NF-kappaB activation prevents dopaminergic neuronal loss in a mouse model of Parkinson's disease. *Proc Natl Acad Sci U S A,* Vol.104, No.47, pp. 18754-18759

Gibbons, H.M. & Dragunow, M. (2006). Microglia induce neural cell death via a proximity-dependent mechanism involving nitric oxide. *Brain Res,* Vol.1084, No.1, pp. 1-15

Graeber, M.B. & Streit, W.J. (2010). Microglia: biology and pathology. *Acta Neuropathol,* Vol.119, No.1, pp. 89-105

Grilli, M., Pizzi, M., Memo, M. & Spano, P. (1996). Neuroprotection by aspirin and sodium salicylate through blockade of NF-kappaB activation. *Science,* Vol.274, No.5291, pp. 1383-1385

Hancock, D.B., Martin, E.R., Stajich, J.M., Jewett, R., Stacy, M.A., Scott, B.L., Vance, J.M. & Scott, W.K. (2007). Smoking, caffeine, and nonsteroidal anti-inflammatory drugs in families with Parkinson disease. *Arch Neurol*, Vol.64, No.4, pp. 576-580

Hanisch, U.K. (2002). Microglia as a source and target of cytokines. *Glia*, Vol.40, No.2, pp. 140-155

He, Y., Appel, S. & Le, W. (2001). Minocycline inhibits microglial activation and protects nigral cells after 6-hydroxydopamine injection into mouse striatum. *Brain Res*, Vol.909, No.1-2, pp. 187-193

Hernan, M.A., Logroscino, G. & Garcia Rodriguez, L.A. (2006). Nonsteroidal anti-inflammatory drugs and the incidence of Parkinson disease. *Neurology*, Vol.66, No.7, pp. 1097-1099

Herrera, A.J., Castano, A., Venero, J.L., Cano, J. & Machado, A. (2000). The single intranigral injection of LPS as a new model for studying the selective effects of inflammatory reactions on dopaminergic system. *Neurobiol Dis*, Vol.7, No.4, pp. 429-447

Hirsch, E.C., Hoglinger, G., Rousselet, E., Breidert, T., Parain, K., Feger, J., Ruberg, M., Prigent, A., Cohen-Salmon, C. & Launay, J.M. (2003). Animal models of Parkinson's disease in rodents induced by toxins: an update. *J Neural Transm Suppl*, Vol.65, No., pp. 89-100

Hirsch, E.C. & Hunot, S. (2009). Neuroinflammation in Parkinson's disease: a target for neuroprotection? *Lancet Neurol*, Vol.8, No.4, pp. 382-397

Hunot, S., Boissiere, F., Faucheux, B., Brugg, B., Mouatt-Prigent, A., Agid, Y. & Hirsch, E.C. (1996). Nitric oxide synthase and neuronal vulnerability in Parkinson's disease. *Neuroscience*, Vol.72, No.2, pp. 355-363

Hunot, S., Brugg, B., Ricard, D., Michel, P.P., Muriel, M.P., Ruberg, M., Faucheux, B.A., Agid, Y. & Hirsch, E.C. (1997). Nuclear translocation of NF-kappaB is increased in dopaminergic neurons of patients with parkinson disease. *Proc Natl Acad Sci U S A*, Vol.94, No.14, pp. 7531-7536

Hunter, R.L., Dragicevic, N., Seifert, K., Choi, D.Y., Liu, M., Kim, H.C., Cass, W.A., Sullivan, P.G. & Bing, G. (2007). Inflammation induces mitochondrial dysfunction and dopaminergic neurodegeneration in the nigrostriatal system. *J Neurochem*, Vol.100, No.5, pp. 1375-1386

Imamura, K., Hishikawa, N., Sawada, M., Nagatsu, T., Yoshida, M. & Hashizume, Y. (2003). Distribution of major histocompatibility complex class II-positive microglia and cytokine profile of Parkinson's disease brains. *Acta Neuropathol*, Vol.106, No.6, pp. 518-526

Jack, C.S., Arbour, N., Manusow, J., Montgrain, V., Blain, M., McCrea, E., Shapiro, A. & Antel, J.P. (2005). TLR signaling tailors innate immune responses in human microglia and astrocytes. *J Immunol*, Vol.175, No.7, pp. 4320-4330

Jang, H., Boltz, D., Sturm-Ramirez, K., Shepherd, K.R., Jiao, Y., Webster, R. & Smeyne, R.J. (2009b). Highly pathogenic H5N1 influenza virus can enter the central nervous system and induce neuroinflammation and neurodegeneration. *Proc Natl Acad Sci U S A*, Vol.106, No.33, pp. 14063-14068

Jang, H., Boltz, D.A., Webster, R.G. & Smeyne, R.J. (2009a). Viral parkinsonism. *Biochim Biophys Acta*, Vol.1792, No.7, pp. 714-721

Jenner, P. (2003). Oxidative stress in Parkinson's disease. *Ann Neurol*, Vol.53 Suppl 3, No., pp. S26-36; discussion S36-28

Johnston, L.C., Su, X., Maguire-Zeiss, K., Horovitz, K., Ankoudinova, I., Guschin, D., Hadaczek, P., Federoff, H.J., Bankiewicz, K. & Forsayeth, J. (2008). Human interleukin-10 gene transfer is protective in a rat model of Parkinson's disease. *Mol Ther*, Vol.16, No.8, pp. 1392-1399

Kettenmann, H., Banati, R. & Walz, W. (1993). Electrophysiological behavior of microglia. *Glia*, Vol.7, No.1, pp. 93-101

Kim, H.J., Hawke, N. & Baldwin, A.S. (2006). NF-kappaB and IKK as therapeutic targets in cancer. *Cell Death Differ*, Vol.13, No.5, pp. 738-747

Kim, H.S. & Suh, Y.H. (2009). Minocycline and neurodegenerative diseases. *Behav Brain Res*, Vol.196, No.2, pp. 168-179

Kim, S.U. & de Vellis, J. (2005). Microglia in health and disease. *J Neurosci Res*, Vol.81, No.3, pp. 302-313

Kim, W.G., Mohney, R.P., Wilson, B., Jeohn, G.H., Liu, B. & Hong, J.S. (2000). Regional difference in susceptibility to lipopolysaccharide-induced neurotoxicity in the rat brain: role of microglia. *J Neurosci*, Vol.20, No.16, pp. 6309-6316

Kim, Y.S., Choi, D.H., Block, M.L., Lorenzl, S., Yang, L., Kim, Y.J., Sugama, S., Cho, B.P., Hwang, O., Browne, S.E., Kim, S.Y., Hong, J.S., Beal, M.F. & Joh, T.H. (2007). A pivotal role of matrix metalloproteinase-3 activity in dopaminergic neuronal degeneration via microglial activation. *FASEB J*, Vol.21, No.1, pp. 179-187

Kim, Y.S., Kim, S.S., Cho, J.J., Choi, D.H., Hwang, O., Shin, D.H., Chun, H.S., Beal, M.F. & Joh, T.H. (2005). Matrix metalloproteinase-3: a novel signaling proteinase from apoptotic neuronal cells that activates microglia. *J Neurosci*, Vol.25, No.14, pp. 3701-3711

Kirik, D., Rosenblad, C. & Bjorklund, A. (1998). Characterization of behavioral and neurodegenerative changes following partial lesions of the nigrostriatal dopamine system induced by intrastriatal 6-hydroxydopamine in the rat. *Exp Neurol*, Vol.152, No.2, pp. 259-277

Knott, C., Stern, G. & Wilkin, G.P. (2000). Inflammatory regulators in Parkinson's disease: iNOS, lipocortin-1, and cyclooxygenases-1 and -2. *Mol Cell Neurosci*, Vol.16, No.6, pp. 724-739

Kohutnicka, M., Lewandowska, E., Kurkowska-Jastrzebska, I., Czlonkowski, A. & Czlonkowska, A. (1998). Microglial and astrocytic involvement in a murine model of Parkinson's disease induced by 1-methyl-4-phenyl-1,2,3,6-tetrahydropyridine (MPTP). *Immunopharmacology*, Vol.39, No.3, pp. 167-180

Konsman, J.P., Parnet, P. & Dantzer, R. (2002). Cytokine-induced sickness behaviour: mechanisms and implications. *Trends Neurosci*, Vol.25, No.3, pp. 154-159

Kopp, E. & Ghosh, S. (1994). Inhibition of NF-kappa B by sodium salicylate and aspirin. *Science*, Vol.265, No.5174, pp. 956-959

Koprich, J.B., Reske-Nielsen, C., Mithal, P. & Isacson, O. (2008). Neuroinflammation mediated by IL-1beta increases susceptibility of dopamine neurons to degeneration in an animal model of Parkinson's disease. *J Neuroinflammation*, Vol.5, No., pp. 8

Kortekaas, R., Leenders, K.L., van Oostrom, J.C., Vaalburg, W., Bart, J., Willemsen, A.T. & Hendrikse, N.H. (2005). Blood-brain barrier dysfunction in parkinsonian midbrain in vivo. *Ann Neurol*, Vol.57, No.2, pp. 176-179

Kurkowska-Jastrzebska, I., Babiuch, M., Joniec, I., Przybylkowski, A., Czlonkowski, A. & Czlonkowska, A. (2002). Indomethacin protects against neurodegeneration caused by MPTP intoxication in mice. *Int Immunopharmacol,* Vol.2, No.8, pp. 1213-1218

Kurkowska-Jastrzebska, I., Litwin, T., Joniec, I., Ciesielska, A., Przybylkowski, A., Czlonkowski, A. & Czlonkowska, A. (2004). Dexamethasone protects against dopaminergic neurons damage in a mouse model of Parkinson's disease. *Int Immunopharmacol,* Vol.4, No.10-11, pp. 1307-1318

Ladeby, R., Wirenfeldt, M., Garcia-Ovejero, D., Fenger, C., Dissing-Olesen, L., Dalmau, I. & Finsen, B. (2005). Microglial cell population dynamics in the injured adult central nervous system. *Brain Res Brain Res Rev,* Vol.48, No.2, pp. 196-206

Langston, J.W., Ballard, P., Tetrud, J.W. & Irwin, I. (1983). Chronic Parkinsonism in humans due to a product of meperidine-analog synthesis. *Science,* Vol.219, No.4587, pp. 979-980

Langston, J.W. & Ballard, P.A., Jr. (1983). Parkinson's disease in a chemist working with 1-methyl-4-phenyl-1,2,5,6-tetrahydropyridine. *N Engl J Med,* Vol.309, No.5, pp. 310

Langston, J.W., Forno, L.S., Tetrud, J., Reeves, A.G., Kaplan, J.A. & Karluk, D. (1999). Evidence of active nerve cell degeneration in the substantia nigra of humans years after 1-methyl-4-phenyl-1,2,3,6-tetrahydropyridine exposure. *Ann Neurol,* Vol.46, No.4, pp. 598-605

Leng, A., Mura, A., Feldon, J. & Ferger, B. (2005). Tumor necrosis factor-alpha receptor ablation in a chronic MPTP mouse model of Parkinson's disease. *Neurosci Lett,* Vol.375, No.2, pp. 107-111

Liberatore, G.T., Jackson-Lewis, V., Vukosavic, S., Mandir, A.S., Vila, M., McAuliffe, W.G., Dawson, V.L., Dawson, T.M. & Przedborski, S. (1999). Inducible nitric oxide synthase stimulates dopaminergic neurodegeneration in the MPTP model of Parkinson disease. *Nat Med,* Vol.5, No.12, pp. 1403-1409

Ling, Z., Gayle, D.A., Ma, S.Y., Lipton, J.W., Tong, C.W., Hong, J.S. & Carvey, P.M. (2002). In utero bacterial endotoxin exposure causes loss of tyrosine hydroxylase neurons in the postnatal rat midbrain. *Mov Disord,* Vol.17, No.1, pp. 116-124

Ling, Z., Zhu, Y., Tong, C., Snyder, J.A., Lipton, J.W. & Carvey, P.M. (2006). Progressive dopamine neuron loss following supra-nigral lipopolysaccharide (LPS) infusion into rats exposed to LPS prenatally. *Exp Neurol,* Vol.199, No.2, pp. 499-512

Ling, Z.D., Chang, Q., Lipton, J.W., Tong, C.W., Landers, T.M. & Carvey, P.M. (2004). Combined toxicity of prenatal bacterial endotoxin exposure and postnatal 6-hydroxydopamine in the adult rat midbrain. *Neuroscience,* Vol.124, No.3, pp. 619-628

Long-Smith, C.M., Collins, L., Toulouse, A., Sullivan, A.M. & Nolan, Y.M. (2010). Interleukin-1beta contributes to dopaminergic neuronal death induced by lipopolysaccharide-stimulated rat glia in vitro. *J Neuroimmunol,* Vol.226, No.1-2, pp. 20-26

Long-Smith, C.M., Sullivan, A.M. & Nolan, Y.M. (2009). The influence of microglia on the pathogenesis of Parkinson's disease. *Prog Neurobiol,* Vol.89, No.3, pp. 277-287

Lyons, A., Downer, E.J., Crotty, S., Nolan, Y.M., Mills, K.H. & Lynch, M.A. (2007). CD200 ligand receptor interaction modulates microglial activation in vivo and in vitro: a role for IL-4. *J Neurosci,* Vol.27, No.31, pp. 8309-8313

McCoy, M.K., Martinez, T.N., Ruhn, K.A., Szymkowski, D.E., Smith, C.G., Botterman, B.R., Tansey, K.E. & Tansey, M.G. (2006). Blocking soluble tumor necrosis factor signaling with dominant-negative tumor necrosis factor inhibitor attenuates loss of dopaminergic neurons in models of Parkinson's disease. *J Neurosci*, Vol.26, No.37, pp. 9365-9375

McCoy, M.K., Ruhn, K.A., Martinez, T.N., McAlpine, F.E., Blesch, A. & Tansey, M.G. (2008). Intranigral lentiviral delivery of dominant-negative TNF attenuates neurodegeneration and behavioral deficits in hemiparkinsonian rats. *Mol Ther*, Vol.16, No.9, pp. 1572-1579

McGeer, E.G. & McGeer, P.L. (2007). The role of anti-inflammatory agents in Parkinson's disease. *CNS Drugs*, Vol.21, No.10, pp. 789-797

McGeer, P.L., Itagaki, S., Boyes, B.E. & McGeer, E.G. (1988). Reactive microglia are positive for HLA-DR in the substantia nigra of Parkinson's and Alzheimer's disease brains. *Neurology*, Vol.38, No.8, pp. 1285-1291

McGeer, P.L. & McGeer, E.G. (2004). Inflammation and the degenerative diseases of aging. *Ann N Y Acad Sci*, Vol.1035, No., pp. 104-116

McGeer, P.L., Schwab, C., Parent, A. & Doudet, D. (2003). Presence of reactive microglia in monkey substantia nigra years after 1-methyl-4-phenyl-1,2,3,6-tetrahydropyridine administration. *Ann Neurol*, Vol.54, No.5, pp. 599-604

McGettrick, A.F. & O'Neill, L.A. (2010). Regulators of TLR4 signaling by endotoxins. *Subcell Biochem*, Vol.53, No.1, pp. 153-171

Misra, U.K. & Kalita, J. (2010). Overview: Japanese encephalitis. *Prog Neurobiol*, Vol.91, No.2, pp. 108-120

Mitchell, J.A., Akarasereenont, P., Thiemermann, C., Flower, R.J. & Vane, J.R. (1993). Selectivity of nonsteroidal antiinflammatory drugs as inhibitors of constitutive and inducible cyclooxygenase. *Proc Natl Acad Sci U S A*, Vol.90, No.24, pp. 11693-11697

Mogi, M., Harada, M., Kondo, T., Riederer, P., Inagaki, H., Minami, M. & Nagatsu, T. (1994a). Interleukin-1 beta, interleukin-6, epidermal growth factor and transforming growth factor-alpha are elevated in the brain from parkinsonian patients. *Neurosci Lett*, Vol.180, No.2, pp. 147-150

Mogi, M., Harada, M., Riederer, P., Narabayashi, H., Fujita, K. & Nagatsu, T. (1994b). Tumor necrosis factor-alpha (TNF-alpha) increases both in the brain and in the cerebrospinal fluid from parkinsonian patients. *Neurosci Lett*, Vol.165, No.1-2, pp. 208-210

Mogi, M., Togari, A., Kondo, T., Mizuno, Y., Komure, O., Kuno, S., Ichinose, H. & Nagatsu, T. (2000). Caspase activities and tumor necrosis factor receptor R1 (p55) level are elevated in the substantia nigra from parkinsonian brain. *J Neural Transm*, Vol.107, No.3, pp. 335-341

Nadeau, S. & Rivest, S. (2003). Glucocorticoids play a fundamental role in protecting the brain during innate immune response. *J Neurosci*, Vol.23, No.13, pp. 5536-5544

Nakajima, K. & Kohsaka, S. (2001). Microglia: activation and their significance in the central nervous system. *J Biochem*, Vol.130, No.2, pp. 169-175

Nakamura, Y. (2002). Regulating factors for microglial activation. *Biol Pharm Bull*, Vol.25, No.8, pp. 945-953

Nimmerjahn, A., Kirchhoff, F. & Helmchen, F. (2005). Resting microglial cells are highly dynamic surveillants of brain parenchyma in vivo. *Science,* Vol.308, No.5726, pp. 1314-1318

NINDS-NET-PD-Investigators. (2006). A randomized, double-blind, futility clinical trial of creatine and minocycline in early Parkinson disease. *Neurology,* Vol.66, No.5, pp. 664-671

NINDS-NET-PD-Investigators. (2008). A pilot clinical trial of creatine and minocycline in early Parkinson disease: 18-month results. *Clin Neuropharmacol,* Vol.31, No.3, pp. 141-150

Nolan, Y., Maher, F.O., Martin, D.S., Clarke, R.M., Brady, M.T., Bolton, A.E., Mills, K.H. & Lynch, M.A. (2005). Role of interleukin-4 in regulation of age-related inflammatory changes in the hippocampus. *J Biol Chem,* Vol.280, No.10, pp. 9354-9362

O'Callaghan, J.P., Miller, D.B. & Reinhard, J.F., Jr. (1990). Characterization of the origins of astrocyte response to injury using the dopaminergic neurotoxicant, 1-methyl-4-phenyl-1,2,3,6-tetrahydropyridine. *Brain Res,* Vol.521, No.1-2, pp. 73-80

Ogata, A., Tashiro, K., Nukuzuma, S., Nagashima, K. & Hall, W.W. (1997). A rat model of Parkinson's disease induced by Japanese encephalitis virus. *J Neurovirol,* Vol.3, No.2, pp. 141-147

Ogata, A., Tashiro, K. & Pradhan, S. (2000). Parkinsonism due to predominant involvement of substantia nigra in Japanese encephalitis. *Neurology,* Vol.55, No.4, pp. 602

Orr, C.F., Rowe, D.B. & Halliday, G.M. (2002). An inflammatory review of Parkinson's disease. *Prog Neurobiol,* Vol.68, No.5, pp. 325-340

Ouchi, Y., Yagi, S., Yokokura, M. & Sakamoto, M. (2009). Neuroinflammation in the living brain of Parkinson's disease. *Parkinsonism Relat Disord,* Vol.15 Suppl 3, No., pp. S200-204

Pankratz, N. & Foroud, T. (2007). Genetics of Parkinson disease. *Genet Med,* Vol.9, No.12, pp. 801-811

Papadopoulos, V., Baraldi, M., Guilarte, T.R., Knudsen, T.B., Lacapere, J.J., Lindemann, P., Norenberg, M.D., Nutt, D., Weizman, A., Zhang, M.R. & Gavish, M. (2006). Translocator protein (18kDa): new nomenclature for the peripheral-type benzodiazepine receptor based on its structure and molecular function. *Trends Pharmacol Sci,* Vol.27, No.8, pp. 402-409

Park, C.H., Carboni, E., Wood, P.L. & Gee, K.W. (1996). Characterization of peripheral benzodiazepine type sites in a cultured murine BV-2 microglial cell line. *Glia,* Vol.16, No.1, pp. 65-70

Perry, V.H. (1998). A revised view of the central nervous system microenvironment and major histocompatibility complex class II antigen presentation. *J Neuroimmunol,* Vol.90, No.2, pp. 113-121

Perry, V.H. (2010). Contribution of systemic inflammation to chronic neurodegeneration. *Acta Neuropathol,* Vol.120, No.3, pp. 277-286

Perry, V.H., Cunningham, C. & Holmes, C. (2007). Systemic infections and inflammation affect chronic neurodegeneration. *Nat Rev Immunol,* Vol.7, No.2, pp. 161-167

Poser, C.M., Huntley, C.J. & Poland, J.D. (1969). Para-encephalitic parkinsonism. Report of an acute case due to coxsackie virus type B 2 and re-examination of the etiologic concepts of postencephalitic parkinsonism. *Acta Neurol Scand,* Vol.45, No.2, pp. 199-215

Pott Godoy, M.C., Tarelli, R., Ferrari, C.C., Sarchi, M.I. & Pitossi, F.J. (2008). Central and systemic IL-1 exacerbates neurodegeneration and motor symptoms in a model of Parkinson's disease. *Brain*, Vol.131, No.Pt 7, pp. 1880-1894

Pranzatelli, M.R., Mott, S.H., Pavlakis, S.G., Conry, J.A. & Tate, E.D. (1994). Clinical spectrum of secondary parkinsonism in childhood: a reversible disorder. *Pediatr Neurol*, Vol.10, No.2, pp. 131-140

Przedborski, S. & Vila, M. (2003). The 1-methyl-4-phenyl-1,2,3,6-tetrahydropyridine mouse model: a tool to explore the pathogenesis of Parkinson's disease. *Ann N Y Acad Sci*, Vol.991, No., pp. 189-198

Qian, L., Hong, J.S. & Flood, P.M. (2006). Role of microglia in inflammation-mediated degeneration of dopaminergic neurons: neuroprotective effect of interleukin 10. *J Neural Transm Suppl*, Vol., No.70, pp. 367-371

Qin, L., Wu, X., Block, M.L., Liu, Y., Breese, G.R., Hong, J.S., Knapp, D.J. & Crews, F.T. (2007). Systemic LPS causes chronic neuroinflammation and progressive neurodegeneration. *Glia*, Vol.55, No.5, pp. 453-462

Quinn, L.P., Crook, B., Hows, M.E., Vidgeon-Hart, M., Chapman, H., Upton, N., Medhurst, A.D. & Virley, D.J. (2008). The PPARgamma agonist pioglitazone is effective in the MPTP mouse model of Parkinson's disease through inhibition of monoamine oxidase B. *Br J Pharmacol*, Vol.154, No.1, pp. 226-233

Rail, D., Scholtz, C. & Swash, M. (1981). Post-encephalitic Parkinsonism: current experience. *J Neurol Neurosurg Psychiatry*, Vol.44, No.8, pp. 670-676

Raivich, G., Bohatschek, M., Kloss, C.U., Werner, A., Jones, L.L. & Kreutzberg, G.W. (1999). Neuroglial activation repertoire in the injured brain: graded response, molecular mechanisms and cues to physiological function. *Brain Res Brain Res Rev*, Vol.30, No.1, pp. 77-105

Ransohoff, R.M. & Cardona, A.E. (2010). The myeloid cells of the central nervous system parenchyma. *Nature*, Vol.468, No.7321, pp. 253-262

Ransohoff, R.M. & Perry, V.H. (2009). Microglial physiology: unique stimuli, specialized responses. *Annu Rev Immunol*, Vol.27, No., pp. 119-145

Reale, M., Iarlori, C., Thomas, A., Gambi, D., Perfetti, B., Di Nicola, M. & Onofrj, M. (2009). Peripheral cytokines profile in Parkinson's disease. *Brain Behav Immun*, Vol.23, No.1, pp. 55-63

Rentzos, M., Nikolaou, C., Andreadou, E., Paraskevas, G.P., Rombos, A., Zoga, M., Tsoutsou, A., Boufidou, F., Kapaki, E. & Vassilopoulos, D. (2007). Circulating interleukin-15 and RANTES chemokine in Parkinson's disease. *Acta Neurol Scand*, Vol.116, No.6, pp. 374-379

Robinson, R.L., Shahida, S., Madan, N., Rao, S. & Khardori, N. (2003). Transient parkinsonism in West Nile virus encephalitis. *Am J Med*, Vol.115, No.3, pp. 252-253

Samii, A., Etminan, M., Wiens, M.O. & Jafari, S. (2009). NSAID use and the risk of Parkinson's disease: systematic review and meta-analysis of observational studies. *Drugs Aging*, Vol.26, No.9, pp. 769-779

Sampaio, E.P., Sarno, E.N., Galilly, R., Cohn, Z.A. & Kaplan, G. (1991). Thalidomide selectively inhibits tumor necrosis factor alpha production by stimulated human monocytes. *J Exp Med*, Vol.173, No.3, pp. 699-703

Sanchez-Pernaute, R., Ferree, A., Cooper, O., Yu, M., Brownell, A.L. & Isacson, O. (2004). Selective COX-2 inhibition prevents progressive dopamine neuron degeneration in a rat model of Parkinson's disease. *J Neuroinflammation*, Vol.1, No.1, pp. 6

Santambrogio, L., Belyanskaya, S.L., Fischer, F.R., Cipriani, B., Brosnan, C.F., Ricciardi-Castagnoli, P., Stern, L.J., Strominger, J.L. & Riese, R. (2001). Developmental plasticity of CNS microglia. *Proc Natl Acad Sci U S A*, Vol.98, No.11, pp. 6295-6300

Sauer, H. & Oertel, W.H. (1994). Progressive degeneration of nigrostriatal dopamine neurons following intrastriatal terminal lesions with 6-hydroxydopamine: a combined retrograde tracing and immunocytochemical study in the rat. *Neuroscience*, Vol.59, No.2, pp. 401-415

Sawada, M., Imamura, K. & Nagatsu, T. (2006). Role of cytokines in inflammatory process in Parkinson's disease. *J Neural Transm Suppl*, Vol., No.70, pp. 373-381

Scheinman, R.I., Gualberto, A., Jewell, C.M., Cidlowski, J.A. & Baldwin, A.S., Jr. (1995). Characterization of mechanisms involved in transrepression of NF-kappa B by activated glucocorticoid receptors. *Mol Cell Biol*, Vol.15, No.2, pp. 943-953

Schintu, N., Frau, L., Ibba, M., Caboni, P., Garau, A., Carboni, E. & Carta, A.R. (2009). PPAR-gamma-mediated neuroprotection in a chronic mouse model of Parkinson's disease. *Eur J Neurosci*, Vol.29, No.5, pp. 954-963

Sedgwick, J.D., Schwender, S., Imrich, H., Dorries, R., Butcher, G.W. & ter Meulen, V. (1991). Isolation and direct characterization of resident microglial cells from the normal and inflamed central nervous system. *Proc Natl Acad Sci U S A*, Vol.88, No.16, pp. 7438-7442

Shan, S., Hong-Min, T., Yi, F., Jun-Peng, G., Yue, F., Yan-Hong, T., Yun-Ke, Y., Wen-Wei, L., Xiang-Yu, W., Jun, M., Guo-Hua, W., Ya-Ling, H., Hua-Wei, L. & Ding-Fang, C. (2011). NEW evidences for fractalkine/CX3CL1 involved in substantia nigral microglial activation and behavioral changes in a rat model of Parkinson's disease. *Neurobiol Aging*, Vol.32, No.3, pp. 443-458

Shoji, H., Watanabe, M., Itoh, S., Kuwahara, H. & Hattori, F. (1993). Japanese encephalitis and parkinsonism. *J Neurol*, Vol.240, No.1, pp. 59-60

Sian, J., Dexter, D.T., Lees, A.J., Daniel, S., Agid, Y., Javoy-Agid, F., Jenner, P. & Marsden, C.D. (1994). Alterations in glutathione levels in Parkinson's disease and other neurodegenerative disorders affecting basal ganglia. *Ann Neurol*, Vol.36, No.3, pp. 348-355

Smithells, R.W. & Newman, C.G. (1992). Recognition of thalidomide defects. *J Med Genet*, Vol.29, No.10, pp. 716-723

Sriram, K., Matheson, J.M., Benkovic, S.A., Miller, D.B., Luster, M.I. & O'Callaghan, J.P. (2006). Deficiency of TNF receptors suppresses microglial activation and alters the susceptibility of brain regions to MPTP-induced neurotoxicity: role of TNF-alpha. *FASEB J*, Vol.20, No.6, pp. 670-682

Stanic, D., Finkelstein, D.I., Bourke, D.W., Drago, J. & Horne, M.K. (2003). Timecourse of striatal re-innervation following lesions of dopaminergic SNpc neurons of the rat. *Eur J Neurosci*, Vol.18, No.5, pp. 1175-1188

Stephenson, D.T., Schober, D.A., Smalstig, E.B., Mincy, R.E., Gehlert, D.R. & Clemens, J.A. (1995). Peripheral benzodiazepine receptors are colocalized with activated microglia following transient global forebrain ischemia in the rat. *J Neurosci*, Vol.15, No.7 Pt 2, pp. 5263-5274

Stone, D.K., Reynolds, A.D., Mosley, R.L. & Gendelman, H.E. (2009). Innate and adaptive immunity for the pathobiology of Parkinson's disease. *Antioxid Redox Signal*, Vol.11, No.9, pp. 2151-2166

Stypula, G., Kunert-Radek, J., Stepien, H., Zylinska, K. & Pawlikowski, M. (1996). Evaluation of interleukins, ACTH, cortisol and prolactin concentrations in the blood of patients with parkinson's disease. *Neuroimmunomodulation*, Vol.3, No.2-3, pp. 131-134

Takahashi, M., Yamada, T., Nakajima, S., Nakajima, K., Yamamoto, T. & Okada, H. (1995). The substantia nigra is a major target for neurovirulent influenza A virus. *J Exp Med*, Vol.181, No.6, pp. 2161-2169

Tansey, M.G. & Goldberg, M.S. (2010). Neuroinflammation in Parkinson's disease: its role in neuronal death and implications for therapeutic intervention. *Neurobiol Dis*, Vol.37, No.3, pp. 510-518

Tansey, M.G., McCoy, M.K. & Frank-Cannon, T.C. (2007). Neuroinflammatory mechanisms in Parkinson's disease: potential environmental triggers, pathways, and targets for early therapeutic intervention. *Exp Neurol*, Vol.208, No.1, pp. 1-25

Teismann, P. & Ferger, B. (2001). Inhibition of the cyclooxygenase isoenzymes COX-1 and COX-2 provide neuroprotection in the MPTP-mouse model of Parkinson's disease. *Synapse*, Vol.39, No.2, pp. 167-174

Teismann, P., Tieu, K., Choi, D.K., Wu, D.C., Naini, A., Hunot, S., Vila, M., Jackson-Lewis, V. & Przedborski, S. (2003). Cyclooxygenase-2 is instrumental in Parkinson's disease neurodegeneration. *Proc Natl Acad Sci U S A*, Vol.100, No.9, pp. 5473-5478

Teo, B.H. & Wong, S.H. (2010). MHC class II-associated invariant chain (Ii) modulates dendritic cells-derived microvesicles (DCMV)-mediated activation of microglia. *Biochem Biophys Res Commun*, Vol.400, No.4, pp. 673-678

Tomas-Camardiel, M., Rite, I., Herrera, A.J., de Pablos, R.M., Cano, J., Machado, A. & Venero, J.L. (2004). Minocycline reduces the lipopolysaccharide-induced inflammatory reaction, peroxynitrite-mediated nitration of proteins, disruption of the blood-brain barrier, and damage in the nigral dopaminergic system. *Neurobiol Dis*, Vol.16, No.1, pp. 190-201

Tomiyama, H., Mizuta, I., Li, Y., Funayama, M., Yoshino, H., Li, L., Murata, M., Yamamoto, M., Kubo, S., Mizuno, Y., Toda, T. & Hattori, N. (2008). LRRK2 P755L variant in sporadic Parkinson's disease. *J Hum Genet*, Vol.53, No.11-12, pp. 1012-1015

Toulouse, A. & Sullivan, A.M. (2008). Progress in Parkinson's disease-where do we stand? *Prog Neurobiol*, Vol.85, No.4, pp. 376-392

Tse, W., Cersosimo, M.G., Gracies, J.M., Morgello, S., Olanow, C.W. & Koller, W. (2004). Movement disorders and AIDS: a review. *Parkinsonism Relat Disord*, Vol.10, No.6, pp. 323-334

Tweedie, D., Sambamurti, K. & Greig, N.H. (2007). TNF-alpha inhibition as a treatment strategy for neurodegenerative disorders: new drug candidates and targets. *Curr Alzheimer Res*, Vol.4, No.4, pp. 378-385

Walters, J.H. (1960). Postencephalitic Parkinson syndrome after meningoencephalitis due to coxsackie virus group B, type 2. *New England Journal of Medicine*, Vol.263, No.15, pp. 744-747

Wang, S., Yan, J.Y., Lo, Y.K., Carvey, P.M. & Ling, Z. (2009). Dopaminergic and serotoninergic deficiencies in young adult rats prenatally exposed to the bacterial lipopolysaccharide. *Brain Res*, Vol.1265, No., pp. 196-204

Wang, X.J., Zhang, S., Yan, Z.Q., Zhao, Y.X., Zhou, H.Y., Wang, Y., Lu, G.Q. & Zhang, J.D. (2011). Impaired CD200-CD200R-mediated microglia silencing enhances midbrain dopaminergic neurodegeneration: Roles of aging, superoxide, NADPH oxidase, and p38 MAPK. *Free Radic Biol Med,* Vol.50, No.9, pp. 1094-1106

Weller, C., Oxlade, N., Dobbs, S.M., Dobbs, R.J., Charlett, A. & Bjarnason, I.T. (2005). Role of inflammation in gastrointestinal tract in aetiology and pathogenesis of idiopathic parkinsonism. *FEMS Immunol Med Microbiol,* Vol.44, No.2, pp. 129-135

Wilms, H., Rosenstiel, P., Sievers, J., Deuschl, G., Zecca, L. & Lucius, R. (2003). Activation of microglia by human neuromelanin is NF-kappaB dependent and involves p38 mitogen-activated protein kinase: implications for Parkinson's disease. *FASEB J,* Vol.17, No.3, pp. 500-502

Wilms, H., Zecca, L., Rosenstiel, P., Sievers, J., Deuschl, G. & Lucius, R. (2007). Inflammation in Parkinson's diseases and other neurodegenerative diseases: cause and therapeutic implications. *Curr Pharm Des,* Vol.13, No.18, pp. 1925-1928

Winkeler, A., Boisgard, R., Martin, A. & Tavitian, B. (2010). Radioisotopic imaging of neuroinflammation. *J Nucl Med,* Vol.51, No.1, pp. 1-4

Wu, D.C., Jackson-Lewis, V., Vila, M., Tieu, K., Teismann, P., Vadseth, C., Choi, D.K., Ischiropoulos, H. & Przedborski, S. (2002). Blockade of microglial activation is neuroprotective in the 1-methyl-4-phenyl-1,2,3,6-tetrahydropyridine mouse model of Parkinson disease. *J Neurosci,* Vol.22, No.5, pp. 1763-1771

Wu, D.C., Teismann, P., Tieu, K., Vila, M., Jackson-Lewis, V., Ischiropoulos, H. & Przedborski, S. (2003). NADPH oxidase mediates oxidative stress in the 1-methyl-4-phenyl-1,2,3,6-tetrahydropyridine model of Parkinson's disease. *Proc Natl Acad Sci U S A,* Vol.100, No.10, pp. 6145-6150

Yamada, T., McGeer, P.L. & McGeer, E.G. (1992). Lewy bodies in Parkinson's disease are recognized by antibodies to complement proteins. *Acta Neuropathol,* Vol.84, No.1, pp. 100-104

Yang, L., Sugama, S., Chirichigno, J.W., Gregorio, J., Lorenzl, S., Shin, D.H., Browne, S.E., Shimizu, Y., Joh, T.H., Beal, M.F. & Albers, D.S. (2003). Minocycline enhances MPTP toxicity to dopaminergic neurons. *J Neurosci Res,* Vol.74, No.2, pp. 278-285

Yasuda, T., Fukuda-Tani, M., Nihira, T., Wada, K., Hattori, N., Mizuno, Y. & Mochizuki, H. (2007). Correlation between levels of pigment epithelium-derived factor and vascular endothelial growth factor in the striatum of patients with Parkinson's disease. *Exp Neurol,* Vol.206, No.2, pp. 308-317

Yirmiya, R., Winocur, G. & Goshen, I. (2002). Brain interleukin-1 is involved in spatial memory and passive avoidance conditioning. *Neurobiol Learn Mem,* Vol.78, No.2, pp. 379-389

Zalcman, S., Green-Johnson, J.M., Murray, L., Nance, D.M., Dyck, D., Anisman, H. & Greenberg, A.H. (1994). Cytokine-specific central monoamine alterations induced by interleukin-1, -2 and -6. *Brain Res,* Vol.643, No.1-2, pp. 40-49

Zhang, F., Qian, L., Flood, P.M., Shi, J.S., Hong, J.S. & Gao, H.M. (2010). Inhibition of IkappaB kinase-beta protects dopamine neurons against lipopolysaccharide-induced neurotoxicity. *J Pharmacol Exp Ther,* Vol.333, No.3, pp. 822-833

Zhang, W., Wang, T., Pei, Z., Miller, D.S., Wu, X., Block, M.L., Wilson, B., Zhou, Y., Hong, J.S. & Zhang, J. (2005). Aggregated alpha-synuclein activates microglia: a process leading to disease progression in Parkinson's disease. *FASEB J*, Vol.19, No.6, pp. 533-542

Zhou, Y., Su, Y., Li, B., Liu, F., Ryder, J.W., Wu, X., Gonzalez-DeWhitt, P.A., Gelfanova, V., Hale, J.E., May, P.C., Paul, S.M. & Ni, B. (2003). Nonsteroidal anti-inflammatory drugs can lower amyloidogenic Abeta42 by inhibiting Rho. *Science*, Vol.302, No.5648, pp. 1215-1217

3

Human Lymphocytes and *Drosophila melanogaster*[1] as Model System to Study Oxidative Stress in Parkinson's Disease

Marlene Jimenez-Del-Rio and Carlos Velez-Pardo
School of Medicine, Medical Research Institute, Neuroscience Research Group,
University of Antioquia,
Medellin,
Colombia

1. Introduction

Parkinson's disease (PD, OMIM entry #168600) is the most common progressive neurodegenerative disorder that not only affects a large group of individuals in Antioquia, Colombia (Pradilla et., 2003; Sanchez et al., 2004) but also affects other regions in the world. Actually, the prevalence of PD is between 0.1% and 0.3% in the general population and between 1% and 2% in persons 65 years of age or older (Alves et al., 2008). Moreover, the number of individuals with PD over age 50 has been projected between 8.7 and 9.3 million in Western countries by 2030 (Dorsey et al., 2007). PD is typified clinically by motor symptoms including bradykinesia, resting tremor, rigidity and gait posture abnormalities followed by postural instability and less frequent non-motor complication such as dementia, depression and autonomic dysfunction (Jancovic, 2008). Pathologically, the disorder is prominently characterized by progressive loss of 50–70% of dopaminergic neurons located in the substantia nigra, decrease of the neurotransmitter dopamine content in striatum (Forno, 1996), cytoplasmic inclusions of insoluble, aggregated proteins, including α-synuclein known as Lewy bodies (Cuervo et al., 2010), elevated levels and/or deposits of iron (Sian-Hülsmann et al., 2010) and selective neuronal vulnerability to oxidative stress (Wang & Michaelis, 2010). The cause of all cases of PD remains unknown. However, in the mid-1990s this situation changed with the identification of a mutation in the α-synuclein gene associated with autosomal dominant PD in Italian kindred (Polymeropoulos et al., 1997). Since then, more than 10 genes have been found either causal of the disease (e.g., *Parkin, DJ-1*, PTEN-induced putative kinase 1 (*PINK-1*), leucine rich region kinase 2 (*LRRK2*), *ATP13A2* (Xiromerisiou et al., 2010; Cookson, 2010; Hardy, 2010)) or as risk factor for PD (e.g. HLA region). Interestingly, the first gene that causes autosomal recessive

---

[1]*Drosophila melanogaster* has misleadingly been known as the fruit fly. Strictly, "...real fruit flies,...attack unblemished fruit and in heavy infestations cause serious economic damage. In contrast, even if present in enormous numbers, *D. melanogaster* is innocuous and of no economic importance" (Green, MM. (2002). It really is not a fruit fly, *Genetics* 162: 1-3). It is therefore most adequate to name *Drosophila melanogaster* as just *Drosophila melanogaster* fly

juvenile Parkinsonism (AR-JP) was reported and named *parkin* in 1998 by Kitada and colleagues. AR-JP maps to the long arm of chromosome 6 (6q25.2-q27). The *parkin* gene is composed of 2,960 base pairs with a 1,395-base-pair open reading frame encoding for a protein of 465 amino acids with moderate similarity to ubiquitin at the amino terminus and a RING-finger motif at the carboxy terminus. The gene spans more than 500 kilobases and has 12 exons (Kitada et al., 1998). Subsequent studies have shown that *parkin* is a RING-finger-containing protein identified as an E3 protein-ubiquitin ligase (Shimura et al., 2000), which is an integral component of the cytoplasmic ubiquitin/ proteosomal degradation pathway (Betarbet et al., 2005). The reaction promoted by E3 ligases is the addition of a lysine-linked chain four or more ubiquitin molecules to the target protein, which is recognised by the subunits in the proteosome. Thus, mutation of the *parkin* gene could result in accumulation of misfolded proteins (Tanaka et al., 2001; Imai and Takahashi, 2004). Therefore, it is hypothesized that mutations in *parkin* gene, which result in loss of function, are unable to remove enough mutated or misfolded proteins leading to nigral neurodegeneration. Moreover, the Parkin protein may play a role in promoting autophagy of dysfunctional mitochondria following loss of mitochondrial membrane potential (Bueler, 2010).

Currently, AR-JP (OMIM entry #600116) is consider a distinct genetic entity characterised by early age at onset (<age 45), dystonia with parkinsonism and improvement of symptoms after sleep, slow disease progression, associated signs such as hyperflexia, dysautonomia, peripheral neuropathy and good response to low doses of L-DOPA (Zhang et al., 2001). Additionally, iron deposits are found in PD (Dexter et al., 1989; Sofic et al., 1991; Riederer et al., 1992; Griffiths et al., 1999) as well as in AR-JP (Takanashi et al., 2001). Why dopaminergic neurons in the substantia nigra are particularly vulnerable to the loss of parkin function and iron deposition is yet unknown. To date, the most common known form of hereditary Parkinsonism, i.e. AR-JP, diagnosed in Antioquia, Colombia is due to the *parkin* C212Y mutation. This mutation is a novel G to A transition in exon 6 at position 736 (G736A) of *parkin* gene. The C212Y mutation was identified in a genetic isolate community from two paisa family groups (PJF-1, PJF-3) by Pineda-Trujillo et al., (2001). Interestingly, the mutation was subsequently observed in a Spanish family, suggesting that it could have been taken to Antioquia by Spanish immigrants. Pineda-Trujillo et al., (2006) screened for the G736A mutation in additional Antioquian early onset PD cases and used haplotype analysis to investigate the relationship between Spanish and Antioquian G736A chromosomes. They confirmed the occurrence of an extensive founder effect in Antioquia. Thirteen individuals (10 homozygotes) from seven nuclear families were identified with the G736A mutation. Genealogical investigations demonstrated the existence of shared ancestors between six of these families four to five generations ago and no evidence of Spanish ancestry during this period. A second parkin mutation (a duplication of exon 3), was detected in the three G736A heterozygote carriers. Haplotype data exclude a recent common ancestry between the Spanish and Antioquian patients studied and are consistent with the introduction of the G736A mutation in Antioquia during early colonial times by about 16 generations ago. Further studies have also confirmed the presence of a GT insertion in exon 3 mutation among Paisa community previously identified in Spanish and French families with juvenile Parkinsonism (Pineda-Trujillo et al., 2001, 2009). Strikingly, the proteins that are reported to be related to familial PD such as PINK1, DJ-1, α-synuclein, LRRK2 and possibly parkin are either mitochondrial proteins or are associated with mitochondria. Interestingly, all those proteins are involved in pathways that elicit oxidative stress or free radical damage (Lin et al., 2009).

Free radials are defined as any atom or molecule that has one or more unpaired electrons in its outer shell such as anion superoxide radical ($\cdot O_2$), hydroxyl radical ($\cdot OH$), nitric oxide ($NO\cdot$) and their products (e.g. H_2O_2). Oxidative stress (OS) refers to a state in which free radicals are in excess of antioxidant defence mechanism (e. g. superoxide dismutase (SOD), glutathion peroxidase (GPx), catalase, vitamin C and E). As a result of this imbalance, the free radicals are capable of reacting with lipids, proteins, nucleic acids, and other molecules altering their structure and function. Accordingly, OS can lead to serious structural modifications in cells by excessive accumulation of oxidized products such as aldehydes and isoprostanes from lipid peroxidation, protein carbonyls from protein oxidation, and base adducts from DNA oxidation. Because the human brain is a high oxygen consumer organ, it is reasonable to assume that, under pathological conditions, it might be a target of permanent OS attack.

Over the last two decade, OS has been proposed to play a critical role in the pathogenesis of PD (Fahn and Cohen, 1992; Jenner & Olanow, 1996; Tsang & Chung, 2009). In fact, several markers of OS have been identified in post-mortem brain tissues including increased levels of DNA and RNA oxidation (e.g. 8-hydroxyl-2-deoxyguanosine and 8-hydroxyl deoxyguanosine), protein carbonyl levels, glycation and glycoxidation, lipid peroxidation and high iron concentration (Zhou et al., 2008). Moreover, given that iron and DA generate reactive oxygen species (ROS), they have been implicated in the OS observed in PD (Asanuma et al., 2004). Not surprisingly, lymphocytes have been used to test for oxidative stress (Battisti et al., 2008) and cell death (Calopa et al., 2010) in PD. For instance, Migliore et al., (2002) has demonstrated an increase in the incidence of spontaneous micronuclei, single strand breaks and oxidized purine bases in PD patients without treatment. These results clearly showed oxidative DNA damage demonstrable in lymphocytes. Moreover, we found that homozygote Cys212Tyr *parkin* mutation in AR-JP patients renders lymphocytes sensitive to dopamine, iron and hydrogen peroxide stimuli (Jimenez-Del-Rio et al., 2004). In agreement with these findings, Prigione and co-workers (2009) have shown increased oxidative stress in lymphocytes from untreated Parkinson's disease patients. Interestingly, Jiang et al., (2004) have shown that parkin protects human dopaminergic neuroblastoma cells against dopamine-induced cell death. Taken together these data suggest that analysis of DNA or lymphocytes response against oxidative stress might be used as an early marker of the OS status in PD patients.

Despite these evidences, there are still major unresolved issues in the understanding of the molecular and cellular biology of PD. Indeed, a complete picture of the precise molecular cascade leading to cell death in a single cellular model in this disorder is still lacking. Therefore, we have been interested in investigating the oxidative stress phenomenon and apoptosis signalling in lymphocytes and *Drosophila melanogaster*.

2. *In vitro* and *In vivo* models

2.1 Human lymphocytes resemble neuronal cells

The brain and the immune system are involved in functionally relevant cross–talk influencing one another's actions, whose main function is to maintain homeostasis. Therefore, to play such a role, lymphocytes are equipped with several biochemical systems that display comparable pathways to neural cells. This unusual characteristic makes lymphocytes an excellent *in vitro* model (Massaud et al., 1998; Kriesberg, 2011) to understand normal and abnormal function from gene to phenotype. Moreover, lymphocytes might provide the basis of biochemical and cytopathological mechanisms for preventive or therapeutic intervention. These cells thus appear to be particularly fascinating cell model for PD at least for three main reasons. First, lymphocytes express six homologous neurochemical systems (Table).

System	Protein Expression
1. Dopaminergic	Tyrosine hydroxylase & monoamine oxidase (Marino et al., 1999 & references within); dopamine transporter (Amenta et al., 2001; Marazziti et al., 2010); dopamine D2-, D3-, D4-, D5-like receptors (Ricci & Amenta, 1994; Ricci et al., 1995, 1997; Amenta et al., 1999; McKenna et al., 2002).
2. Serotonergic	Serotonin transporter (SERT, Faraj et al., 1991; Marazziti et al., 2010); serotonin receptors (Stefulj et al, 2000); tryptophan hydroxylase (Carrillo-Vico et al., 2004).
3. Cholinergic	Acetylcholine (Ach), muscarinic and nicotinic Ach receptors (mAChRs and nAChRs), choline acetyltransferase (ChAT), high affinity choline transporter and acetylcholinesterase (Kawashima & Fujii, 2004).
4. Glutamatergic	Ionotrophic glutamate receptors (Lombardi et al., 2001, 2004); group I metabotropic glutamate receptors (Miglio et al., 2005).
5. Adrenergic	β-2 adrenergic receptors (Sanders, 1998).
6. Gabaergic	γ-aminobutiric acid (GABA) receptors (Tillakaratne et al., 1995).

Table 1. Neuronal Molecular systems expressed in lymphocytes.

Second, lymphocytes express similar molecular death machinery leading to typical morphologic and biochemical features of apoptosis. Apoptosis is a type of programmed cell death initially defined by Kerr and co-workers in 1972 and recently refined by several others (Kerr et al., 1995; Xu & Shi, 2007; Kroemer et al., 2009). Apoptosis is originally a morphological phenomenon characterised by chromatin condensation and nuclear fragmentation, plasma membrane blebbing, cell shrinkage and preservation of organelles such as mitochondria. These characteristics can be recognised in lymphocytes under fluorescent microscopy (Fig. 1) or electron microscopy (Sakahira et al., 1999; Marini et al., 2001). Noticeably, what causes these morphological changes that we recognize as apoptosis occurs through multiple independent pathways that are initiated either from triggering events within the cell (i.e the "intrinsic pathway") or from outside the cell (i.e. the "extrinsic pathway"). The "intrinsic pathway" involves the release of mitochondrial proteins such as cytochrome C, second mitochondrial-derived activator of caspase/direct IAP-associated binding protein with low PI (Smac/DIABLO), apoptosis inducing factor (AIF) and Endonuclease G (Endo G). The "extrinsic pathway" involves Fas/FasL pathway, caspase-8 activation, bid degradation and releasing cytochrome C. Strikingly, both pathways converge on a common machinery of cell dismantling executed by a family of cysteine proteases known as Caspases. Indeed, caspases cleavage at aspartate residues of targeted proteins (Chowdhury et al., 2008). Particularly, caspase-3 degrades the inhibitor of caspase-activated DNase (ICAD/ DNA fragmentation Factor-45, DFF-45) protein releasing the caspase-activated DNase (CAD/ DFF-40) that result in DNA degradation ("DNA ladder pattern") from mouse T-cell lymphoma (Enari et al., 1998; Sakahira et al. 1998), Jurkat T cells (Liu et al, 1997) and HeLa cells (Halenbeck et al., 1998) under pro-apoptotic treatments. It is worth to mention that almost 18-years passed before an explanation could be drawn for one of the earliest well-recognized biochemical characteristics of apoptosis i.e. "DNA ladder pattern", from the time when Wyllie reported glucocorticoid-induced thymocytes apoptosis associated with endonuclease activation (Wyllie, 1980). Unquestionably, morphological and biochemical data have helped considerably to enlighten, yet unsettled, the mechanism of neural cell death in PD (Levy et al., 2009).

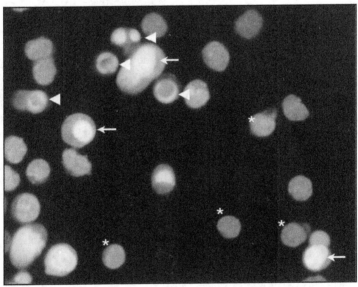

Fig. 1. **Human lymphocytes treated with xenobiotic paraquat, PQ for 24h.** Figure shows typical nuclear apoptotic morphology such as highly condensed chromatin (arrows) and nuclear fragmentation (arrowheads) from lymphocytes treated with PQ compared to normal nuclei (asterisk) stained with acridine orange/ ethidium bromide. A similar apoptotic morphology can be observed with dopamine, DA; 6-hydroxydopamine, 6-OHDA; 5,6 & 5,6 dihydroxydopamine, 5,6 & 5,7-DHT; rotenone, ROT. Jimenez-Del-Rio & Velez-Pardo, 2008. Reproduced with permission from Informa Healtcare UK Ltd.

Third, lymphocytes and neurons are post-mitotic cells, i.e. they become locked in a G_0 phase of the cell cycle. This is a remarkable biological feature to be cautiously considered when interpreting experimental data since evidence has accumulated that a cell division forced on a mature neuron leads to apoptosis rather than division (Herrup et al., 2004), but cell division is induced in lymphocytes. In other words, the use of cell lines instead of primary cultures could be confusing and /or misleading. For instance, NF-κB is a transcriptional factor composed of a p50/p65 heterodimer protein that upon activation binds to specific DNA sequences in target genes, designated as κB-elements. This factor is involved in both cell cycle-regulation and cell death processes. In dividing cells, NF-κB transcribes cyclin D1, which in association with cyclin-dependent kinases, CDK4 and CDK6, promotes G1/S phase transition through CDK-dependent phosphorilation of retinoblastoma protein (pRb), thereby releasing the transcription factor E2F, required from the activation of S phase-specific genes. Indeed, constitutive activation of NF-κB is intimately intertwined with cancer growth and metastasis (Prasad et al., 2010). On the other hand, the regulatory roles of NF-κB on apoptosis suggest that NF-κB is acting on the upstream pathways of apoptosis, either negatively or positively (Shishodia & Aggarwal, 2004; Qin et al., 2007). Noticeably, in non-dividing cells, these confounding matters connected with the role of NF-κB in apoptosis and cell-cycle control might not be an important issue given that NF-κB function can eventually be studied independently from the cell cycle function. Thus, G_0 represents not simply the absence of signals for mitosis but an active repression of the genes needed for mitosis.

2.1.1 Human lymphocytes as cellular model to study oxidative stress and apoptosis in PD.

Deciphering the Parkinson's disease cascade(s) is one of the ultimate research goals in the PD field not only because it offers the possibility to scrutinize a basic cellular machinery of response to different deleterious stimuli, but also because it brings the possibility to predict novel therapies. Accordingly, we postulated a unified molecular cascade model wherein H_2O_2 is definitely a paramount molecule involved in intracellular signalisation that induces neuronal loss in PD (Jimenez-Del-Rio & Velez-Pardo, 2000, 2004a & Fig. 2). Effectively, we were able to clarify the major signalling events by which DA (Jimenez-Del-Rio et al., 2004), monoamine related toxins (e.g. 6-OHDA; 5,6-DHT; 5,7-DHT: Jimenez-Del-Rio & Velez-Pardo, 2002), redox metals such as Fe^{2+}, Cu^{2+}, Mn^{2+}, Zn^{2+} (Jimenez-Del-Rio & Velez-Pardo, 2004b & Fig. 3) and H_2O_2 (Jimenez-Del-Rio & Velez-Pardo, 2006) might induced cell death in normal and/or mutated lymphocytes (e. g. C212Y in parkin) PD.

During the last few years, several reports have been published supporting our findings. Liang et al., (2007) have found that NF-κB contributes to 6-OHDA-induced apoptosis of nigral dopaminergic neurons through p53. Bernstein and co-worker (2011) have shown that 6-OHDA generated ROS induces DNA damage and p53- and PUMA-dependent cell death. Bilobalide, which is a constituent of *Ginkgo biloba* 761, inhibits 6-OHDA-induced activation of NF-κB and loss of dopaminergic neurons in rat substantia nigra (Li et al., 2008). Importantly, Aleyasin et al., (2004) have shown that acute inhibition of NF-κB via expression of a stable IκB mutant, down-regulation of the p65 NF-κB subunit by RNA interference (RNAi), or pharmacological NF-κB inhibitors significantly protected against DNA damage-induced neuronal death. NF-κB inhibition also reduced p53 transcripts and p53 activity as measured by the p53-inducible messages, Puma and Noxa, implicating the p53 tumor suppressor in the mechanism of NF-κB-mediated neuronal death. Takada et al. (2003) have shown that H_2O_2 activates NF-kappa B through tyrosine phosphorylation of IκBα and serine phosphorylation of p65 by IκBα kinase and Syk protein-tyrosine kinase. Prabhakaran et al., (2008) have shown that NF-κB induction and the activation of nitric oxide synthase through ROS represents a proximate mechanism for Mn-induced neurotoxicity. Therefore, we conclude that NF-κB, p53 and caspase-3 are crucial signalling molecules involved in H_2O_2-induced cell death. Based on this model, we predicted that molecules capable of generating

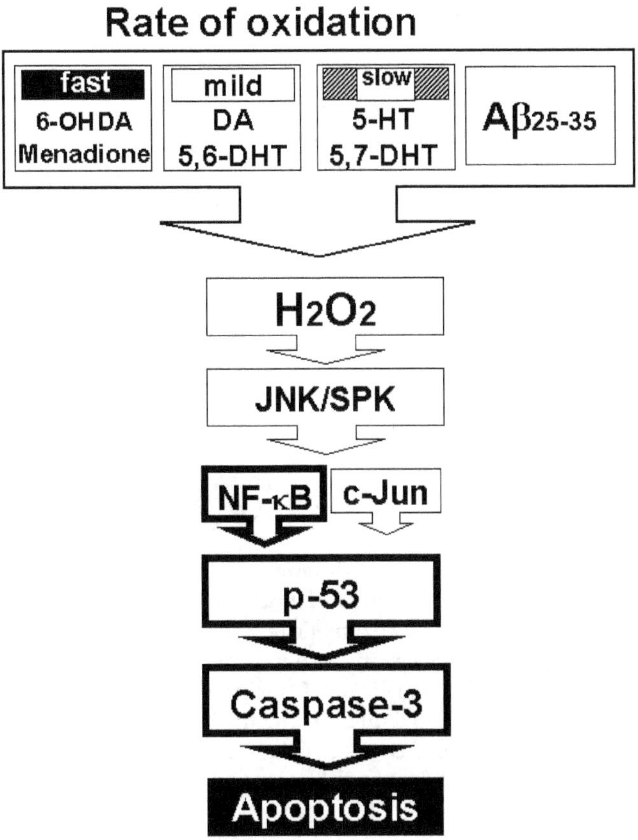

Rate of oxidation

fast	mild	slow	
6-OHDA	DA	5-HT	$A\beta_{25-35}$
Menadione	5,6-DHT	5,7-DHT	

↓

H2O2

↓

JNK/SPK

↓

NF-κB **c-Jun**

↓

p-53

↓

Caspase-3

↓

Apoptosis

Fig. 2. **Schematic model of dopaminergic and serotonergic related toxins-induced apoptosis by an oxidative stress mechanism in PBL.** 6-OHDA; 5,6-& 5,7-DHT or protein fragment Aβ generate H_2O_2. This last compound might activates JNK/SAPK kinases pathway, which in turn activate in parallel both NF-κB and c-Jun transcription factors. NF-κB is able to activate the transcriptional factor p53 and subsequently it may activate the pro-apoptotic Bax protein, which induces cytochrome C release from mitochondria to activate the apoptosome complex leading to caspase-3 activation and apoptosis. Jimenez Del Rio and Velez-Pardo, 2002. Reproduced with permission from Elsevier.

H_2O_2 might induce a mechanism resembling the one depicted in Fig. 2. To further test our model, we used paraquat (PQ), also known as methyl viologen dichloride or 1,1'-dimethyl-4,4'-bipyridinium dichloride, and rotenone (ROT), a redox cycling herbicide and a mitochondrial complex I inhibitor as xenobiotic compound generally used to model PD (Bové et al., 2005). We concluded that both PQ-and ROT-induced time- and concentration-dependent apoptosis in lymphocytes which was mediated by anion superoxide radicals ($O_2\bullet$)) / hydrogen peroxide, depolarization of mitochondria, caspase-3 activation, concomitantly with the nuclear translocation of transcription factors such as NF-κB, p53, c-Jun and nuclei fragmentation (Fig. 4-5, Jimenez-Del-Rio & Velez-Pardo, 2008; Avila-Gomez

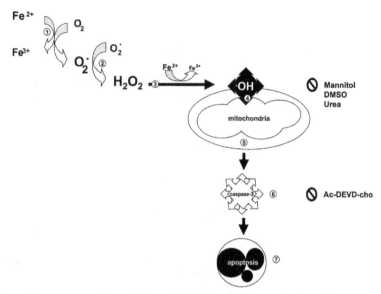

Fig. 3. **Schematic representation of the major molecular events induced by metals in lymphocytes.** Fe^{2+}-metal ions in the presence of molecular dioxygen (1) generate superoxide radicals (2), which dismutate either by enzymatic (e.g., superoxide dismutase, SOD) or spontaneously into H_2O_2 (3). This last compound in turn may react with Fe^{2+} to produce hydroxyl radicals (4) (OH·) by Fenton reaction. Over-production of (OH·) may alter the mitochondria transmembrane potential (5) inducing the liberation of different apoptogenic factors and subsequent activation of caspase-3 (6) resulting in disassembly and fragmentation of nuclear chromatin leading PBL to apoptosis (7). The symbol ( ) represents the inhibition (by indicated compound) of the critical steps of the molecular cascade leading to apoptosis by metal ions. Jimenez-Del-Rio & Velez-Pardo, 2004b. Reproduced with permission from Elsevier.

et al., 2010). Interestingly, Choi et al., (2010) have shown that JNK3 mediates PQ- and ROT-induced dopaminergic neuron death. Remarkably, the cell death routine depicted in Fig. 3 can be reversed by the action of cannabinoids (Jimenez-Del-Rio & Velez-Pardo, 2008), IGF-1 (Avila-Gomez et al., 2010) and glucose (Jimenez-Del-Rio & Velez-Pardo, 2008; Avila-Gomez et al., 2010). These data may provide innovating therapeutic strategies to intervene environmentally or genetically susceptible PD population to oxidative stress.

2.1.2 Alternative therapies for parkinson's diseases: a mechanistic igf-1, cannabinoids and glucose proposal

Based on recent progress in delineating the disease cascade and cell death process (Jenner & Olanow, 1998; Blum et al., 2001; Wirths et al., 2004; Jimenez-Del-Rio & Velez-Pardo; 2004a; Green & Kroemer, 2005; Przedborski, 2005; Jimenez-Del-Rio & Velez-Pardo, 2008; Avila-Gomez et al., 2010), discrete types of potentially disease modifying treatment could be administered for PD. In this regard, our data have highlighted the potential use of lymphocytes as a model to screen antioxidant strategies designed to remove $(Fe^{2+})/(O_2\cdot)/(H_2O_2)/(OH\cdot)$, signalling inhibitors and/or restorative approaches as promising

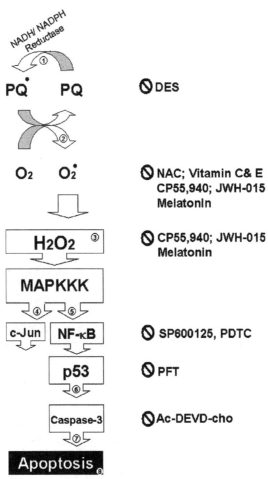

Fig. 4. **Schematic model of the major molecular events induced by PQ in lymphocytes.**
PQ in the presence of NADH/NADPH reductases (1) is converted into monocationic radical compound which readily react with molecular dioxygen to generate superoxide radicals (2), which dismutase either by enzymatic (e.g. superoxide dismutase, SOD) or spontaneously into H_2O_2 (3) This last compound in turn may activate the mitogen-activated protein kinase kinase kinase (e.g. MEKK1) which can activate both c-Jun (4) via activation of MKK4/JNK, and NF-κB activation (5) via phosphorylation of the IκBa (i.e. the repressor of NF-κB) by the IKK complex. The NF-κB translocates into the nucleus and transcribes p53 protein (6). Consequently, this protein transcribes pro-apoptotic proteins (e.g. Bax) which are able to permeabilize mitochondria, thus, promoting the activation of caspase-3 (7) which signals chromatin fragmentation, typical of apoptotic morphology (8). The symbol ( ) represents the inhibition (by indicated compound) of the critical step of the molecular cascade leading to apoptosis by PQ. Jimenez Del Rio & Velez-Pardo, 2008. Reproduced with permission from Informa Healtcare UK Ltd.

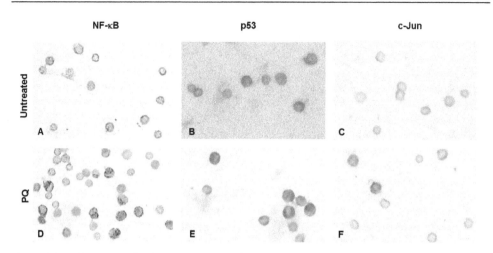

Fig. 5. PQ induces simultaneous activation of the transcription factors in lymphocytes. PBL cells were left untreated (A–C) or exposed to 1mMPQ (D–F) for 24 h. After this time of incubation, cells were stained with anti-NF-κB-p65 (A and D), anti-p53 (B and E) and anti-c-Jun (C and F) antibodies according to procedure described in Materials and methods. Notice that NF-κB, p53 and c-Jun positive-nuclei (dark brown color) reflect their nuclear translocation/activation and appear to correlate with the apoptotic nuclear morphology, i.e. condensed/fragmented nuclei when compared with untreated cells (A–C). Magnification 400 x (A–F). Jimenez-Del-Rio & Velez-Pardo, 2008. Reproduced with permission from Informa Healtcare UK Ltd.

therapy for PD. As depicted in Figs. 2-4, these mechanistic pathways may be of potential use for screening pharmacologically chemical libraries containing hundreds to thousands of compounds each that could modulate or control sensible molecules critical in cell fate (e. g., H_2O_2, NF-κB, p53, c-Jun, caspases). Recently, neurotrophic factors have come into focus as potential therapy in PD (Evans et al., 2008). One clue of its neuroprotective capability comes from the fact that IGF-1 is able to activate NF-κB against H_2O_2 oxidative stress (Heck et al., 1999). However, it has also been shown that NF-κB activation is involved in H_2O_2-induced apoptosis (Kutuk & Basaga, 2003). Therefore, the molecular mechanism(s) that explain the dual role of NF-κB as attenuator or promoter of apoptosis and the IGF-1's molecular mechanism of neuroprotection still remain to be established.

Taken advantage of the fact that human PBL express IGF-1 receptors (Tapson et al., 1988; Kooijman et al., 1992) and IGF-1 appears to be of potential therapeutic use against PD (Quesada et al., 2008), we were interested in the understanding of the molecular events that are thought to be downstream of IGF-1, in relation to the role played by NF-κB in survival and death-signalisation against PQ, ROT and H_2O_2 in lymphocytes, as a single cell model. We found that (100 nM) IGF-1 protects lymphocytes from (1 mM) PQ, (250 μM) ROT and (25, 50, 100μM) H_2O_2-induced apoptosis through NF-κB activation and p53 down regulation involving the phosphoinositide 3-kinase (PI-3K)–dependent pathway. Interestingly, IGF-1, PDTC (a NF-κB inhibitor) and pifithrin-α (PFT, a p53 inhibitor) were able to protect and rescue lymphocytes pre-exposed to PQ even when the three compounds were added up-to 6 h post-PQ exposure. Overall these observations suggest that survival and rescue of lymphocytes from PQ and ROT toxicity is determined by p53 inactivation via IGF-1/ PI-3K pathway (Jimenez Del Rio & Velez-Pardo, 2008; Avila-Gomez et al., 2010).

Which molecular mechanism(s) explain the dual role of NF-κB as an attenuator or promoter of apoptosis? NF-κB has been reported to activate both pro-apoptotic genes such as p53 transcription factor (Wu & Lozano, 1994; Hellin et al., 1998; Jimenez Del Rio & Velez-Pardo, 2002; Velez-Pardo et al., 2002; Aleyasin et al., 2004), which in turn activates the expression of several genes that directly control or regulate the process of apoptosis such as Bax, which is a pro-apoptotic Bcl-2 protein family (Xiang et al., 1998), and anti-apoptotic genes such as Bcl-2, Bcl-X$_L$, X-linked inhibitor of apoptosis (Kairisalo et al., 2009). Therefore, one prevailing model proposes that when the molecular ratio of pro-survival (e.g. Bcl-2, Bcl-xL, Bcl-w) to pro-death Bcl-2 family members (e.g. Bax, Bad, Bak, Bid) is biased towards pro-death Bcl-2 family members either through changes in expression level, localization or activity, the outer mitochondrial membrane becomes permeable to apoptogenic proteins resulting in the activation of a cascade of effector caspases, such as caspase-3, that kill the cells by irreversible proteolysis of critical nuclear and cytoplasmic constituents. In this vein, our data suggest that IGF-1 might promote gene transcription of survival genes via NF-κB activation (Kane et al., 1999) and suppresses gene transcription of pro-apoptotic proteins through p53 inactivation. How then p53 turn-off could be related with IGF-1 citoprotection? One possible explanation for this phenomenon comes from the work by Ogawara and colleagues (2002) who showed that Akt enhances the ubiquitinization-promoting function of Mdm2 (murine double minute) by phosphorylation of S^{186}, which results in reduction of p53 protein. Furthermore, Feng and colleagues (2004) showed that PKB/Akt induces phosphorylation of Mdm2 at Ser^{166} and Ser^{188} resulting in Mdm2 protein stabilization. Based on this information and our data, it is reasonable to assume that p53 is modulated by IGF-1 through PI3K-Akt pathway. In fact, our findings reveal that p53 but not NF-κB is the critical transcription factor that may possibly balances the expression of pro-death proteins towards intracellular death decision under oxidative noxious stimuli (Lu, 2005). Therefore, an ideal natural or synthetic pharmacological compound would be one that efficiently function as an antioxidant (e.g. 17β-estradiol (Jimenez-Del-Rio & Velez-Pardo, 2001; vitamin E) and simultaneously act as a survival signalling molecule (e.g. IGF-1). To our surprise, the molecules exhibiting both features might come from the glandular hairs of *Cannabis sativa* or marijuana, actually known as cannabinoids.

2.1.2.1 Cannabinoids

Cannabinoids are a group of C$_{21}$ terpenophenolic compounds (Elsohly & Slade, 2005), which exert their effects by binding to specific plasma membrane G-protein-couple receptors, termed CB1 (Matsuda et al., 1990) and CB2 (Munro et al., 1993) receptors. Activation of these receptors has been shown to trigger several G$_{i/o}$-protein-mediated signalling pathways (Turu & Hunyady, 2010). Although, it is currently accepted that CB1 receptors are specially abundant in basal ganglia, hippocampus, cerebellum and cortical structures; and CB2 receptors are restricted to cell types related to the immune function such as spleen macrophages, tonsils, B cells and natural killer cells, monocytes, neutrophils, and T cells (Pazos et al., 2005), it has also been demonstrated the existence of CB2 receptors in purkinje cerebellar neurons (Skaper et al., 1996), microglia (Klegeris et al., 2003), oligodendrocytes (Molina-Holgado et al., 2002) and brainstem neurons (Van Sickle et al., 2005). Moreover, both receptors elicit similar signalling pathways such as inhibition of adenylate cyclase, stimulation of extracellular-signal-regulated kinase (Demuth & Molleman, 2006) and activation of phosphoinositide 3-kinase/PKB (Gomez Del Pulgar et al., 2000; 2002; Molina-Holgado et al., 2002; Sanchez MG et al., 2003). The physiological significance of these common characteristics is still unknown.

Cannabinoids have been proposed as potential therapeutic agents against PD (García-Arencibia et al., 2009) thanks to their involvement in control of cell death/ survival decision and in neuroprotection (van der Stelt & Di Marzo, 2005). However, the mechanism of both actions by cannabinoids is far from clear. Moreover, cannabinoids have been shown to function as antioxidant compounds via receptor-independent (Hampson et al., 1998; Chen et al., 2000; Marsicano et al., 2002) or receptor-dependent mechanisms (Nagayama et al., 1999; Kim et al., 2005) or both mechanisms (Kaplan et al., 2003). Although CB antagonists (v. gr. SR141716A) have been used to elucidate the neuroprotective mechanism of cannabinoids, they have not been conclusive (see Marsicano et al., 2002 versus Nagayama et al., 1999; Kim et al., 2005). Therefore, the molecular mechanism(s) of cannabinoids effect on cells is a complex and still controversial issue.

Despite intense investigation, the detailed intracellular mechanism(s) involved in cannabinoids survival effect remains to be elucidated. Because CB2 cannabinoid receptor is linked to activation of PI3K (Sanchez MG et al., 2003), and the non-classical cannabinoid (-)-CP55,940 (a CB1 and CB2 agonist) and JWH-015 (a CB2 agonist) are commercially available, we wanted to elucidate the molecular signalling downstream of CB2 receptor linked to the role played by NF-κB and p53 in survival and death-signalisation against oxidative stress stimuli. We found that both synthetic agonists protect and rescue PBL against Aβ$_{25-35}$- and PQ-induced apoptosis by receptor-independent and receptor-dependent pathway (Velez-Pardo & Jimenez-Del-Rio, 2006; Jimenez Del Rio & Velez-Pardo, 2008). In agreement with our previous observations with IGF-1, these results suggest that CP55,940 /(JWH-015) protective and rescue effect on PBL from noxious stimuli is determined by p53 inactivation.

Recently, we investigated the ability of CP55,940 and JWH-015 to scavenge reactive oxygen species and their effect on mitochondria permeability transition (MPT) in either a mitochondria-free superoxide anion generation system, intact rat brain mitochondria or in sub-mitochondrial particles (SMP) treated with PQ. Oxygen consumption, mitochondrial membrane potential ($\Delta\psi_m$) and MPT were determined as parameters of mitochondrial function. It was found that both cannabinoids effectively attenuate mitochondrial damage against PQ-induced oxidative stress by scavenging anion superoxide radical ($O_2^{\bullet-}$) and hydrogen peroxide (H_2O_2), maintaining $\Delta\psi_m$ and by avoiding Ca^{2+}-induced mitochondrial swelling (Velez-Pardo et al., 2010). Understanding the mechanistic action of cannabinoids on mitochondria might provide new insights into more effective therapeutic approaches for oxidative stress related disorders (Fig. 6). Further investigation is needed to classify cannabinoids molecules (Padgett, 2005; Thakur et al., 2005) with effective anti-oxidant from those with pro-oxidant actions.

2.1.2.2 Glucose

Glucose is a soluble sugar added to all cell culture media. In fact, glucose entry to the cell is facilitated by glucose transporters (GLUTs 1-13) (Manolescu et al., 2007) and depending on cell type, the amount of glucose in cell culture formulations ranges from 1 g/L (5.5 mM) to as high as 10 g/L (55 mM). This is an important consideration to take into account because the same processes that can affect cells and molecules *in vitro* can occur *in vivo*. Lymphocytes are ideal for learning about glucose metabolism and resistance against oxidative stress for several reasons. First, these cells express GLU-1 and GLU-3 transporter proteins

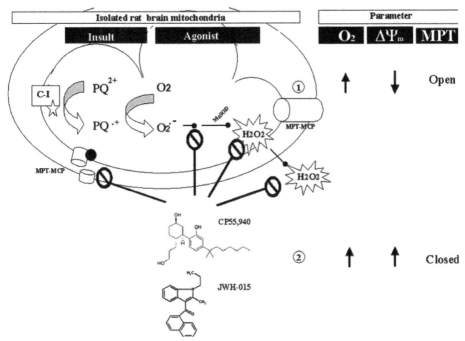

Fig. 6. Scheme of proposed cannabinoid mechanism of action against Paraquat-induced mitochondrial oxidative stress. High mitochondrial membrane potential ($\Delta\psi_m$) in intact rat brain mitochondria drives PQ compound into the mitochondrial matrix. Once inside, (1) PQ is reduced to the monocation radical $PQ\bullet-$ at complex I in the respiratory chain by electrons donated from NADH. $PQ\bullet-$ reacts rapidly with O_2 to produce superoxide ($O_2\bullet-$), thereby consuming high amount of oxygen. In turn, the ($O_2\bullet-$) is enzymatically dismutated by MnSOD into H_2O_2. Then, H_2O_2 induces mitochondrial permeability transition pore (MPT) and decreases $\Delta\psi_m$. Interestingly, when cannabinoids are present (2), they can remove both $O_2\bullet-$ and H_2O_2 thereby blocking further ROS signaling. Most interestingly, cannabinoids inhibit MPT probably through interactions with the cyclosporine A-binding cyclophilin-D protein (black circle). As a result, cannabinoids maintain the MPT-multiprotein complex (MPC) in a close-stated, high ($\Delta\psi m$) but O_2 consumption is still high. Taken in conjunction these actions, cannabinoids thus protect mitochondria from further damage. Velez-Pardo et al., 2010. Reproduced with permission from Springer Publishers Ltd.

(Piatkiewicz et al., 2007). Second, glucose metabolism in lymphocytes is a regulated process. Indeed, glucose can enter glycolytic, pentose phosphate and Krebs cycle pathways (Maciver et al., 2008). Therefore, these cells represent a remarkable non-neural cell model to understanding metabolic regulation of apoptosis and cell survival signaling against stressful stimuli.

Previously, we have demonstrated that PQ- and ROT-induce apoptosis in lymphocytes cultured in standard RPMI 1640 culture medium, which contains 11 mM glucose (11G), via a cascade of molecular events involving $O_2\cdot-$ and H_2O_2, as prime death signals (Jimenez-De-Rio & Velez-Pardo, 2008; Avila-Gomez et al., 2010). Interestingly, by increasing the concentration of glucose to 55 mM (55G) in RPMI 1640 culture medium, it has been shown that glucose almost completely protected lymphocytes against PQ-and ROT-induced apoptotic cell death (Jimenez-De-Rio & Velez-Pardo, 2008; Avila-Gomez et al., 2010). These data thus suggest that the predominance of PQ- and ROT-induced oxidative stress damage may be adjusted by decreasing or increasing the concentration of glucose in the cell culture media. By using biochemical analysis and pharmacological inhibition, we found that 55G was effective in suppressing rotenone-induced apoptosis in lymphocytes via four acting pathways which involve the pentose phosphate pathway (PPP-II), glutathione pathway, SOD and CAT antioxidant system and PI3-K signalling. Moreover, it is shown for the first time that glucose induced lymphocyte survival by NF-κB activation and down-regulation of p53 and caspase-3 (Bonilla-Ramirez, L., Jimenez-De-Rio, M. & Velez-Pardo, C. (2011). Unpublished observations). Taken altogether these results suggest that antioxidants (e.g. cannabinoids), growth factors (e.g. IGF-1) and environmental factor (e.g. glucose) might regulate cell death in lymphocytes upon oxidative stress. Unfortunately, lymphocytes as *in vitro* model of PD do not provide information about executive functions (i.e. cognitive process), kinesthesia (i.e. physical movement) and/or diet-related to PD. To further study the effect of xenotoxicity, diet and movement alterations, we therefore turn out our attention to *Drosophila melanogaster*.

2.2 *Drosophila melanogaster*: an unexpected invertebrate in scene
During the last few years, *Drosophila melanogaster* has been recognized as a valuable model to study neurodegenerative diseases (Lu, 2009; Hirth, 2010), especially PD (Botella et al., 2009; Guo, 2010; Whitworth, 2011) for three main reasons. First, some genes implicated as causative of PD have at least one homolog in the fly (e.g. *parkin*, *DJ-1*, *PINK*::see htpp://superfly.ucsd.edu for further information). This unique feature has facilitated the functional interpretation of these genes in the human (Park et al., 2009; Bayersdorfer et al., 2010). Second, the expression of PD related genes in *Drosophila* can be performed by using the binary GAL-4-dependent upstream activating sequence (GAL4/UAS) system (Phelps & Brand, 1998), thus providing an excellent tool to express pathological proteins in the fly's brain (e.g. α-synuclein, Feany & Bender, 2000). Third, the dopaminergic system of the fly is well characterised (Mao & Davis, 2009; White et al., 2010). Furthermore, comparable to the human condition, the *Drosophila* DA system is also involved in locomotor control (Riemensperger et al., 2011). Therefore, the similarity between the dopaminergic network, mode of drug action and behaviour in *D. melanogaster* and mammalian systems, has made the fly a very attractive model for anti-parkinsonism drug discovery (Whitworth et al., 2006). Additionally, *Drosophila* offers the power of rapid drug screening (Pendleton et al., 2002a; Faust et al., 2009). Amazingly, a variety of approaches have been used to model Parkinson's-like motor dysfunction in *Drosophila*, including specific genetic alterations (Feany & Bender, 2000; Pendleton et al., 2002b; Wang et al., 2007; Sang et al., 2007); pharmacological inhibition of crucial proteins in the dopamine system (Pendleton et al., 2002 a, b) or pharmacological insult (Coulom et al., 2004; Chaudhuri et al., 2007). Indeed, previous studies have demonstrated that paraquat (PQ) induces selective cell death of dopaminergic neurons (Chaudhuri et al., 2007) through interaction with complex I of the mitochondrial respiratory chain (Cocheme & Murphy, 2008) and oxidative stress (Bonilla et al., 2006). Therefore, on the understanding that the causes of PD are mainly oxidative stress and mitochondrial dysfunction, antioxidants, free radical scavengers, monoamine oxidase inhibitors, iron-chelators, and other such drugs are expected to be used. The study of

antioxidants is becoming one of the most important subjects in PD research. Based on our *in vitro* data, we investigated the effect of cannabinoids and polyphenols, which are defined as a group of chemical substances present in plants, fruits and vegetables characterized by the presence of one or more than one phenol unit per molecule with several hydroxyl groups on aromatic rings, in *Drosophila melanogaster* against PQ-induced oxidative stress.

Recently, we have shown for the first time that CP55,940, a non-selective CB1/CB2 cannabinoid receptor agonist, significantly protects and rescues *Drosophila* against PQ toxicity via a receptor-independent mechanism (Fig. 7). Interestingly, CP55,940 restores the negative geotaxis activity (i.e., climbing capability) of the fly exposed to PQ. Moreover, *Drosophila* fed with (1–200 µM) SP600125, a specific inhibitor of the stress responsive Jun-N-terminal kinase (JNK) signalling, and 20 mM PQ increased survival percentage and movement function (i.e., climbing capability) when compared to flies only treated with PQ. Taken together our results suggest that exogenous antioxidant cannabinoids can protect against and rescue from locomotor dysfunction in wild type (Canton-S) *Drosophila* exposed to stress stimuli (Jimenez-Del-Rio et al., 2008). Therefore, cannabinoids may offer promising avenues for the design of molecules to prevent, delay, or ameliorate the treatment of population at high risk of suffering Parkinson disease.

Polyphenols are a group of chemical substances found in plants classified according to their chemical structural as (i) phenolic acids such as gallic (GA), caffeic (CA), coumaric (CouA), ferulic acid (FA), propyl gallate (PG); (ii) flavonoids, which are the largest group of polyphenols, and (iii) non-flavonoid polyphenols. Flavonoids involve anthocyanins and anthoxantins. The latter group is divided into flavonols, flavans, flavanols such as epicatechin (EC), epigallocatechin (EGC) and epigallocatechin-3-gallate (EGCG), flavones and isoflavones (D'Archivio et al., 2007). Numerous studies in the past decade have shown that polyphenols have *in vitro* and *in vivo* activity by preventing or reducing the deleterious effects of ROS associated with oxidative stress and neurodegeneration not only because of their strong antioxidant and metal-chelating properties (Sestili et al., 2002; Melidou et al., 2005; Perron & Brumaghim, 2009), but also because of their capability to induce intracellular signalling pathways associated with cell survival and gene expression (Ramassamy, 2006; Zaveri, 2006). We demonstrated for the first time that pure polyphenols GA, FA, CA, CouA, PG, EC, EGC, and EGCG protect, rescue and, most importantly, restore the impaired movement activity (i.e., climbing capability) induced by paraquat in *Drosophila melanogaster* (Fig. 8). We also showed for the first time that high concentrations of iron (e.g. 15 mM $FeSO_4$) were able to diminish fly survival and movement to a similar extent as (20 mM) paraquat treatment. Moreover, paraquat and iron synergistically affect both survival and locomotor function. Remarkably, propyl gallate and epigallocatechin gallate protected and maintained movement abilities in flies co-treated with paraquat and iron. Our findings indicate that pure polyphenols might be potent neuroprotective agents for the treatment of PD against stressful stimuli (Jimenez-Del-Rio et al., 2010).

It is generally accepted that the causes of PD are mainly oxidative stress, abnormal protein aggregation and mitochondrial dysfunction. Furthermore, substantial evidence suggests diet (Chen et al., 2007) and environmental risk factors such as pesticides (Dick et al., 2007) and heavy metals (Jones & Miller, 2008), in particular iron intake (Logroscino et al., 2008), as causative of PD. However, how genetic and environmental factors are related to the nutritional status of PD patients is still unknown. Moreover, it has not yet been definitively established whether the nutritional status of PD patients might contribute to the

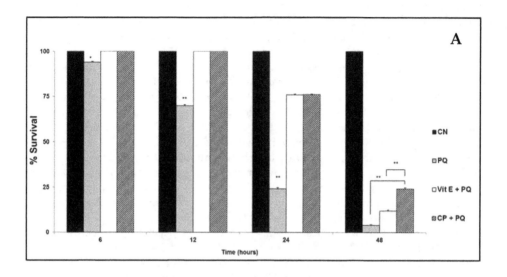

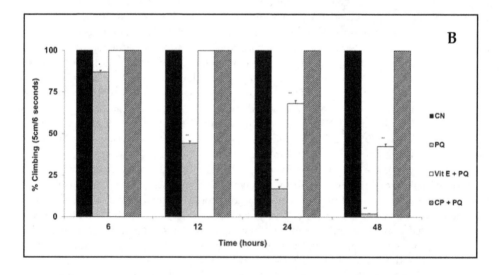

Fig. 7. **Protective effect of antioxidants in** *Drosophila m.* **exposed to paraquat.**
Female flies were pre-fed with either 1% glucose alone, 0.5 mM CP55,940 or 0.5 mM vitamin
E with 1% glucose in dW for 72 h. Then, flies were left untreated (GLU) or treated with 20
mMparaquat (PQ; vit E + PQ; CP + PQ) for 6, 12, 24 and 48 h. (A) Survival rate (%) and (B)
locomotion assay were recorded at the indicated time. *p < 0.05, **p < 0.001. Jimenez-Del-
Rio et al., 2008. Reproduced with permission from Elsevier.

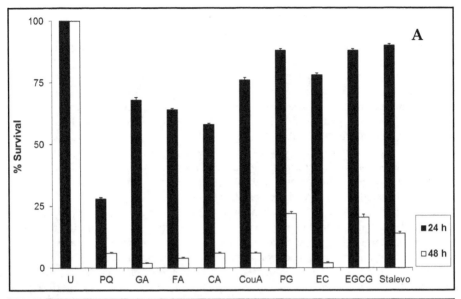

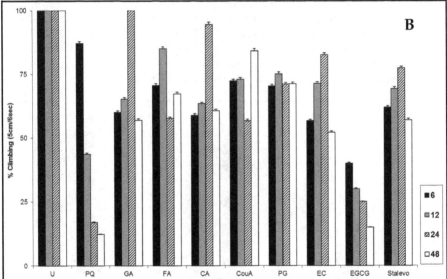

Fig. 8. **Protective effect of polyphenols in** *D. melanogaster* **exposed to paraquat.**
(A) Female flies were pre-fed with either 1% glucose alone or with 0.1 mM gallic acid (GA), ferulic acid (FA), caffeic acid (CA), coumaric acid (CouA), propyl gallate (PG), epicatecin (EC), epigallocatechin (EGC), epigallocatechin gallate (EGCG) polyphenols and 0.1 mg/ml Stalevo® with 1% glucose in distilled water (dW) for 72 h. Then, flies were left untreated (U) or treated with 20mM paraquat (PQ) for 24 and 48 h. Survival rate (%) and (B) locomotion assay were recorded at the indicated time. *p<0.05, ** p<0.001. Jimenez-Del-Rio et al., 2010. Reproduced with permission from Elsevier.

development of the disorder. Therefore, we investigated the effect of glucose in *Drosophila melanogaster* under oxidative stress stimuli.

We have shown that female *D. melanogaster* fed acutely with 20mM PQ in high concentration of glucose (e.g. 10%), as the sole energetic source, not only prolonged survival but also the locomotor activity remained unaltered when compared to fly fed with low concentration of glucose (e.g. 1%) and PQ over a period of 24-48 h (Fig. 9). Additionally, we found that polyphenols protect, rescue and restore the impaired movement activity in *Drosophila* induced by 20 mM PQ in 1% glucose for 24 h exposure (Fig. 8). We also showed that high concentrations of iron (e.g. 10-20 mM FeSO₄) were able to diminish fly survival and locomotor activity over a period of 120 h (5 days). Taken together these findings suggest that either glucose or polyphenols might modulate life span and movement capabilities in *D. melanogaster* exposed to PQ and iron in short time frame. Since there is compelling evidence that shows that the pre-clinical period of PD extends at least 20 years before the motor manifestations (Savica et al., 2010), it is necessary to establish a close parallel with the fly to better understand antioxidant therapy approaches over long period of time. Therefore, we studied the life span and locomotor activity (i.e. climbing capability) of *D. melanogaster* chronically exposed to increasing concentrations of PQ and iron alone or in combination upon 1% or 10% glucose feeding regimen for 15 days and determined whether polyphenols such as GA, PG, EC and EGCG affect the life span and locomotor activity of the fly exposed to PQ for 15 days. It is known that protein aggregation is associated to PD (Tan et al., 2009). Interestingly, high expression levels of the transcription GAL4 protein in *D. melanogaster* have been shown to result in reduced life span (Haywood et al., 2002). Therefore, by using *Ddc-GAL4 Drosophila melanogaster* line, we also investigated whether genetically altered *Ddc-GAL4* flies renders them sensitive to PQ-induced oxidative stress and whether glucose and polyphenols might modulate life span and/or locomotor activity in this line of *Drosophila melanogaster*.

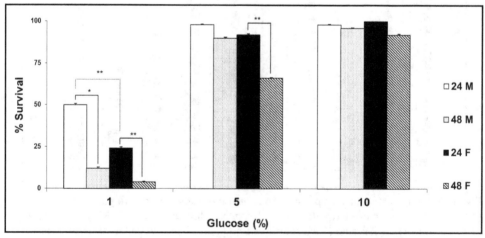

Fig. 9. Effect of glucose concentration in *Drosophila m.* exposed to paraquat.
Male (M) and female (F) were either pre-fed with 1, 5 or 10% glucose (GLU) in distilled water for 72 h. Then, flies were treated with 20 mM paraquat (PQ) for 24 and 48 h. Survival rate (%) weas recorded at the indicated time. *p < 0.05, **p < 0.001. Jimenez-Del-Rio et a., 2008. Reproduced with permission from Elsevier.

We found for the first time that polyphenols exposure prolong life span (P<0.05 by log-rang test) and restore locomotor activity (i.e., climbing capability, P<0.05 by χ^2 test) of *Drosophila melanogaster* chronically exposed to paraquat compared to flies treated with paraquat alone in 1% glucose (Fig. 10). We found that (10%) glucose partially prolongs life span and climbing in *Drosophila* exposed to iron, PQ or in combination, suggesting that both stimuli enhance a movement disorder in a concentration-dependent and temporal-related fashion. Moreover, chronic exposure of (1 mM) PQ/ (0.5 mM) iron synergistically affect both survival and locomotor function independently of the temporal order of the exposure to the toxicants, but the survival is modulated in a concentration and temporal fashion by glucose. This investigation is the first to report that *Ddc-GAL4* transgenic flies chronically fed with polyphenols increase life span (P<0.05 by log-rang test) and enhance movement abilities (P<0.05 by χ^2 test) compared to untreated *Ddc-GAL4* or treated with paraquat in 1% glucose. Our present findings support the notion that *Drosophila melanogaster* might be a suitable model to study genetic, environmental and nutritional factors as causal and/or modulators in the development of PD. Most importantly, according to our model, we have demonstrated for the first time chronic polyphenols exposure as potential therapeutic compounds in the treatment of PD. These findings altogether open new avenues for the screening, testing and development of novel antioxidant drugs against oxidative stress stimuli (Ortega-Arellano et al., 2011).

3. Conclusion

As noted by the Nobel Prize laureate Dr. S. Brenner (2002) "...choosing the right organism for one's research is as important as finding the right problems to work on..." In this regard, human peripheral blood lymphocytes and *Drosophila melanogaster* as model system are well validated and permit totally controlled experiments, are relatively low cost and ease to use, but most importantly, they resemble neuronal cells and clinical manifestation from PD patients, respectively. As any other model (e.g. animal or human tissue and cell lines), their limitation is your removal from the reality of the whole, integrated physiologic system. Despite this drawback, it turns out that their use in complex biologic investigations such as the one presented in this chapter, introduce lymphocytes and *Drosophila* as a unique opportunity to integrate oxidative stress, cell death, cell survival signalling and therapeutic pathways signalling in a single-cell and organism model.

Our present data support the notion that *Drosophila melanogaster* might be a suitable model to study genetic, environmental and nutritional factors as causal and/or modulators in the development of PD. Most importantly, according to our model, we have demonstrated for the first time that acute cannabinoids or chronic polyphenols exposure as potential therapeutic compounds in the treatment of PD.

These findings altogether open new avenues for the screening, testing, monitoring and development of novel antioxidant drugs against oxidative stress stimuli. Furthermore, based on our present findings, we propose that a combined therapy with antioxidant and high energetic agents should provide to pre-clinical genetically individuals at risk to suffer PD a means to delay or to prevent motor symptoms and/or frank PD-ARJP disorders, as those encounter in Antioquia, Colombia (Pineda-Trujillo et al., 2001, 2006, 2009). These data may contribute to a better understanding of the inherent nutritional status, genetic predisposition and environmental agents as causative factors of PD. However, further studies are needed to fully determine target selection and validation, pharmacology, measurement of efficacy

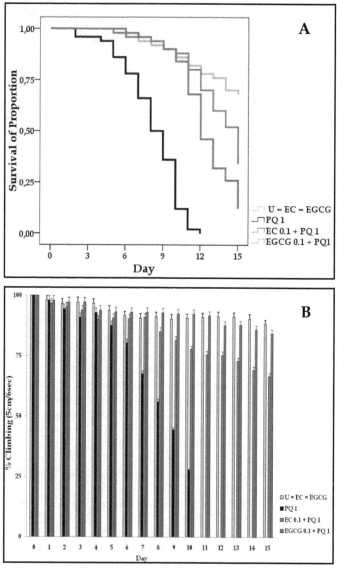

Fig. 10. **Survival (A) and locomotor activity (B) of** *Drosophila melanogaster* **in absence (0, gray bar) or presence of paraquat (1mM) alone (black bar) or in combination of polyphenols (epicathecin (EC, 0.1 mM, red bar) or epigallocathecin gallete, EGCG gallate (0.1 mM, blue bar) in 1% glucose.** Female flies (n= 50 per treatment) were treated as described in *Materials and Methods* section. The graphs show that the proportion of survival and climbing performance dramatically increased in flies exposed to polyphenols compared to PQ treatment alone. Statistical comparisons between treated flies with PQ and polyphenols and PQ alone showed (A) a P<0.001 by log-rank test and (B) a P<0.05 by χ^2 test. Ortega-Arellano et al., 2011. Reproduced with permission from Elsevier.

(Kieburtz & Ravina, 2007) and bioavailability (D'Archivio et al., 2010) of potential antioxidant molecules, particularly cannabinoids and polyphenols, before one can envision a preventive and effective neuroprotectant therapy against PD.

4. Acknowledgements

This work was supported by Colciencias grants #1115-343-19119 & #1115-408-20504; Programa Jovenes Investigadores from Colciencias #8790-018-2011; "Proyecto Investigaciones Enfermedades Neurodegenerativas" grants #8780, and "Programa de Sostenibilidad grants 2007/2008/2009/2010" to CV-P and MJ-Del-Rio.

5. References

Aleyasin, H., Cregan, SP., Lyirhiaro, G., O'Hare, MJ., Callaghan, SM., Slack, RS. & Park, DS. (2004). Nuclear factor-(kappa)B modulates the p53 response in neurons exposed to DNA damage, *J Neurosci* 24: 2963-2973.

Alves, G., Forsaa, EB., Pedersen, KF., Dreetz-Gjerstad, M. & Larsen, JP. (2008). Epidemiology of Parkinson's disease, *J Neurol* 255 Suppl 5:18-32.

Amenta, F., Bronzetti, E., Felici, L., Ricci, A. & Tayebati, SK. (1999). Dopamine D2-like receptors on human peripheral blood lymphocytes: a radioligand binding assay and immunocytochemical study, *J Auton Pharmacol* 19:151-159.

Amenta, F., Bronzetti, E., Cantalamessa, F., El-Assouad, D., Felici, L., Ricci, A. & Tayebati, SK. (2001). Identification of dopamine plasma membrane and vesicular transporters in human peripheral blood lymphocytes, *J Neuroimmunol* 117 (1-2):133-142.

Asanuma, M., Miyazaki, I., Diaz-Corrales, FJ. & Ogawa, N. (2004). Quinone formation as dopaminergic neuron-specific oxidative stress in the pathogenesis of sporadic Parkinson's disease and neurotoxin-induced parkinsonism, *Acta Med Okayama* 58: 221-233.

Avila-Gomez, I.C., Velez-Pardo, C. & Jimenez-Del-Rio, M. (2010). Effects of insulin-like growth factor-1 on rotenone-induced apoptosis in lymphocyte cells, *Basic Clin Pharmacol Toxicol* 106(1): 53-61.

Bayersdorfer, F., Voigt, A., Schneuwly, S. & Botella, JA. (2010). Dopamine-dependent neurodegeneration in Drosophila models of familial and sporadic Parkinson's disease, *Neurobiol Dis* 40(1):113-119.

Betarbet, R; Sherer, TB & Greenamyre, JT. (2005). Ubiquitin-proteasome system and Parkinson's disease, *Exp Neurol* 191 Suppl 1: S17-S27.

Battisti, C., Formichi, P., Radi, E. & Federico, A. (2008). Oxidative-stress-induced apoptosis in PBLs of two patients with Parkinson disease secondary to alpha-synuclein mutation, *J Neurol Sci* 267(1-2):120-124.

Bernstein, AI., Garrison, SP., Zambetti, GP. & O'Malley, KL. (2011). 6-OHDA generated ROS induces DNA damage and p53- and PUMA-dependent cell death, *Mol Neurodegener* 6(1):2.

Bonilla, E., Medina-Leendertz, S., Villalobos, V., Molero, L. & Bohórquez, A. (2006). Paraquat-induced oxidative stress in drosophila melanogaster: effects of melatonin, glutathione, serotonin, minocycline, lipoic acid and ascorbic acid, *Neurochem Res* 31(12):1425-1432.

Botella, JA., Bayersdorfer, F., Gmeiner, F. & Schneuwly, S. (2009). Modelling Parkinson's disease in Drosophila, *Neuromolecular Med* 11(4):268-280.

Bove, J., Prou, D., Perier, C. & Przedborski, S. (2005). Toxin-induced Models of Parkinson' disease, *NeuroRx* 2:484-494.

Blum, D., Torch, S., Lambeng, N., Nissou, M., Benabid, AL., Sadoul, R. & Verna, JM. (2001). Molecular pathways involved in the neurotoxicity of 6-OHDA, dopamine and MPTP: contribution to the apoptotic theory in Parkinson's disease, *Prog Neurobiol* 65:135-172.

Brenner, S. (2002). Nature's gift to science. Nobel lecture, December 8, (*www.nobelprize.com*).

Büeler, H. (2010). Mitochondrial dynamics, cell death and the pathogenesis of Parkinson's disease, *Apoptosis* 15(11):1336-1353.

Calopa, M., Bas, J., Callén, A. &, Mestre, M. (2010). Apoptosis of peripheral blood lymphocytes in Parkinson patients, *Neurobiol Dis* 38(1):1-7.

Carrillo-Vico, A., Calvo, JR., Abreu, P., Lardone, PJ., Garcia-Maurino, S., Reiter, RJ. & Guerrero, JM. (2004). Evidence of melatonin synthesis by human lymphocytes and its physiological significance: possible role as intracrine, autocrine, and/or paracrine substance, *FASEB J* 18: 537-539.

Cocheme, HM. & Murphy, MP. (2008). Complex I is the major site of mitochondrial superoxide production by paraquat, *J Biol Chem* 283: 1786–1798.

Cookson, MR. (2010). Unravelling the role of defective genes, *Prog Brain Res* 183:43-57.

Coulom, H. & Birman, S. (2004). Chronic exposure to rotenone models sporadic Parkinson's disease in Drosophila melanogaster, *J Neurosci* 24:10993–10998.

Chaudhuri, A., Bowling, K., Funderburk, C., Lawal, H., Inamdar, A., Wang, Z. & O'Donnell, JM. (2007). Interaction of genetic and environmental factors in a Drosophila parkinsonism model, *J Neurosci* 27:2457–2467.

Chen, Y. & Buck, J. (2000). Cannabinoids protect cells from oxidative cell death: a receptor-independent mechanism, *J Pharmacol Exp Ther* 293: 807-812.

Chen, H., O'Reilly, E., McCullough, ML., Rodriguez, C., Schwarzschild, MA., Calle, EE., Thun, MJ. & Ascherio, A. (2007). Consumption of dairy products and risk of Parkinson's disease, *Am J Epidemiol* 165(9):998-1006.

Choi, WS., Abel, G., Klintworth, H., Flavell, RA. & Xia, Z. (2010). JNK3 mediates paraquat- and rotenone-induced dopaminergic neuron death, *J Neuropathol Exp Neurol* 69(5):511-520.

Chowdhury, I., Tharakan, B. & Bhat, GK. Caspases- an update, *Comp Biochem Physiol B Biochem Mol Biol* 2008;151(1):10-27.

Cuervo, AM., Wong, ES. & Martinez-Vicente, M. (2010). Protein degradation, aggregation, and misfolding, *Mov Disord* 25 Suppl 1:S49-S54.

D'Archivio, M., Filesi, C., Di Benedetto, R., Gargiulo, R., Giovannini, C. & Masella, R. (2007). Polyphenols, dietary sources and bioavailability, *Ann Ist Super Sanita* 43(4):348-361.

D'Archivio, M., Filesi, C., Varì, R., Scazzocchio, B. & Masella R. (2010). Bioavailability of the polyphenols: status and controversies, *Int J Mol Sci* 11(4):1321-1342.

Demuth, DG. & Molleman, A. (2006). Cannabinoid signalling, *Life Sci* 78: 549-563.

Dexter, DT., Wells, FR., Lees, AJ., Agid, F., Agid, Y., Jenner, P. & Marsden, CD. (1989). Increased nigral iron content and alterations in other metal ions occurring in brain in Parkinson's disease, *J Neurochem* 52:1830-1836.

Dick, FD., De Palma, G., Ahmadi, A., Scott, NW., Prescott, GJ., Bennett, J., Semple, S., Dick, S., Counsell, C., Mozzoni, P., Haites, N., Wettinger, SB., Mutti, A., Otelea, M., Seaton, A., Soderkvist, P., Felice A, & Geoparkinson study group. (2007). Environmental risk factors for Parkinson's disease and parkinsonism: the Geoparkinson study, *Occup Environ Med* 64:666–672.

Dorsey, ER., Constantinescu, R., Thompson, JP., Biglan, KM., Holloway, RG., Kieburtz, K., Marshall, FJ., Ravina, BM., Schifitto, G., Siderowf, A. & Tanner CM. (2007). Projected number of people with Parkinson disease in the most populous nations, 2005 through 2030, *Neurology* 68(5):384-386.

Elsohly, MA. & Slade, D. (2005). Chemical constituents of marijuana: the complex mixture of natural cannabinoids, *Life Sci* 78: 539-548.

Enari, M., Sakahira, H., Yokoyama, H., Okawa, K., Iwamatsu, A. & Nagata, S. (1998). A caspase-activated DNase that degrades DNA during apoptosis, and its inhibitor ICAD. *Nature* 391: 43-50. Erratum in: *Nature* 1998; 393:396.

Evans, JR. & Barker, RA. (2008). Neurotrophic factors as a therapeutic target for Parkinson's disease, *Expert Opin Ther Targets* 12(4):437-447.

Fahn, S. & Cohen, G. (1992). The oxidant stress hypothesis in Parkinson's disease: evidence supporting it, *Ann Neurol* 32: 804-812.

Faraj, BA., Olkowski, ZL. & Jackson, RT. (1991). Binding of [3H]-dopamine to human lymphocytes: possible relationship to neurotransmitter uptake sites, *Pharmacology* 42:135-141.

Faust, K., Gehrke, S., Yang, Y., Yang, L., Beal, MF. & Lu, B. (2009). Neuroprotective effects of compounds with antioxidant and anti-inflammatory properties in a Drosophila model of Parkinson's disease, *BMC Neurosci* 10:109.

Feany, MB. & Bender, WW. (2000). A Drosophila model of Parkinson's disease, *Nature* 404:394–398.

Feng, J., Tamaskovic, R., Yang, Z., Brazil, DP., Merlo, A., Hes, D. & Hemmings, BA. (2004). Stabilization of Mdm2 via decreased ubiquitination is mediated by protein Kinase/Akt-dependent phosphorylation. *J Biol Chem* 279: 35510-35517.

Forno, LS. (1996). Neuropathology of Parkinson's disease, *J Neuropathol Exp Neurol* 55:259-272.

García-Arencibia, M., García, C. & Fernández-Ruiz, J. (2009). Cannabinoids and Parkinson's disease, *CNS Neurol Disord Drug Targets* 8(6):432-439.

Gomez Del Pulgar, T., Velasco, G. & Guzman, M. (2000). The CB 1 cannabinoid receptor is coupled to the activation of protein kinase B/Akt, *Biochem J* 347: 369-373.

Gomez Del Pulgar, T., de Ceballos, ML., Guzman, M. & Velasco, G. (2002). Cannabinoids protect astrocytes from ceramide-induced apoptosis through the phosphatidylinositol 3-kinase/protein kinase B pathway, *J Biol Chem* 277: 36527-36533.

Guo, M. (2010). What have we learned from Drosophila models of Parkinson's disease? *Prog Brain Res* 184:3-16.

Griffiths, PD., Dobson, BR., Jones, GR. & Clarke, DT. (1999). Iron in the basal ganglia in Parkinson's disease. An in vitro study using extended X-ray absorption fine structure and cryo-electron microscopy, *Brain* 122 (Pt 4):667-673.

Halenbeck, R., MacDonald, H., Roulston, A., Chen, TT., Conroy, L. & Williams, LT. (1998). CPAN, a human nuclease regulated by the caspase-sensitive inhibitor DFF45, *Curr Biol* 8: 537-540.

Hampson, AJ., Grimaldi, M., Axelrod, J. & Wink, D. (1998). Cannabidiol and (-) Delta9-tetrahydrocannabinol are neuroprotective antioxidants, *Proc Natl Acad Sci USA* 95: 8268-8273.

Hardy, J. (2010). Genetic analysis of pathways to Parkinson disease, *Neuron* 68(2):201-206.

Haywood, A.F.M., Saunders, LD. & Staveley, BE. (2002). Dopa decarboxylase (Ddc)-GAL4 dramatically reduces life span, *Dros Inf Serv* 85: 42-45.

Heck, S., Lezoualc'h, F., Engert, S. & Behl, C. (1999). Insulin-like growth factor-1-mediated neuroprotection against oxidative stress is associated with activation of nuclear factor κB, *J Biol Chem* 274:9828–9835.

Herrup, K., Neve, R., Ackerman, SL & Copani, A. (2004). Divide and die: cell cycle events as triggers of nerve cell death, *J Neurosci* 24:9232-9239.

Hirth, F. (2010). Drosophila melanogaster in the study of human neurodegeneration, *CNS Neurol Disord Drug Targets* 9(4):504-523.

Imai, Y., Soda, M. & Takahashi, R. (2000). Parkin suppresses unfolded protein stress-induced cell death through its E3 ubiquitin-protein ligase activity, *J Biol Chem* 275: 35661-35664.

Jankovic, J. (2008). Parkinson's disease: clinical features and diagnosis, *J Neurol Neurosurg Psychiatry* 79(4):368-376.

Jenner, P. & Olanow, W. (1996). Oxidative stress and the pathogenesis of Parkinson's disease. *Neurology* 47 (Suppl. 3):S161-S170.

Jenner, P. & Olanow, CW. (1998). Understanding cell death in Parkinson's disease. *Ann Neurol.* 44 (3 Suppl 1):S72-S84.

Jiang, H., Ren, Y., Zhao, J. & Feng, J. (2004). Parkin protects human dopaminergic neuroblastoma cells against dopamine-induced apoptosis, *Human Mol Genet* 13:1745–1754.

Jimenez-Del-Rio, M. & Velez-Pardo, C. (2000). Molecular mechanism of monoamine toxicity in Parkinson's disease: A hypothetical cell death model, *Medic Hypotheses* 54: 269-274.

Jimenez-Del-Rio, M & Velez-Pardo, C. (2001). 17β-Estradiol protects lymphocytes against dopamine and iron-induced apoptosis by a genomic-independent mechanism Implication in Parkinson's disease, *Gen Pharmacol* 35: 1– 9.

Jimenez-Del-Rio, M. & Velez-Pardo, C. (2002). Monoamine neurotoxin-induced apoptosis in lymphocytes by a common mechanism: involvement of hydrogen peroxide (H_2O_2), caspase-3, and nuclear factor kappa-B (NF-κB), p53, c-Jun transcription factor, *Biochem Pharmacol* 63: 677-688.

Jimenez-Del-Rio, M., Moreno, S., Garcia-Ospina, G., Buritica, O., Uribe, CS., Lopera, F. & Velez-Pardo, C. (2004). Autosomal recessive juvenile parkinsonism Cys212Tyr mutation in parkin renders lymphocytes susceptible to dopamine and iron-mediated apoptosis, *Mov Disord* 19: 324-330.

Jimenez-Del-Rio, M. & Velez-Pardo, C. (2004a). The hydrogen peroxide and its importance in the Alzheimer's and Parkinson's disease, *Current Medical Chemistry- Central Nervous System Agents* 4: 279-285.

Jimenez-Del-Rio, M. & Velez-Pardo, C. (2004b). Transition metals-induced apoptosis in lymphocytes via hydroxyl radical generation, mitochondria dysfunction and caspase-3 activation: an *in vitro* model for neurodegeneration, *Arch Medic Res* 35:185-193.

Jimenez-Del-Rio, M. & Velez-Pardo, C. (2006). Insulin-like growth factor-1 prevents $A\beta_{[25-35]}$ /(H_2O_2)-induced apoptosis in lymphocytes by reciprocal NF-κB activation and p53 inhibition via PI3K-dependent pathway. *Growth Factors* 24: 67-78.

Jimenez-Del-Rio, M. & Velez-Pardo, C. (2008). Paraquat induces apoptosis in human lymphocytes: Protective and rescue effects of glucose, cannabinoids and Insulin-like growth factor-1, *Growth Factors* 26(1): 49-60.

Jimenez-Del-Rio, M., Daza-Restrepo, A. & Velez-Pardo, C. (2008). The cannabinoid CP55, 940 prolongs survival and improves locomotor activity in Drosophila melanogaster against paraquat: implications in Parkinson's disease, *Neurosci Res* 61:404–411.

Jimenez-Del-Rio, M., Guzman-Martinez, C. & Velez-Pardo, C. (2010). The effects of polyphenols on survival and locomotor activity in Drosophila melanogaster exposed to iron and paraquat, *Neurochem Res* 35(2):227-238.

Jones, DC. & Miller, GW. (2008). The effects of environmental neurotoxicants on the dopaminergic system: a possible role in drug addiction, *Biochem Pharmacol* 76:569–581.

Kairisalo, M., Korhonen, L., Blomgren, K. & Lindholm, D. (2007). X-linked inhibitor of apoptosis protein increases mitochondrial antioxidants through NF-kappaB activation, *Biochem Biophys Res Commun* 364(1):138-144.

Kane, LP., Shapiro, VS., Stokoe, D. & Weiss, A. (1999). Induction of NF-kappaB by the Akt/PKB kinase. *Curr Biol.* 9: 601-604.

Kawashima, K. & Fujii, T. (2004). Expression of non-neuronal acetylcholine in lymphocytes and its contribution to the regulation to the regulation of immune function, *Frontiers Biosci* 9:2063-2085.

Kerr, JFR., Wyllie, AH. & Currie, AR. (1972). Apoptosis: a basic biological phenomenon with wide ranging implications in tissue kinetics, *Br J Cancer* 26: 239-257.

Kerr, JFR., Gobe, GC., Winterford, CM. & Harmon, BV. Anatomical methods in cell death. In: Schwartz, LM. & Osborne, BA; editors. *Methods in cell biology: cell death*. New York: Academic Press; 1995; pp. 1–27.

Kim, SH., Won, SJ., Mao, XO., Jin, K. & Greenberg, DA. (2005). Involvement of protein kinase A in cannabinoid receptor-mediated protection from oxidative neuronal injury, *J Pharmacol Exp Ther* 313: 88-94.

Kitada, T., Asakawa, S., Hattori, N., Matsumine, H., Yamamura, Y., Minoshima, S., Yokochi, M., Mizuno, Y. & Shimizu, N. (1998). Mutations in the parkin gene cause autosomal recessive juvenile parkinsonism, *Nature* 392:605-608.

Kooijman, R., Willems, M., DeCarla, HJC., Rijkers, GT., Schuurmans, ALG., Van Buul-Offers, SC., Heijnen, CJ. & Zegers, BJM. (1992). Expression of type I insulin-like growth factor receptors on human peripheral blood mononuclear cells, *Endocrinol* 131: 2244-2250.

Kutuk, O. & Basaga, H. (2003). Aspirin prevents apoptosis and NFkappaB activation induced by H_2O_2 in HeLa cells, *Free Radic Res* 37:1267–1276.

Kaplan, BL., Rockwell, CE. & Kaminski, NE. (2003). Evidence for cannabinoid receptor-dependent and -independent mechanisms of action in leukocytes, *J Pharmacol Exp Ther* 306(3):1077-1085.

Kieburtz, K. & Ravina, B. (2007). Why hasn't neuroprotection worked in Parkinson's disease? Nat Clin Pract Neurol 3(5):240-241.

Kriesberg, N. (2011). Animals as models. (http://ori.dhhs.gov/education/products/ncstate/models.htm, available in April, 2011).

Klegeris, A., Bissonnette, CJ. & McGeer, PL. (2003). Reduction of human monocytic cell neurotoxicity and cytokine secretion by ligands of the cannabinoid-type CB2 receptor. *Br J Pharmacol.* 139: 775-786.

Kroemer, G., Galluzzi, L., Vandenabeele, P., Abrams, J., Alnemri, ES., Baehrecke, EH., Blagosklonny, MV., El-Deiry, WS., Golstein, P., Green, DR., Hengartner, M., Knight, RA., Kumar, S., Lipton, SA., Malorni, W., Nuñez, G., Peter, ME., Tschopp, J., Yuan, J., Piacentini, M., Zhivotovsky, B., Melino, G. & Nomenclature Committee on Cell Death 2009. (2009. Classification of cell death: recommendations of the Nomenclature Committee on Cell Death 2009, *Cell Death Differ* 16(1):3-11.

Levy, OA., Malagelada, C. & Greene, LA. (2009). Cell death pathways in Parkinson's disease: proximal triggers, distal effectors, and final steps, *Apoptosis* 14(4):478-500.

Liang, ZQ., Li, YL., Zhao, XL., Han, R., Wang, XX., Wang, Y., Chase, TN., Bennett, MC. & Qin, ZH. (2007). NF-κB contributes to 6-hydroxydopamine-induced apoptosis of nigral dopaminergic neurons through p53. *Brain Res* 1145:190-203.

Li, LY., Zhao, XL., Fei, XF., Gu, ZL., Qin, ZH. & Liang, ZQ. (2008). Bilobalide inhibits 6-OHDA-induced activation of NF-kappaB and loss of dopaminergic neurons in rat substantia nigra, *Acta Pharmacol Sin* 29(5):539-547.

Lin, TK., Liou, CW., Chen, SD., Chuang, YC., Tiao, MM., Wang, PW., Chen, JB. & Chuang, JH. (2009). Mitochondrial dysfunction and biogenesis in the pathogenesis of Parkinson's disease, *Chang Gung Med J* 32(6):589-599.

Liu, X., Zou, H., Slaughter, C. & Wang, X. (1997). DFF, a heterodimeric protein that functions downstream of caspase-3 to trigger DNA fragmentation during apoptosis, *Cell.* 89:175-184.

Logroscino, G., Gao, X., Chen, H., Wing A. & Ascherio, A. (2008). Dietary iron intake and risk of Parkinson's disease, *Am J Epidemiol* 168(12):1381-1388.

Lombardi, G., Dianzani, C., Miglio, G., Canonico, PL. & Fantozzi, R. (2001). Characterization of ionotropic glutamate receptors in human lymphocytes, *Br J Pharmacol* 133: 936-944.

Lombardi, G., Miglio, G., Dianzani, C., Mesturini, R., Varsaldi, F., Chiocchetti, A., Dianzani, U., Fantozzi, R. (2004). Glutamate modulation of human lymphocyte growth: in vitro studies, *Biochem Biophys Res Commun.* 28; 318: 496-502.

Lu, Y. (2005). p53: a heavily dictated dictator of life and death, *Curr Opin Genet Dev* 15: 27-33.

Lu, B. (2009). Recent advances in using Drosophila to model neurodegenerative diseases, *Apoptosis* 14(8):1008-1020.

Maciver, NJ., Jacobs, SR., Wieman, HL., Wofford, JA., Coloff, JL. & Rathmell, JC. (2008). Glucose metabolism in lymphocytes is a regulated process with significant effects on immune cell function and survival, *J. Leukoc. Biol.* 84,949-957.

Manolescu, AR., Witkowska, K., Kinnaird, A., Cessford T., Cheeseman, C. (2007). Facilitated hexose transporters: new perspectives on form and function, *Physiology (Bethesda)* 22, 234-240.

Mao, Z. & Davis, RL. (2009). Eight different types of dopaminergic neurons innervate the Drosophila mushroom body neuropil: anatomical and physiological heterogeneity, *Front Neural Circuits* 3:5.

Marazziti, D., Consoli, G., Masala, I., Catena Dell'Osso, M. & Baroni, S. (2010). Latest advancements on serotonin and dopamine transporters in lymphocytes, *Mini Rev Med Chem* 10(1):32-40.

Marini, M., Frabetti, F., Canaider, S., Dini, L., Falcieri, E. & Poirier, GG. (2001). Modulation of caspase-3 activity by zinc ions and by the cell redox state, *Exp Cell Res* 266:323-332.

Marino, F., Cosentino, M., Bombelli, R., Ferrari, M., Lecchini, S. & Frigo, G. (1999). Endogenous catecholamine synthesis, metabolism, storage, and uptake in human peripheral blood mononuclear cells, *Exp Hematol* 27:489-495.

Marsicano, G., Moosmann, B., Hermann, H., Lutz, B. & Behl, C. (2002). Neuroprotective properties of cannabinoids against oxidative stress: role of the cannabinoid receptor CB1, *J Neurochem* 80: 448-456.

Massoud, TF., Hademenos, GJ., Young, WL., Gao, E., Pile-Spellman, J., Viñuela, F. (1998). Principles and philosophy of modeling in biomedical research,*FASEB J* 12(3):275-285.

Matsuda, LA., Lolait, SJ., Brownstein, M., Young, A. & Bonner, TI. (1990). Structure of a cannabinoid receptor and functional expression of the cloned cDNA, *Nature* 346: 561-564.

Melidou, M., Riganakos, K. & Galaris, D. (2005). Protection against nuclear DNA damage offered by flavonoids in cells exposed to hydrogen peroxide: the role of iron chelation, *Free Radic Biol Med* 39:1591–1600.

Miglio, G., Varsaldi, F., Dianzani, C., Fantozzi, R. & Lombardi, G. (2005). Stimulation of group I metabotropic glutamate receptors evokes calcium signals and c-jun and c-fos gene expression in human T cells, *Biochem Pharmacol* 70:189-199.

Migliore, L., Petrozzi, L., Lucetti, C., Gambaccini, G., Bernardini, S., Scarpato, R., Trippi, F., Barale, R., Frenzilli, G., Rodilla, V. & Bonuccelli, U. (2002). Oxidative damage and cytogenetic analysis in leukocytes of Parkinson's disease patients, *Neurology* 58: 1809-1815.

Miyashita, T. & Reed, JC. (1995). Tumor suppressor p53 is a direct transcriptional activator of the human bax gene, *Cell* 80: 293–299.

Molina-Holgado, E., Vela, J.M., Arevalo-Martin, A., Almazan, G., Molina-Holgado, F., Borrell, J. & Guaza, C. (2002). Cannabionoids promote oligodendrocyte progenitor survival: involvement of cannabinoid receptors and phospahatidylinositol-3 kinase/Akt signaling, *J Neurosc* 22: 9742-9753.

Munro, S., Thomas, KL. & Abu-Shaar, M. (1993). Molecular characterization of a peripheral receptor for cannabinoids, *Nature* 365: 61-65.

McKenna, F., McLaughlin, PJ., Lewis, BJ., Sibbring, GC., Cummerson, JA., Bowen-Jones, D. & Moots, RJ. (2002). Dopamine receptor expression on human T- and B-lymphocytes, monocytes, neutrophils, eosinophils and NK cells: a flow cytometric study, *J Neuroimmunol.* 132 (1-2):34-40.

Nagayama, T., Sinor, AD., Simon, RP., Chen, J., Graham, SH., Jin, K. & Greenberg, DA. (1999). Cannabinoids and neuroprotection in global and focal cerebral ischemia and in neuronal cultures, *J Neurosci* 19: 2987-2995.

Ogawara, Y., Kishishita, S., Obata, T., Isazawa, Y., Suzuki, T., Tanaka, K., Masuyama, N. & Gotoh, Y. (2002). Akt enhances Mdm2-mediated Ubiquitination and degradation of p53, *J Biol Chem* 277: 21843-21850.

Ortega-Arellano, HF., Jimenez-Del-Rio, M. & Velez-Pardo, C. (2011). Life span and locomotor activity modification by glucose and polyphenols in *Drosophila melanogaster* chronically exposed to oxidative stress-stimuli: Implications in Parkinson's disease, *Neurochem Res* 36: 1073-1086.

Padgett, LW. (2005). Recent developments cannabinoid ligands, *Life Sci* 77: 1767-1798.

Pendleton, RG., Parvez, F., Sayed, M., Hillman, R. (2002a). Effects of pharmacological agents upon a transgenic model of Parkinson's disease in Drosophila melanogaster, *J Pharmacol Exp Ther* 300:91–96.

Pendleton, RG., Rasheed, A., Sardina, T., Tully, T. & Hillman, R. (2002b). Effects of tyrosine hydroxylase mutants on locomotor activity in Drosophila: a study in functional genomics, *Behav Genet* 32: 89–94.

Park, J., Kim, Y., Chung, J. (2009). Mitochondrial dysfunction and Parkinson's disease genes: insights from Drosophila, *Dis Model Mech* 2(7-8):336-340.

Pazos, MR., Nunez, E., Benito, C., Tolon, RM. & Romero, J. (2005). Functional neuroanatomy of the endocannabinoid system, *Pharmacol Biochem Behav* 81:239-247.

Perron, NR. & Brumaghim, JL. (2009). A review of the antioxidant mechanisms of polyphenol compounds related to iron binding, *Cell Biochem Biophys* 53:75–100.

Phelps, CB. & Brand, AH. (1998). Ectopic gene expression in Drosophila using GAL4 system, *Methods* 14(4):367-379.

Piatkiewicz, P., Czech, A. & Tatoń, J. (2007). Glucose transport in human peripheral blood lymphocytes influenced by type 2 diabetes mellitus, *Arch. Immunol. Ther. Exp. (Warsz)* 55,119-126.

Pineda-Trujillo, N., Carvajal-Carmona, LG., Buritica, O., Moreno, S., Uribe, C., Pineda, D., Toro, M., Garcia, F., Arias, W., Bedoya, G., Lopera, F. & Ruiz-Linares, A. (2001). A novel Cys212Tyr founder mutation in parkin and allelic heterogeneity of juvenile Parkinsonism in a population from North West Colombia, *Neurosci Lett* 298: 87-90.

Pineda-Trujillo, N., Apergi, M., Moreno, S., Arias, W., Lesage, S., Franco, A., Sepulveda-Falla, D., Cano, D., Buritica, O., Pineda, D., Uribe, CS., de Yebenes, JG., Lees, AJ., Brice, A., Bedoya, G., Lopera, F. & Ruiz-Linares, A. (2006). A genetic cluster of early onset Parkinson's disease in a Colombian population, *Am J Med Genet B Neuropsychiatr Genet* 141B(8):885-888.

Pineda-Trujillo, N., Dulcey-Cepeda, A., Arias-Pérez, W., Moreno-Masmela, S., Saldarriaga-Henao, A., Sepúlveda-Falla, D., Bedoya-Berrío, G., Lopera-Restrepo F. & Ruiz-Linares, A. (2009). Una mutación en el gen *PARK2* causa enfermedad de Parkinson juvenil en una extensa familia colombiana, *IATREIA* 22(2): 122-131.

Polymeropoulos, MH., Lavedan, C., Leroy, E., Ide, SE., Dehejia, A., Dutra, A., Pike, B., Root, H., Rubenstein, J., Boyer, R., Stenroos, ES., Chandrasekharappa, S., Athanassiadou, A., Papapetropoulos, T., Johnson, WG., Lazzarini, AM., Duvoisin, RC., Di Iorio G., Golbe LI. & Nussbaum, RL. (1997). Mutation in the alpha-synuclein gene identified in families with Parkinson's disease, *Science* 27; 276:2045-2047.

Prabhakaran, K., Ghosh, D., Chapman, GD. & Gunasekar, PG. (2008). Molecular mechanism of manganese exposure-induced dopaminergic toxicity, *Brain Res Bull* 76(4):361-367.

Pradilla, AG., Vesga, ABE., León-Sarmiento, FE; GENECO. (2003). [National neuroepidemiological study in Colombia (EPINEURO)], *Rev Panam Salud Publica* 14(2):104-11.

Prasad, S., Ravindran, J. & Aggarwal, BB. (2010). NF-kappaB and cancer: how intimate is this relationship, *Mol Cell Biochem* 336(1-2):25-37.

Przedborski, S. (2005). Pathogenesis of nigral cell death in Parkinson's disease, *Parkinsonism Relat Disord* 11 Suppl 1:S3-S7.

Prigione, A., Isaias, IU., Galbussera, A., Brighina, L., Begni, B., Andreoni, S., Pezzoli, G., Antonini, A., Ferrarese, C. (2009). Increased oxidative stress in lymphocytes from untreated Parkinson's disease patients, *Parkinsonism Relat Disord* 15(4):327-328.

Qin, ZH., Tao, LY. & Chen, X. (2007). Dual roles of NF-kappaB in cell survival and implications of NF-kappaB inhibitors in neuroprotective therapy, *Acta Pharmacol Sin* 28(12):1859-72.

Quesada, A., Lee, BY. & Micevych, PE. (2008). PI3 kinase/Akt activation mediates estrogen and IGF-1 nigral DA neuronal neuroprotection against a unilateral rat model of Parkinson's disease, *Dev Neurobiol* 68(5):632-644.

Ramassamy, C. (2006). Emerging role of polyphenolic compounds in the treatment of neurodegenerative diseases: a review of their intracellular targets, *Eur J Pharmacol* 545:51-64.

Ricci, A. & Amenta, F. (1994). Dopamine D5 receptors in human peripheral blood lymphocytes: a radioligand binding study, *J Neuroimmunol* 53: 1-7.

Ricci, A., Veglio, F. & Amenta, F. (1995). Radioligand binding characterization of putative dopamine D3 receptor in human peripheral blood lymphocytes with {3H} 7OH-DPAT, *J Neuroimmunol* 58: 139-144.

Ricci, A., Bronzetti, E., Felici, L., Tayebati, SK. & Amenta, F. (1997). Dopamine D4 receptor in human peripheral blood lymphocytes: a radioligand binding assay study, *Neurosci Lett* 229: 130-134.

Riederer, P., Dirr, A., Goetz, M., Sofic, E., Jellinger, K. & Youdim, MB. (1992). Distribution of iron in different brain regions and subcellular compartments in Parkinson's disease, *Ann Neurol* 32 Suppl: S101-S104.

Riemensperger, T., Isabel, G., Coulom, H., Neuser, K., Seugnet, L., Kume, K., Iché-Torres, M., Cassar, M., Strauss, R., Preat, T., Hirsh, J. & Birman, S. (2011). Behavioral consequences of dopamine deficiency in the Drosophila central nervous system, *Proc Natl Acad Sci U S A* 108(2):834-839.

Sanchez, MG., Ruiz-Llorente, L., Sanchez, AM. & Diaz-Leviada, I. (2003). Activation of phosphoinositide 3-kinase/PKB pathway by CB(1) and CB(2) cannabinoid receptors expressed in prostate PC-3 cells. Involvement in Raf-1 stimulation and NGF induction, *Cell Signal* 15: 851-859.

Sanchez, JL., Buritica-Henao, O., Pineda Salazar, DA., Ribe, CS. & Palacio-Baena, LG. (2004). Prevalence of Parkinson´s disease and Parkinsonism in a Colombian population using the capture recapture methods. *Int J Neurosci* 113:175-182.

Sanders, VM. (1998). The role of norepinephrine and beta-2 adrenergic receptor stimulation in the modulation of Th1, Th2, and B lymphocyte function, *Adv Exp Med Biol* 437:269-278.

Sang, TK., Chang, HY., Lawless, GM., Ratnaparkhi, A., Mee, L., Ackerson, LC., Maidment, NT., Krantz, DE. & Jackson, GR. (2007). A Drosophila model of mutant human parkin-induced toxicity demonstrates selective loss of dopaminergic neurons and dependence on cellular dopamine, *J Neurosci* 27:981–992.

Sakahira, H., Enari, M. & Nagata, S. (1998). Cleavage of CAD inhibitor in CAD activation and DNA degradation during apoptosis, *Nature* 391: 96-99.

Sakahira, H., Enari, M., Ohsawa, Y., Uchiyama, Y. & Nagata, S. (1999). Apoptotic nuclear morphological change without DNA fragmentation, *Curr Biol* 9: 543-546.

Savica, R., Rocca, WA. & Ahlskog, JE. (2010). When does Parkinson disease start? *Arch Neurol* 67(7):798-801.

Sestili, P., Diamantini, G., Bedini, A., Cerioni, L., Tommasini, I., Tarzia, G. & Cantoni, O. (2002). Plant-derived phenolic compounds prevent the DNA single-strand breakage and cytotoxicity induced by tertbutylhydroperoxide via an iron-chelating mechanism, *Biochem J* 364(Pt 1):121–128.

Sian-Hülsmann, J., Mandel, S., Youdim, HMB. & Riederer, P. (2010). The Relevance of iron in the pathogenesis of Parkinson's Disease, *J Neurochem* doi: 10.1111/j.1471-4159.2010.07132.x.

Sofic, E., Paulus, W., Jellinger, K., Riederer, P. & Youdim, MB. (1991). Selective increase of iron in substantia nigra zona compacta of parkinsonian brains, *J Neurochem*. 56: 978-982.

Shishodia, S. & Aggarwal, BB. (2004). Nuclear factor kB: a friend or a foe in cancer? *Biochem Pharmacol* 68: 1071-1080.

Shimura, H., Hattori, N., Kubo, S., Mizuno, Y., Asakawa, S., Minoshima, S., Shimizu, N., Iwai, K., Chiba, T., Tanaka, K. & Suzuki, T. (2000). Familial Parkinson disease gene product, parkin is an ubiquitin-protein ligase, *Nat Genet* 25:302-305.

Skaper, SD., Buriani, A., Dal Toso, R., Petrelli, L., Romanello, S., Facci, L. & Leon, A. (1996). The Aliamide palmitoylethanolamine and cannabinoids, but not anandamide, are protective in a delayed postglutamate paradigm of exocitotoxic death in cerebellar granule neurons, *Proc Natl Acad Sci USA* 93: 3984-3989.

Stefulj, J., Jernej, B., Cicin-Sain, L., Rinner, I. & Schauenstein K. (2000). mRNA expression of serotonin receptors in cells of the immune tissues of the rat, *Brain Behav Immun* 14(3):219-224.

Tan, JM., Wong, ES. & Lim, KL. (2009). Protein misfolding and aggregation in Parkinson's disease, *Antioxid Redox Signal* 11(9):2119-2134.

Takada, Y., Mukhopadhyay, A., Kundu, GC., Mahabeleshwar, GH., Singh, S. & Aggarwal, BB. (2003). Hydrogen peroxide activates NF-kappa B through tyrosine hosphorylation of I kappa B alpha and serine phosphorylation of p65: evidence for the involvement of I kappa B alpha kinase and Syk protein-tyrosine kinase, *J Biol Chem* 278: 24233-24241.

Takanashi, M., Mochizuchi, H., Yokomizo, K., Hattori, N., Mori, H., Yamamura, Y. & Mizuno, Y. (2001). Iron accumulation in the substantia nigra of autosomal recessive juvenile parkinsonism (ARJP), *Parkinsonism Relat Disord* 7: 311–314.

Tanaka, K., Suzuki, T., Chiba, T., Shimura, H., Hattori, N. & Mizuno, Y. (2001). Parkin is linked to the ubiquitin pathway, *J Mol Med* 79: 482-494.

Tapson, VF., Schenetzler, B., Pilch, PF., Center, DM. & Berman, JS. (1988). Structural and functional characterization of the human T lymphocyte receptor for insulin-like growth factor I in vitro, *J Clin Invest* 82: 950-957.

Tillakaratne, NJ., Medina-Kauwe, L. & Gibson, KM. (1995). Gamma Aminobutyric acid (GABA) metabolism in mammalian neural and non-neural tissues, *Comp Biochem Physiol A Physiol* 112(2):247-263.

Thakur, GA., Duclos, RI Jr. & Makriyannis, A. (2005). Natural cannabinoids: Templates for drug discovery, *Life Sci* 78: 454-466.

Tsang, AH. & Chung, KK. (2009). Oxidative and nitrosative stress in Parkinson's disease, *Biochim Biophys Acta* 1792(7):643-650.

Turu, G. & Hunyady, L. (2010). Signal transduction of the CB1 cannabinoid receptor, *J Mol Endocrinol* 44(2):75-85.

Van der Stelt, M. & Di Marzo, V. (2005). Cannabinoid receptors and their role in neuroprotection, *Neuromolecular Med.* 7(1-2):37-50.

Van Sickle, MD., Duncan, M., Kingsley, PJ., Mouihate, A., Urbani, P., Mackie, K., Stella, N., Makriyannis, A., Piomelli, D., Davison, JS., Marnett, LJ., Di Marzo, V., Pittman, QJ., Patel, KD. & Sharkey, KA. (2005). Identification and functional characterization of brainstem cannabinoid CB2 receptors, *Science* 310:329-332.

Velez-Pardo, C. & Jimenez-Del-Rio, M. (2006). Avoidance of Aβ[25-35] /(H₂O₂)-induced apoptosis in lymphocytes by the cannabinoid agonists CP55,940 and JWH-015 via receptor-independent and PI3K-dependent mechanisms: Role of NF-κB and p53, *Medicinal Chemistry* 2: 471-479.

Velez-Pardo, C., Jimenez-Del-Rio, M., Lores-Arnaiz, S. & Bustamante, J. (2010). Protective effects of the synthetic cannabinoids CP55,940 and JWH-015 on rat brain mitochondria upon paraquat exposure, *Neurochemical Research* 35:1323-1332.

Wang, C., Lu, R., Ouyang, X., Ho, M.W., Chia, W., Yu, F., & Lim, K.L. (2007). Drosophila overexpressing parkin R275W mutant exhibits dopaminergic neuron degeneration and mitochondrial abnormalities, *J Neurosci* 27:8563-8570.

White, KE., Humphrey, DM., Hirth, F. (2010). The dopaminergic system in the aging brain of Drosophila, *Front Neurosci* 4:205.

Wu, H; Lozano, G. (1994). NF-κB activation of p53, *J Biol Chem* 269: 20067-20074.

Wyllie, AH. (1980). Glucocorticoid-induced thymocytes apoptosis associated with endogenous endonuclease activation, *Nature* 284: 555-556.

Wang, C., Lu, R., Ouyang, X., Ho, M.W., Chia, W., Yu, F., & Lim, K.L. (2007). Drosophila overexpressing parkin R275W mutant exhibits dopaminergic neuron degeneration and mitochondrial abnormalities, *J Neurosci* 27:8563-8570.

Wang, X. & Michaelis, EK. (2010) Selective neuronal vulnerability to oxidative stress in the brain, *Front Aging Neurosci* 2:12.

Whitworth, AJ., Wes, PD. & Pallanck, LJ. (2006). Drosophila models pioneer a new approach to drug discovery for Parkinson's disease, *Drug Discov Today* 11(3-4):119-126.

Whitworth, AJ. (2011). Drosophila models of Parkinson's disease, *Adv Genet* 73:1-50.

Xiang, H., Kinoshita, Y., Knudson, CM., Korsmeyer, SJ., Schwartzkroin, PA. & Morrison, RS. (1998). Bax involvement in p53-mediated neuronal cell death, *J Neurosci* 18(4):1363-1373.

Xiromerisiou, G., Dardiotis, E., Tsimourtou, V., Kountra, PM., Paterakis, KN., Kapsalaki, EZ., Fountas, KN. & Hadjigeorgiou, GM. (2010). Genetic basis of Parkinson disease, *Neurosurg Focus* 28(1):E7.

Xu, G. & Shi, Y. (2007). Apoptosis signaling pathways and lymphocyte homeostasis, *Cell Res* 17(9):759-771.

Zaveri, NT. (2006). Green tea and its polyphenolic catechins: medicinal uses in cancer and noncancer applications, *Life Sci* 78:2073-2080.

Zhang, Y., Dawson, VL. & Dawson, TM. (2001). Parkin: clinical aspects and neurobiology, *Clin Neurosci Res* 1: 467- 482.

Zhou, C., Huang, Y., Przedborski, S. (2008). Oxidative stress in Parkinson's disease: a mechanism of pathogenic and therapeutic significance, *Ann N Y Acad Sci* 1147:93-104.

4

Application of Embryonic Stem Cells in Parkinson's Disease

Hassan Niknejad

Nanomedicine and Tissue Engineering Research Center,
Shahid Beheshti University of Medical Sciences, Tehran,
Iran

1. Introduction

The nervous system is a stimulating target for regenerative medicine. Parkinson's disease (PD), which afflicts over a 1 million people in the US, is a chronic neurodegenerative disorder characterized by the degeneration and death of midbrain neurons that produce the neurotransmitter dopamine (DA), resulting in tremors at rest, an inability to initiate or complete routine movements, muscle rigidity, postural instability, and lack of facial expression. Although the etiology of idiopathic PD is not known, several predisposing factors for the dopaminergic depletion associated with the disease have been suggested, including programmed cell death, viral infection, and environmental toxins.

DA neurons, in the substantia nigra pars compacta, play a prominent role in the control of many brain functions, such as voluntary movements and many behavioral processes (Maxwell & Li, 2005). These neurons can be identified via the expression of some specific transcription factors, including Engrailed 1 (EN1), PITX3, NURR1, and LMX1b, which are also very important in the development of DA neurons (Smidt et al., 2003).

2. Current therapeutic strategies for PD

2.1 Drug therapy and DBS

Current established therapeutic strategies for PD patients comprise drug treatments such as L-dopa (a precursor of dopamine), DA agonists, enzyme inhibitors and deep brain stimulation in the thalamus, subthalamic nucleus and globus pallidus (Figure 1). However, these treatments are effective in early stage and can temporarily ameliorate symptoms and cannot cure the disease. Therefore, there is a need for novel therapeutic approaches which one of them is to regenerate the damaged tissue. Since direct regeneration of brain tissues is difficult to achieve, an alternate supply of neural cells is required in order to attain any therapeutic goal. Cell replacement therapy (neurotransplantation) has been suggested to have a great potential for restorative therapy in PD (Freed et al., 2001; Hagell & Brundin, 2001; Olanow et al., 2003).

2.2 Cell replacement therapy
2.2.1 Foetal mesencephalic tissue

Transplantation of human foetal ventral mesencephalic tissues into the putamen or caudate nucleus of PD patients has been adopted as a potentially curative cell replacement therapy

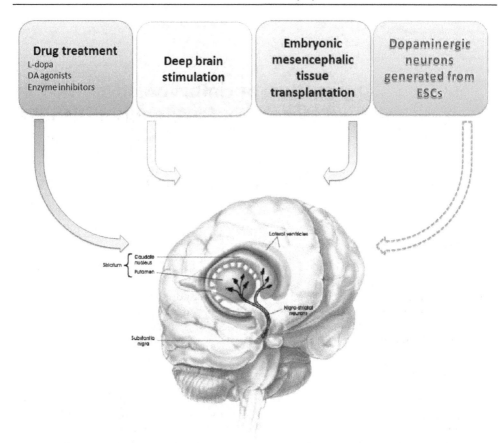

Fig. 1. In the normal brain, DA neurons located in the substantia nigra send their axons to the striatum (i.e. the putamen and caudate nucleus). In the PD brain, the main pathology leading to motor symptoms is a degeneration of these neurons causing a loss of DA in the striatum. Drug treatment, deep brain stimulation and embryonic mesencephalic tissue transplantation are current therapeutic approaches for PD. Transplantation of DA neurons generated from embryonic stem cells has been suggested to restore striatal dopaminergic innervation thereby alleviating PD symptoms.

with long term survival of grafted cells (Kordower et al., 2008a; Li et al., 2008; Mendez et al., 2008). A bulk of experimental and clinical studies have shown functional efficacy of grafting of embryonic mesencephalic tissue into the striatum and a biological mechanism underlying the observed improvement. In spite of promising results of foetal mesencephalic cells transplantation, so far numerous unresolved problems remain to be addressed, such as ethical and religious questions and logistics of acquiring foetal tissues, graft-induced off-medication dyskinesias in up to 56% of transplanted patients (Freed et al., 2001; Hagell et al., 2002; Olanow et al., 2003) and inadequate foetal tissues for transplantation (since treatment of a single PD patient requires DA neurons from six to ten human aborted foetuses). To bypass these difficulties, neurons with a DA phenotype generated from embryonic stem cells (ESCs) could be employed as a practical and effective alternative for foetal brain tissues for transplantation.

2.2.2 Embryonic stem cells

ESCs, derived from the inner cell mass of early post-fertilization blastocysts, are capable of unlimited cell expansion *in vitro* while maintaining their pluripotency. These characteristics of ESCs make them an excellent source of functional differentiated cells for cell replacement therapy of neurodegenerative medicine such as PD, provided that reliable means of inducing differentiation to specific cell types can be achieved. After differentiation, ESCs-derived neurons have to work at least similar to those in embryonic mesencephalic transplantations. Therefore, these neurons have to achieve the following requirements to improve PD markedly after grafting: (i) release DA and exhibit the molecular, morphological and electrophysiological properties of midbrain DA neurons (Mendez et al., 2005; ,Isacson et al., 2003); (ii) reverse motor deficits in animal models resembling the symptoms in patients; (iii) enable 100000 or more grafted DA neurons to survive long term in each human putamen (Hagell & Brundin, 2001); (iv) re-establish a dense terminal network throughout the striatum; and (v) become functionally integrated into host neural circuitries (Piccini et al., 2000).

Two basic strategies can be employed to use ESCs as a cell source for cell replacement therapy: they can be used without any previous in vitro differentiation based on the hypothesis that regional microenvironment is the best inductive cue to obtain the required cell type. An alternative strategy would be to partly or totally differentiate ESCs into the desired cells based on the hypothesis that the host tissue-derived inductive cues are not sufficient to achieve this and to avoid tumor formation at the same time.

Although it has been reported that transplantation of undifferentiated ESCs into the midbrain parkinsonian rats resulted in dopaminergic differentiation of these cells, high rate of differentiated cells were serotonergic neurons (a relation of 2:1 of dopaminergic to serotonergic neurons). Due to this fact that serotonergic neurons in grafts are responsible for off-medication dyskinesias in clinical transplantation studies (Carlsson et al., 2007), it is rather unlikely that the resulting cell composition is well suited for successful transplantation. A more limiting issue was that 20% of the grafted animals had to be sacrificed before the defined study endpoint because of teratoma formation. Although several strategies have been employed to reduce the risk of tumor formation (Chung et al., 2006; Li et al., 1998; Schuldiner et al., 2003), the use of undifferentiated ESCs remains an unsafe strategy.

3. In vitro neural differentiation of ESCs

The in vitro differentiation of ESCs toward dopaminergic neurons has followed different culture protocols in the presence of various combinations of growth factors and signaling molecules. By studying these signaling molecules present in the midbrain microenvironment during development and in the adult, and which key regulatory transcription factors the cells express, protocols for controlling *ex vivo* dopaminergic neurons differentiation can be achieved.

3.1 The major signaling molecules

Retinoic acid (RA) is one of the most important signaling molecules that promote neuralization in embryos and later in development (Bain et al., 1996; Guan et al., 2001; Diez del Corral & Storey, 2004). All-trans RA, which can bind to both RAR subtypes, is commonly employed to induce neuronal differentiation *in vitro*. RA induces a pan-neuronal differentiation and the cell population obtained after application of this differentiation factor is relatively heterogeneous (Carpenter et al., 2001, Schuldiner et al., 2000). Takahashi *et al* showed that cells cultured with RA and fetal bovine serum (FBS) expressed markers for GABAergic, dopaminergic, and cholinergic neuronal phenotypes at low levels (Takahashi et al., 1999).

Wnt3a is another signaling molecule recently shown to play a key role in regulating neurogenesis in the adult brain. *In vivo* expression of a Wnt3a inhibitor reduced neurogenesis in the adult hippocampus. By contrast, Wnt3 overexpression *in vivo* and *in vitro* increased neuronal differentiation (Lie et al., 2005). However, Wnt3's overexpression *in vitro* resulted in a mixed culture of glia and neurons. Also, it is yet to be determined whether Wnt signaling induces a specific neuronal phenotype or serves as a nonspecific, pan-neuronal signal.

BMP is another inhibitory signal found within neural differentiation. It has been shown that the overexpression of the BMP antagonist Noggin increased neural differentiation in neurosphere culture (Setoguchi et al., 2004). BMP signaling activation in undifferentiated cells can result in extraembryonic endoderm committed cells and epidermogenesis. In addition, it has been reported that BMP4 can induce mesodermal differentiation. Noggin is a well characterized BMP2 and BMP4 antagonist and has been shown as neural inducer in *Xenopus* embryos (Niknejad et al., 2010). Since ESCs are pluripotent and susceptible to give rise to all three germ layers, blocking BMP signaling using its antagonist noggin can induce neuronal differentiation by its inhibitory effects on the mesodermal, endodermal, and epidermal fate of ESCs (Gerrard et al., 2005). In addition, inhibiting Notch and BMP-2 signaling may synergistically enhance neuronal differentiation more than suppressing either alone.

However, using these signaling molecules solely result in the mixed population of neural cells, indicating that there are most likely other signals found within the *in vivo* microenvironment that work in conjunction with each other to ensure a neuronal cell fate commitment.

3.2 Current protocols for DA differentiation

Numerous methods have been employed to differentiate mouse and human ESCs into neural cells. Mouse ESCs can be induced into neural progenitors by several methods, such as the use of retinoic acid (RA) treatment of embryoid body (EB) (Bain et al., 1995; Wichterle et al., 2002), a multistep-induction and selection culture (Lee et al., 2000), an adherent monoculture system in serum-free medium (Ying et al., 2003), and a co-culture with stromal cell types (Kawasaki et al., 2000, Barberi et al., 2003). Human ESCs can be induced into the neural lineages using similar methodologies: through the formation of EBs in suspension (Zhang et al., 2006), an adherent monoculture system (Benzing et al., 2006), with co-culture (Ueno et al., 2006) and through spontaneous differentiation of human ESCs (Zhang et al., 2001, Reubinoff et al., 2001). Each of these protocols has its pros and cons. In the following part, the most used procedures for neural differentiation of ESCs will be described.

3.2.1 Embryoid body formation

The well-studied system for neuronal differentiation of ESCs involves the formation of three-dimensional structures called embryoid bodies (EBs) that, to a limited extent, simulates embryonic development *in vivo* (Itskovitz-Eldor et al., 2000). EBs are spontaneously generated when ESCs are cultured in suspension cultures without LIF or serum, in either non-adhesive dishes or hanging drops. The cells in EB begin to differentiate into a heterogeneous

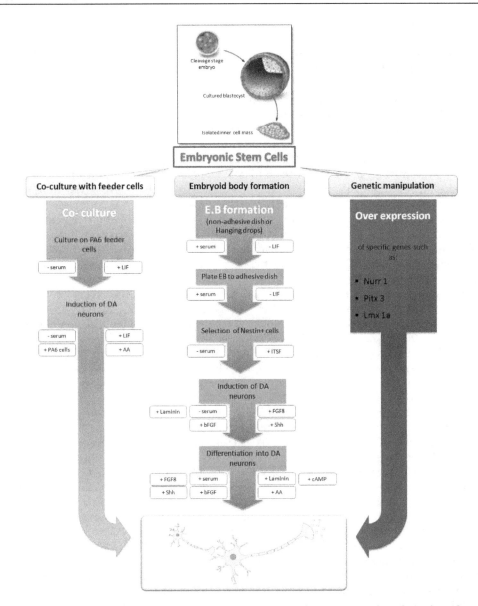

Fig. 2. Schemata depicting steps of three protocols by which ESCs are induced to adopt the DA Lineage.

population of progenitor cells that can form all cell types from the three germ layers, such as skeletal muscle, cardiac, hematopoietic and neuron-like cells. Therefore, spontaneous differentiation of EBs yields only a small fraction of cells with neural lineages. By using different morphogens and growth factors during EB formation, a higher fraction of neural cells can be produced (Figure 2).

After transfer of EBs from a low attachment plate into a normal adhesion plate, the EBs form neuroepithelial cells that organize into neural tube like rosettes. After dissociation of neuroepithelial cells and addition of neural differentiation medium, which consists of BDNF, GDNF, AMP, and ascorbic acid, DA differentiation begins 3–4 weeks after the initial treatment of ESCs (Yan et al., 2005).

EB formation method is still commonly used with the addition of the other supplementary to media such as growth factors. Bain *et al* were the first to show that RA can induce neural differentiation in EBs derived from mouse ESCs, i.e. a high proportion of the resulting cells expressed neuronal markers and had neuronal properties (Bain et al., 1995). In this work, EBs were cultured with RA for 4 days and then plated on laminin-coated dishes. The cells expressed neuronal markers beta-tubulin III and NF-M as well as neural-related genes such as transmitter synthesizing genes glutamic acid decarboxylase (GAD), TH, transmitter receptor subunits GluRs, and a cytoskeletal subunit, NF-L.

RA applied to ESCs can induce concentration-dependent differentiation of neural cells. Okada *et al* tested the effects of different concentrations of RA on the neural differentiation of mouse ESCs (Okada et al., 2004). Lower RA levels (10^{-8}M) were found to induce neural progenitor cells from ESCs, indicated by the high protein expression of the neural precursor marker nestin and low expression of neuronal and glial markers beta-tubulin III and GFAP, respectively. In contrast, high levels of RA (2×10^{-6} M) decreased the expression of nestin while increasing beta-tubulin III and GFAP levels. These results are consistent with other studies demonstrating differentiation of neural progenitors at high RA concentrations (Wichterle., 2002, Bain et al., 1996). RA also directs neural differentiation in human ESCs derived-EB cultures (Guan et al., 2001). The addition of RA and nerve growth-factor (NGF) increased the rate of neuronal cells that formed within human ESC-derived EBs (Schuldiner et al., 2001). However, RA is a strong teratogen and should therefore be used at lower doses to prevent toxicity.

One strategy to direct mouse and human ESCs into "midbrain dopaminergic" neurons is through formation of EBs, followed by the combined addition of Shh and FGF-8 and at a later stage ascorbic acid (AA) (Lee et al., 2000). Using this method, 34% of the resulting beta-tubulin III positive neurons derived from mouse ESCs were TH positive. To shorten induction protocol time, Lau *et al* cultured EBs in KO DMEM supplemented with EGF, FGF-2, and ascorbic acid (Lau et al., 2006). After 3 days, EBs were plated on gelatin-coated dishes and cultured with DMEM/F12 containing EGF, FGF-8, Shh, and ascorbic acid. Cells were subsequently cultured in Neurobasal medium with ascorbic acid. This method generated approximately 40% DA neurons, characterized by their expression of dopamine transporter DAT in 14 days. This chemically defined system for ESCs derivation of DA neurons may be advantageous compared to the co-culturing method, which will be discussed in the next part, as it reduces exposure to animal-derived components and allows for easier determination of factors that influence cell fate.

Another strategy to obtain "midbrain dopaminergic" neurons is the growth of EBs in a conditioned medium with a human hepatocarcinoma cell line followed by conventional serum- free culture in a medium containing bFGF (Schulz et al., 2004, Schulz et al., 2003), or by co-culturing them with telomerase-immortalized fetal midbrain astrocytes (Roy et al., 2006). EBs plated on tissue culture dishes and in the presence of serum-free ITSF medium showed induced differentiation toward dopaminergic precursors within 10 days. In the next step, the cells were transferred to polyornithine/laminin-coated dishes and exposed to a new medium supplemented with FGF2 and Shh (Roy et al., 2006). Withdrawal of these factors, but the addition of BDNF, GDNF, and FBS, yields dopaminergic neurons that are TH positive. The majority of TH positive cells expressed simultaneously G-protein gated inwardly rectifying potassium channel type 2 (Sonntag et al., 2007), which is almost exclusively expressed in the membrane of DA neurons projecting to the dorsolateral putamen, and are functionally linked to dopamine D2 and GABAB receptors (Sonntag et al., 2007).

3.2.2 Co-culture with feeder cells

Another important strategy to enhance the differentiation toward neuron lineage is co-culture of ESCs with stromal cell lines such as PA6 (Kawasaki et al., 2000) and MS5 (Barberi et al., 2003). This effect of PA6 cells has been named the inductive factor stromal cell-derived inducing activity (SDIA) (Mizusekiet et al., 2003; Kawasaki et al., 2000). After screening various cell lines, Kawasaki *et al* found that PA6 stromal cells derived from mouse skull bone marrow is a potent inducer of neural differentiation from ESCs (Figure 2). In contrast to EB formation protocol, this method does not require growth in serum, the formation of EBs, or the selection of neural precursor cells. In this method, ESCs were co-cultured without serum on PA6 cells for 8 days in differentiation medium and for an additional 6-12 days in G-MEM supplemented with N2 and other components. Ninety-two percent of the colonies contained differentiated neurons positive for neural markers NCAM, nestin, and beta-tubulin III and MAP2 and only less than 2% of the colonies were positive for mesodermal and glial markers.

Co-culturing with stromal cell lines with some modifications has become a common strategy to differentiate ESCs into neural cells. In comparison to EB formation protocol, this method has fewer steps and is relatively easier and more reproducible for the generation of neural precursors and neuronal subtypes (Figure 2). Due to the risk of contamination with animal-derived components (Martin et al., 2005), some alternative approaches were recently developed to use instead of stromal feeders. Human amniotic membrane, the innermost layer of placenta has been used as an alternative (Ueno et al., 2006; Niknejad et al., 2008). This approach involves the co-culture of matrix layers of human amniotic membrane with human ESCs for neural induction. Fifteen days after culturing on amniotic membrane, human ESCs produced a population of cells that were greater than 85% nestin positive, and many of these formed rosette-like clusters. While this method eliminates the introduction of animal-derived products, identification of the factors involved in the regulation of neural differentiation, and overcoming inherent limitations in the scale up of processes involving cell co-cultures, need to be further addressed.

Kitajima *et al* devised a co-culture method for producing neurospheres using PA6 stromal cells (Kitajima et al., 2005). To induce neural spheres, ESCs were differentiated on PA6 stroma for 7 days, detached, dissociated, and cultured in growth medium with FGF-2 and EGF. The resulting neurospheres expressed multiple neural markers such as nestin, MAP2 and GFAP, indicative of a heterogeneous population of neural progenitors, mature neurons, and glial cells. Co-culture with PA6 cells for 0-13 days progressively increased the number of spheres generated in a time-dependent manner until day 11. The resulting neurospheres could be further propagated when switched to a serum-free culture and then differentiated into all three neural types. By changing the time of co-culture with PA6 cells, it was also possible to induce different proportions of neuronal and glial precursor cells. This system thus enabled the production of large numbers of spheres without utilizing EB formation.

Also, using MS5 instead of PA6 stromal cells efficiently induced neural differentiation of mouse ES cells, and the resulting cells were able to differentiate into more neuronal types (GABAergic, sertonergic, dopaminergic and cholinergic neurons) (Barberi et al., 2003).

Yue *et al* showed that primate ESCs can differentiate into dopaminergic neurons by coculture of ESCs with sertoli cells. Neurons that had been differentiated on sertoli cells were positive for Pax2, En1, and AADC; midbrain related markers and negative for dopamine-β-hydroxylase, a marker of noradrenergic neurons and could release dopamine *in vitro* when depolarized by KCL (Yue et al., 2006).

3.2.3 Genetic manipulation

At this time, EB formation protocol and co-culture with feeder cells typically lead to a mixed population of cell types. Moreover, to effectively use this approaches *in vitro* the dose, order of addition, and time of exposure to growth factors are all important parameters that must be optimized. This is a difficult task since many of the signals involved in regulating neuronal differentiation are only now being elucidated. It seems transfection of key genes such as important transcription factors (using conventional DNA delivery, lentiviral and adenoviral vectors, and homologous recombination) to ESCs is capable of inducing a specific neural lineage and can potentially increase the homogeneity of differentiated cells (Figure 2).

To enhance TH expression in neural stem cells, Sakurada *et al* used a retrovirus to overexpress Nurr1, a transcription factor belonging to the nuclear receptor super family that is expressed in midbrain DA neurons. This approach induced TH expression in nearly all infected cells *in vitro*. However, infected cells did not express detectable levels of DOPA, the dopamine precursor whose production is catalyzed by TH, and functional production of DOPA was only detected when the cells were differentiated with retinoic acid. Even though the resulting population uniformly expressed TH, the frequency of neuronal markers within these TH positive cells was still low (Sakurada et al., 1999). These results implicate a need for additional manipulations to increase neuronal maturation and the functional production of dopamine.

Similar results were observed in neural stem cells derived from E13/E14 rat foetal brain tissue, in which Nurr1 overexpression led to an increase in TH expression (Kim et al., 2003). However, infected cells did not mature. Park *et al* used retroviral vectors that co-expressed Nurr1 and a second transcription factor to force neuronal differentiation. They examined the bHLH transcription factors Mash1, Ngn1, Ngn2 and NeuroD1, all known to induce neuronal differentiation (Kageyama& Nakanishi, 1997), and they reported that the induction of TH expression depended on which bHLH transcription was co-expressed with Nurr1. Ngn1, Ngn2 and NeuroD1 decreased the Nurr1-induced expression of TH, whereas Mash1 overexpression not only maintained expression but also increased the fraction of cells that expressed the neuronal marker Map2ab. Importantly, they showed that the combined expression of Mash1 and Nurr1 yielded neurons with electrophysiological properties similar to those of mature DA neurons (Park et al., 2006a).

Furthermore, Park *et al* showed that when grafted into Parkinsonian rats, cells co-expressing Nurr1 and Mash1 reversed behavioral deficits. Intriguingly, a retrovirus encoding Shh, the anti-apoptotic protein Bcl-xl, and Nurr1 produced functionally mature dopaminergic neurons similar to the Mash1 vector studies (Park et al., 2006b). These studies demonstrate the potency of genetic manipulation and highlight the fact that significant additional work will be needed to explore whether extracellular signal combinations can achieve similar results.

In addition to its role in directing differentiation towards a DA phenotype, Nurr1 synergizes with Pitx3 to promote terminal maturation of midbrain DA neurons from both mouse and human ESCs (Martinat et al., 2006). Lentiviral vectors carrying Nurr1, Pitx3, Lmx1b, or En1 were introduced at the neural precursor stage after induction into EBs from mouse ESCs. The combined transduction of Nurr1 and Pitx3 dramatically induced the expression of the late marker DAT (dopamine transporter), but not TH. Only Nurr1 alone induced expression of TH.

The two predominant methods developed on mouse cells, transfection of mouse ESCs with specific factors such as Nurr-1 and Lmx1a as well as co-cultures with stromal cells, have been translated to human ESCs to direct DA neuron differentiation. Similar results were found after human ES cells were transduced with lentiviral vectors carrying both Nurr1 and Pitx3 at the neural precursor stage as well as co-cultured with stromal cells (Martinat et al., 2006). Nurr1 and Pitx3 together promoted the maturation of midbrain DA neurons and led to an increase in TH positive cells. In electrophysiological analysis, differentiated human ESCs displayed basic neuronal characteristics such as action potentials, burst firing, and miniature spontaneous excitatory postsynaptic currents. Transplantation of these cells into a mouse model of PD improved some motor ability 6 weeks post-transplantation; however, there was limited maturation of the engrafted human ES-derived cells, as assessed by low expression of TH

4. ESCs in PD: hype or hope

Despite all of the advantages of ESCs for cell replacement therapy, some pitfalls must be overcome before ESCs are used therapeutically for PD. The major limitation is ethical issues concerning to their embryonic origin. Human embryos are most often destroyed as the stem cells are harvested. Hence the question: Can we intentionally kill a developing human being at this stage to expand scientific knowledge and potentially provide medical benefit to others? As a result, some regulations limit funding of research to the initial set of derived human ESCs, strictly withholding support for the study and derivation of new stem cells lines. However, creating new stem lines by deriving human ESCs from single blastomeres (Klimanskaya et al., 2006), without destroying the embryo was a promising result to bypass the ethical problem of ESCs.

The other challenge in employing ESCs for developmental biology research and their possible application in cell replacement therapy is to direct their wide differentiation potential into specific neural cell lineages. The most important concern of the mentioned protocols of ESCs differentiation toward specific neural lineages is the nonspecific generation of cell populations derived from the three germ layers in the total cell population. In all protocols, the presence of mesodermal- and endodermal-originated cell lineages is unavoidable, which is undesirable for further application in regenerative medicine. Hence, understanding the coordination and roles of intrinsic factors with extrinsic factors will be a critical step to direct ESCs differentiation into dopaminergic neuronal cells.

In addition to mesodermal and endodermal lineages, current protocols result in heterogonous population of glia and neural cells, such as serotonergic, GABAergic and noradrenergic. To date, it is uncertain which of these ingredients are of positive or negative impact on the clinical effectiveness of the transplants. For example in transplantation of foetal mesencephalon which is a mixture of all neural cell types homing to the foetal midbrain, containing serotonergic neurons might be responsible for dyskinetic side effects. On the other hand, it has been shown that foetal midbrain-derived astrocytes have beneficial effects on in vitro differentiation of ESCs into DA neurons. Transplanting a mixture of dopaminergic precursors/neurons and midbrain-specific astrocytes might thus be more effective than a purified DA cell source. No information is available on the effect of GABAergic or noradrenergic neurons also present in midbrain transplants. Therefore, further studies will be required to investigate the effects of the other constituents of neural cells other than DA neurons on dopaminergic differentiation of ESCs and after grafting in the animal model of PD.

As mentioned, current differentiation protocols rely on the use of animal products (e.g. PA6 is a mouse stromal cell line) and thus carry the potential to induce disease transmission through contamination with bacteria, viruses or other infectious agents, such as those responsible for transmissible spongiform encephalopathy. Therefore, animal products should, where possible, be replaced by components of human origin and defined and feeder-free conditions should be developed for differentiation of ESCs into dopaminergic neurons if the cells are going to be implanted in patients.

The other unresolved problem is whether the grafts will be affected by the PD process. The results of foetal mesencephalic tissue transplantations provide evidence that PD pathology might propagate from host to graft (Kordower et al., 2008a; Li et al., 2008; Brundin et al., 2008, Kordower et al., 2008b). However, it seems that at least one decade is required for the development of Lewy bodies (LBs) in the grafted cells (Kordower et al., 2008a; Mendez et al., 2008). This issue should be noticed in the animal model of PD.

Rejection of grafts is an important issue in cell replacement therapy, particularly for ESCs which are transplanted as an allograft. Although immune responses to brain allografts are moderate and survival can be obtained even without immunosuppression (Freed et al., 2001), most investigators prefer to use immunosuppressive agents for 6 to 12 months after transplantation (Brundin etal., 2000, Mendez et al., 2005; Olanow et al., 2003). Another way to keep away from immune reactions after transplantation is the using of therapeutic cloning. It has been shown that genetically identical ESCs derived DA neurons, generated by transfer of autologous nuclei from fibroblasts, improve functional deficits without immune reaction in PD mice (Tabar et al. 2008). However, it should be evaluated whether genetically modified cells would be acceptable in a clinical protocol.

Tumor formation remains another obstacle concerning the transplantation of ESCs that has to be eliminated before human ESCs can be safely applied in PD. Because life expectancy is almost normal in PD patients, even a minor risk of tumor formation associated with cell replacement therapy is unacceptable in this disorder. To improve safety, it might be necessary to engineer ESCs with regulated suicide genes or to use cell sorting to eliminate cells that could give rise to tumors.

In the end, on the basis of the available experimental data, ESCs are promising source for the cell replacement therapy. Although much more studies will be required to overcome the mentioned challenging issues, it seems it is now possible to start defining a road map including the main steps towards clinical application of ESCs in PD.

5. Acknowledgment

Author would like to thank Prof. H. Peirovi, Prof M. Jorjani, Prof. A. Ahamdiani, B.J. Nooshin and Dr. Tina Deihim for their critical comments.

6. References

Bain G, Kitchens D, Yao M, Huettner JE & Gottlieb DI. (1995). Embryonic stem cells express neuronal properties *in vitro*. *Dev Biol*, 168, pp. 342-57

Bain G., Ray W. J., Yao M. & Gottlieb DI. (1996). Retinoic acid promotes neural and represses mesodermal gene expression in mouse embryonic stem cells in culture. *Biochem Biophys Res Commun*, 223, pp. 691-4

Barberi T, Klivenyi P, Calingasan NY, Lee H, Kawamata H, Loonam K., Perrier AL, Bruses J, Rubio ME, Topf N, Tabar V, Harrison NL, Beal MF, Moore MA & Studer L. (2003). Neural subtype specification of fertilization and nuclear transfer embryonic stem cells and application in parkinsonian mice. *Nat Biotechnol*, 21, pp. 1200-7

Benzing C, Segschneider M, Leinhaas A, Itskovitz-Eldor J & Brustle O. (2006). Neuralconversion of human em bryonic stem cell colonies in the presence of fibroblast growth factor-2. *Neuroreport*, 17, pp. 1675-81

Brundin P, Pogarell O, Hagell P, Piccini P, Widner H, Schrag A, Kupsch A, Crabb L, Odin P, Gustavii B, Björklund A, Brooks DJ, Marsden CD, Oertel WH, Quinn NP, Rehncrona S & Lindvall O. (2000). Bilateral caudate and putamen grafts of embryonic mesencephalic tissue treated with lazaroids in Parkinson's disease. *Brain*, 123, 1380-1390

Carlsson T, Carta M, Winkler C, Bjorklund A & Kirik D. (2007). Serotonin neuron transplants exacerbate L-DOPA-induced dyskinesias in a rat model of Parkinson's disease. *J Neurosci*, 27, pp. 8011-8022

Carpenter MK, Inokuma MS, Denham J, Mujtaba T, Chiu CP & Rao MS. (2001). Enrichment of neurons and neural precursors from human embryonic stem cells. *Exp Neurol*, 172, pp. 383-397

Chung S, Shin BS, Hedlund E, Pruszak J, Ferree A, Kang UJ, Isacson O & Kim KS. (2006). Genetic selection of sox1GFPexpressing neural precursors removes residual tumorigenic pluripotent stem cells and attenuates tumor formation after transplantation. *J Neurochem*, 97, pp. 1467-1480

Diez del Corral, R. & Storey K. G. (2004). Opposing FGF and retinoid pathways: a signalling switch that controls differentiation and patterning onset in the extending vertebrate body axis. *Bioessays*, 26, pp. 857-69

Freed CR, Greene PE, Breeze RE, Tsai WY, Du Mouchel W, Kao R, Dillon S, Winfield H, Culver S, Trojanowski JQ, Eidelberg D & Fahn S. (2001). Transplantation of embryonic dopamine neurons for severe Parkinson's disease. *N Engl J Med*, 344, pp. 710-719

Gerrard L, Rodgers L & Cui W. (2005). Differentiation of human embryonic stem cells to neural lineages in adherent culture by blocking bone morphogenetic protein signaling. *Stem Cells*, 23(9), pp. 1234-41

Guan K., Chang H, Rolletschek A & Wobus AM. (2001). Embryonic stem cell derived neurogenesis. Retinoic acid induction and lineage selection of neuronal cells. *Cell Tissue Res*, 305, pp. 171-6

Hagell P & Brundin P. (2001). Cell survival and clinical outcome following intrastriatal transplantation in Parkinson disease. *J Neuropathol Exp Neurol*, 60, pp.741-752

Hagell P, Piccini P, Bjorklund A, Brundin P, Rehncrona S, Widner H, Crabb L, Pavese N, Oertel WH, Quinn N, Brooks DJ & Lindvall O. (2002). Dyskinesias following neural transplantation in Parkinson's disease. *Nat Neurosci*, 5, pp. 627-628

Isacson O. Bjorklund LM &Schumacher JM. (2003). Toward full restoration of synaptic and terminal function of the dopaminergic system in Parkinson's disease by stem cells. *Ann Neurol*, 53 (Suppl. 3), pp. S135–S146

Itskovitz-Eldor J, Schuldiner M, Karsenti D, Eden A, Yanuka O, Amit M, Soreq H & Benvenisty N. (2000). Differentiation of human embryonic stem cells into embryoid bodies compromising the three embryonic germ layers. *Mol Med*, 6 pp. 88 –95

Kageyama R & Nakanishi S. (1997). Helix-loop-helix factors in growth and differentiation of the vertebrate nervous system. *Curr Opin Genet Dev*, 7, pp.659-65

Kawasaki H, Mizuseki K, Nishikawa S, Kaneko S, Kuwana Y, Nakanishi S, Nishikawa SI & Sasai Y. (2000). Induction of midbrain dopaminergic neurons from ES cells by stromal cell-derived inducing activity. *Neuron*, 28, pp. 31-40

Kim JY, Koh HC, Lee JY, Chang MY, Kim YC, Chung HY, Son H, Lee YS, Studer L, McKay R & Lee SH. (2003). Dopaminergic neuronal differentiation from rat embryonic neural precursors by Nurr1 overexpression. *J Neurochem*, 85, pp. 1443-54

Kitajima H, Yoshimura S, Kokuzawa J, Kato M, Iwama T, Motohashi T, Kunisada T & Sakai N. (2005). Culture method for the induction of neurospheres from mouse embryonic stem cells by coculture with PA6 stromal cells. *J Neurosci Res*, 80, pp. 467-74

Klimanskaya I, Chung Y, Becker S, Lu SJ & Lanza R. (2006). Human embryonic stem cell lines derived from single blastomeres. *Nature*, 444, pp. 481-5

Kordower JH, Chu Y, Hauser RA, Freeman TB & Olanow CW. (2008a). Lewy body like pathology in long-term embryonic nigral transplants in Parkinson's disease. *Nat Med*, 14, pp. 504–6

Kordower JH Chu Y, Hauser RA, Olanow CW & Freeman TB. (2008b). Transplanted dopaminergic neurons develop PD pathologic changes: a second case report. *Mov Disord*, 23, pp. 2303–2306

Lau T, Adam S & Schloss P. (2006). Rapid and efficient differentiation of dopaminergic neurons from mouse embryonic stem cells. *Neuroreport*, 17, pp. 975-9

Lee SH, Lumelsky N, Studer L, Auerbach JM & McKay RD. (2000). Efficient generation of midbrain and hindbrain neurons from mouse embryonic stem cells. *Nat Biotechnol*, 18, pp. 675-9

Li JY, Englund E, Holton JL, Soulet D, Hagell P, Lees AJ, Lashley T, Quinn NP, Rehncrona S, Björklund A, Widner H, Revesz T, Lindvall O & Brundin P. (2008). Lewy bodies in grafted neurons in subjects with Parkinson's disease suggest host-to-graft disease propagation. *Nat Med*, 14, pp. 501–3

Li M, Pevny L, Lovell-Badge R & Smith A. (1998). Generation of purified neural precursors from embryonic stem cells by lineage selection. *Curr Biol*, 8, pp. 971–974

Lie DC, Colamarino SA, Song HJ, Desire L, Mira H, Consiglio A, Lein ES, Jessberger S, H. Lansford, Dearie AR & Gage FH. (2005). Wnt signalling regulates adult hippocampal neurogenesis. *Nature*, 437, pp. 1370-5

Maxwell SL & Li M. (2005). Midbrain dopaminergic development in vivo and in vitro from embryonic stem cells. *J Anat*, 207, pp. 209 –218

Martin MJ, Muotri A, Gage F & Varki A. (2005). Human embryonic stem cells express an immunogenic nonhuman sialic acid. *Nat Med*, 11, pp. 228-32

Martinat C, Bacci JJ, Leete T, Kim J, Vanti WB, Newman AH, Cha JH, Gether U, Wang H & Abeliovich A. (2006) Cooperative transcription activation by Nurr1 and Pitx3 induces embryonic stem cell maturation to the midbrain dopamine neuron phenotype. *Proc Natl Acad Sci U S A*, 103, pp. 2874-9

Mendez, I, Sanchez-Pernaute R, Cooper O, Viñuela A, Ferrari D, Björklund L, Dagher A & Isacson O. (2005). Cell type analysis of functional fetal dopamine cell suspension transplants in the striatum and substantia nigra of patients with Parkinson's disease. *Brain*, 128, pp. 1498–1510

Mendez I, Vinuela A, Astradsson A, Mukhida K, Hallett P, Robertson H, Tierney T, Holness R, Dagher A, Trojanowski JQ & Isacson O. (2008). Dopamine neurons implanted into people with Parkinson's disease survive without pathology for 14 years. *Nat Med*, 14, pp. 507–9

Mizuseki K, Sakamoto T, Watanabe K, Muguruma K, Ikeya M, Nishiyama A, Arakawa A, Suemori H, Nakatsuji N, Kawasaki H, Murakami F & Sasai Y. (2003).Generation of neural crest-derived peripheral neurons and floor plate cells from mouse and primate embryonic stem cells. *Proc Natl Acad Sci U S A*, 100, pp. 5828–5833

Niknejad H, Peirovi H, Jorjani M, Ahmadiani A, Ghanavi J & Seifalian AM. (2008). Properties of the amniotic membrane for potential use in tissue engineering. *Eur Cell Mater*, 15, pp. 88-99

Niknejad H, Peirovi H, Ahmadiani A, Ghanavi J & Jorjani M. (2010). Differentiation factors that influence neuronal markers expression in vitro from human amniotic epithelial cells. *Eur Cell Mater*, 19, pp. 22-9

Okada Y, Shimazaki T, Sobue G & Okano H. (2004) Retinoic-acid-concentration-dependent acquisition of neural cell identity during *in vitro* differentiation of mouse embryonic stem cells. *Dev Biol*, 275, pp.124-42

Olanow CW, Goetz CG, Kordower JH, Stoessl AJ, Sossi V, Brin MF, Shannon KM, Nauert GM, Perl DP, Godbold J & Freeman TB. (2003). A double-blind controlled trial of bilateral fetal nigral transplantation in Parkinson's disease. *Ann Neurol*, 54, pp. 403–414

Park CH, Kang JS, Kim JS, Chung S, Koh JY, Yoon EH, Jo AY, Chang MY, Koh HC, Hwang S, Suh- Kim H, Lee YS, Kim KS & Lee SH. (2006a). Differential actions of the proneural genes encoding Mash1 and neurogenins in Nurr1- induced dopamine neuron differentiation. *J Cell Sci*, 119, pp. 2310-20

Park CH, Kang JS, Shin YH, Chang MY, Chung S, Koh HC, Zhu MH, Oh SB, Lee YS, Panagiotakos G, Tabar V, Studer L & Lee SH. (2006b). Acquisition of *in vitro* and *in vivo* functionality of Nurr1-induced dopamine neurons. *Faseb J*,20, pp. 2553-5

Piccini P, Lindvall O, Björklund A, Brundin P, Hagell P, Ceravolo R, Oertel W, Quinn N, Samuel M, Rehncrona S, Widner H & Brooks DJ. (2000). Delayed recovery of movement-related cortical function in Parkinson's disease after striatal dopaminergic grafts. *Ann Neurol*, 48, pp. 689–695

Reubinoff BE, Itsykson P, Turetsky T, Pera MF, Reinhartz E, Itzik A & Ben-Hur T. (2001). Neural progenitors from human embryonic stem cells. *Nat Biotechnol*, 19, pp. 1134-40

Roy NS, Cleren C, Singh SK, Yang L, Beal MF & Goldman SA. (2006). Functional engraftment of human ES cell-derived dopaminergic neurons enriched by coculture with telomerase-immortalized midbrain astrocytes. *Nat Med*,12, pp. 1259 –1268

Sakurada K, Ohshima-Sakurada M, Palmer TD & Gage FH. (1999). Nurr1, an orphan nuclear receptor, is a transcriptional activator of endogenous tyrosine hydroxylase in neural progenitor cells derived from the adult brain. *Development*, 126, pp. 4017-26

Schuldiner M, Eiges R, Eden A, Yanuka O, Itskovitz-Eldor J, Goldstein RS & Benvenisty N. (2001). Induced neuronal differentiation of human embryonic stem cells. *Brain Res*, 913, pp.201-5

Schuldiner M, Itskovitz-Eldor J & Benvenisty N. (2003). Selective ablation of human embryonic stem cells expressing a "suicide" gene. *Stem Cells*, 21, pp. 257–265

Schuldiner M, Yanuka O, Itskovitz-Eldor J, Melton DA & Benvenisty N. (2000). Effects of eight growth factors on the differentiation of cells derived from human embryonic stem cells. *Proc Natl Acad Sci U S A*, 97, pp. 11307–11312

Schulz TC, Noggle SA, Palmarini GM, Weiler DA, Lyons IG, Pensa KA, Meedeniya AC, Davidson BP, Lambert NA & Condie BG. (2004). Differentiation of human embryonic stem cells to dopaminergic neurons in serum-free suspension culture. *STEM CELLS*, 22:1218 –1238.

Schulz TC, Palmarini GM, Noggle SA, Weiler DA, Mitalipova MM & Condie BG. (2003). Directed neuronal differentiation of human embryonic stem cells. *BMC Neurosci*, 4, pp.27

Setoguchi T., Nakashima K, Takizawa T, Yanagisawa M, Ochiai W, Okabe M, Yone K, Komiya S & Taga T. (2004). Treatment of spinal cord injury by transplantation of fetal neural precursor cells engineered to express BMP inhibitor. *Exp Neurol*, 189, pp. 33-44

Smidt MP, Smits SM & Burbach JP. (2003) Molecular mechanisms underlying midbrain dopamine neuron development and function. *Eur J Pharmacol*, 480, pp. 75– 88

Sonntag KC, Pruszak J, Yoshizaki T, van Arensbergen J, Sanchez-Pernaute R & Isacson O. (2007). Enhanced yield of neuroepithelial precursors and midbrain-like dopaminergic neurons from human embryonic stem cells using the bone morphogenic protein antagonist noggin. *STEM CELLS*, 25, pp. 411– 418

Tabar V. Tomishima M, Panagiotakos G, Wakayama S, Menon J, Chan B, Mizutani E, Al-Shamy G, Ohta H, Wakayama T, & Studer L. (2008). Therapeutic cloning in individual parkinsonian mice. *Nat Med*, 14, pp. 379–381

Takahashi J., Palmer T D & Gage FH. (1999). Retinoic acid and neurotrophins collaborate to regulate neurogenesis in adultderived neural stem cell cultures. *J neurobiol*, 38, pp. 65-81

Ueno M, Matsumura M, Watanabe K, Nakamura T, Osakada F, Takahashi M, Kawasaki H, Kinoshita S & Sasai Y. (2006). Neural conversion of ES cells by an inductive activity on human amniotic membrane matrix. *Proc Natl Acad Sci U S A*, 103, pp. 9554-9

Wichterle H, Lieberam I, Porter JA& Jessell TM. (2002). Directed differentiation of embryonic stem cells into motor neurons. *Cell*, 110, pp. 385-97

Yan Y, Yang D, Zarnowska ED, Du Z, Werbel B, Valliere C, Pearce RA, Thomson JA & Zhang SC. (2005). Directed differentiation of dopaminergic neuronal subtypes from human embryonic stem cells. *STEM CELLS*, 23 pp.781–790

Ying QL, Stavridis M, Griffiths D, Li M & Smith A. (2003). Conversion of embryonic stem cells into neuroectodermal precursors in adherent monoculture. *Nat Biotechnol*, 21, pp. 183-6

Yue F, Cui L, Johkura K, Ogiwara N & Sasaki K. (2006). Induction of midbrain dopaminergic neurons from primate embryonic stem cells by coculture with sertoli cells. *Stem Cells*, 24(7), pp. 1695-706.

Zhang SC, Wernig M, Duncan ID, Brustle O. & Thomson JA. (2001). *In vitro* differentiation of transplantable neural precursors from human embryonic stem cells. *Nat Biotechnol*, 19, pp. 1129-33

Zhang X, Cai J., Klueber KM, Guo Z, Lu C, Winstead WI, Qiu M & Roisen FJ. (2006). Role of transcription factors in motoneuron differentiation of adult human olfactory neuroepithelial-derived progenitors. *Stem Cells*, 24, pp. 434-42

5

The Role of the Neuropeptide Substance P in the Pathogenesis of Parkinson's Disease

Emma Thornton and Robert Vink
University of Adelaide
Australia

1. Introduction

Parkinson's disease (PD) was first described by James Parkinson in 1815 as "shaking palsy syndrome". Today, it is the second most common neurodegenerative disorder, with a lifetime risk of 1 in 45 of developing the debilitating disease and currently affecting 1% of the population over the age of 65 (G. Alves, et al., 2008).

PD is characterized by a slow and progressive loss of the pigmented dopaminergic neurons of the substantia nigra pars compacta (SNc). This loss of dopaminergic neurons is often accompanied by a loss of the noradrenergic pigmented neurons of the locus ceruleus, and in the later stages of the disease, both the cholinergic neurons of the nucleus basalis of Meynert and the serotoninergic neurons of the dorsal raphe nucleus may also degenerate (Marey-Semper, et al., 1995). In remaining DA neurons proteinaceous cytoplasmic inclusions called Lewy bodies (LBs) are found. They are filamentous in nature and predominantly contain alpha-synuclein and ubiquitin proteins (Bennett, 2005). Although LBs are also found in other diseases, such as diffuse Lewy body dementia and incidental Lewy body disease, they are considered to be the pathological hallmark of PD (Greenfields, 1992).

The dopaminergic neurons of the SNc are part of the basal ganglia (BG), an integral part of the brain that ensures smooth execution of movement. Accordingly motor symptoms such as resting tremor, bradykinesia, akinesia, rigidity and postural instability are most common. Degeneration of dopaminergic neurons is slow, with progressive loss of about 5% per year (Blum, et al., 2001), suggesting that a therapy could halt or slow down the progression of the disease, but to date no known neuroprotective therapy exists. Instead, current treatment involves managing patients' symptoms. Normally this treatment is L-DOPA, the precursor to DA. The rationale for this therapy is to restore DA levels to near normal and therefore restore normal function of the basal ganglia for a period of time. Unfortunately, following prolonged use many patients fail to maintain a good response and often experience "wearing off" effects, which is a reduction in the length of time that L-DOPA effectively alleviates symptoms (Krasnova, et al., 2000). Furthermore, motor complications like dyskinesia, or involuntary movements, occur in approximately 50-80% of PD patients who have been on L-DOPA for more than 5-10 years. These side effects are often more debilitating than the original motor deficits (Chen, et al., 2004).

In addition to the loss of dopaminergic neurons, there is also a reduction in the expression of the neuropeptide, substance P (SP), an important neurotransmitter in the BG, which is essential for proper execution of function. However, this loss of SP has been observed in animal and human studies under conditions that represented end-stage PD. We suggest that this late loss of SP content is an event secondary to dopamine neuronal death. In the early phase of the disease, we propose that SP expression may actually be increased, and that this increase in SP may contribute to dopaminergic cell death through its effects on inflammatory processes and blood brain barrier (BBB) dysfunction. This review critically analyses the evidence that SP contributes to the pathogenesis of PD.

2. The basal ganglia

The BG is a group of nuclei located within the midbrain whose primary function is the smooth execution of movement. Apart from the substantia nigra, which also contains the pars reticulta (SNr), the BG nuclei include the striatum (caudate/putamen), the globus pallidus, both internal (GPi) and external segments (GPe), and the subthalamic nucleus (STN). Although the thalamus is not strictly part of the BG, it is fundamental to its function. In order for the BG to function correctly, it requires the two main signalling pathways, the direct and indirect pathway, to act in concert.

The direct signalling pathway involves an excitatory glutamatergic signal being sent from the cortex to striatal GABAergic projection neurons that project to the GPi and SNr resulting in inhibition of these nuclei. These nuclei also send inhibitory GABAergic signals, the inhibition of GPi/SNr neurons results in decreased inhibitory output to the thalamus. Consequently, the activity of thalamic neurons are increased causing excitatory glutamatergic signals to be sent back to the cortex, reinforcing cortical activity. The direct pathway therefore provides positive feedback for the cortex to allow movement (Silkis, 2001). Alternatively, the indirect pathway involves an excitatory signal being sent from the cortex to striatal inhibitory GABAergic neurons that project to the GPe, resulting in increased inhibition of the GPe neurons. As these neurons send an inhibitory GABAergic signal to the STN, the inhibition of these neurons leads to increased glutamatergic excitatory output from the STN. Subsequently, the STN sends excitatory signals to the inhibitory GPi and SNr neurons increasing their inhibitory output to the thalamus ensuring inhibition of the thalamic neurons and thus inhibition of cortical activity. The indirect pathway is therefore involved in negative feedback to the cortex and inhibition of the posture keeping the limb there (Sil'kis, 2002). These signalling pathways are kept in balance to ensure the almost simultaneous inhibition of the original position and initiation of the new required movement.

The direct and indirect signalling pathways are kept in balance by the dopaminergic input from the SNc to the striatum, known as the nigrostriatal pathway. The striatal GABAergic projection neurons express both DA receptors, namely D1 and D2 (Yelnik, 2002), although there are higher numbers of D1 receptors on the projections neurons involved in the direct pathway and D2 receptors for the indirect pathway (Aizman, et al., 2000). Through binding to D1 receptors, DA increases cAMP production, thereby reinforcing the activity of the direct pathway. In contrast, when DA binds to D2 receptors, cAMP production is reduced, creating a reversal of the activity of the nuclei within the indirect pathway and a decrease in its activity. As the indirect pathway is involved in negative feedback to the cortex, DA causes increased activity of the cortical neurons and reinforcement of cortical activity (van der Stelt and Di Marzo, 2003). Thus, the release of striatal DA within the nigrostriatal pathway of the BG allows fine-tuning of movement control and smooth execution of movement.

2.1 Basal ganglia function in Parkinson's disease

The initial loss of dopaminergic neurons in early PD does not decrease striatal DA activity due to pre- and post-synaptic compensatory responses of the dopaminergic system. These include upregulation of D1 and D2 dopamine receptor expression, which have a lower threshold for activation than normal, and an increase in activity of the surviving dopaminergic neurons (Deumens, et al., 2002). These compensatory mechanisms are able to sustain normal activity until approximately 50% of DA neurons and 80% of the total striatal DA is lost. Once this threshold level of striatal DA is reached, the direct and indirect signalling pathways become imbalanced producing a subsequent increase in the indirect signalling pathway and a decrease in the direct signalling pathway (Contreras-Vidal and Stelmach, 1996, Wardas, et al., 2003). Although these pathways also control the limbic system, the deficiency of DA in PD is heterogenous and DA is predominantly lost in the putamen area of the striatum, which is mainly involved in motor function of the BG. Therefore, PD is a hypokinetic disorder where the decreased activity of the direct pathway and increased activity of the indirect pathway results in a lack of movement as the common symptom (Silkis, 2001).

The BG does not only contain classical neurotransmitters such as glutamate, GABA and DA, but it also involves neuropeptides such as SP, neurokinin A (NKA) and the opioids enkephalin and dynorphin that act together for the fine-tuning of BG pathways (Graybiel, 1990, Hauber, 1998). These neurotransmitters can be segregated into the two pathways, with SP, NKA and dynorphin located in the GABAergic projection neurons of the direct pathway, whereas enkephalin is found within the striatal GABAergic projections neurons of the indirect pathway. Accordingly, in PD the change in activity of signalling pathways creates abnormal levels of these neurotransmitters. Changes in SP may be particularly important with respect to PD.

3. Substance P

Substance P was first discovered in 1934 by Gaddum and Schild, as the active principle in a stable dry powder. In 1936, Von Euler suggested the peptidergic nature of SP as its activity was stopped following digestion with trypsin, although later it was discovered that the degradation of SP was due to chymotrypsin as SP is trypsin-resistant (Leeman and Ferguson, 2000). Consequently it became part of the tachykinin family of which NKA and neurokinin B (NKB) are also members. Tachykinins are located in capsaicin-sensitive neurons, also known as primary sensory neurons, within the CNS, peripheral tissue and non-neuronal cells including endothelial cells and inflammatory cells (Hokfelt, et al., 2001). Within the brain there is a heterogeneous distribution of SP, with higher levels found in the grey matter. The highest concentration of SP is actually found within the SN (Ribeiro-da-Silva and Hokfelt, 2000), where SP immunoreactivity in the SNc is 25% higher than that in the SNr (Sutoo, et al., 1999). Also, within the BG SP expression is high within the internal segment of the globus pallidus.

Tachykinins share a common terminal sequence, Phe-X-Gly-Leu-Met-NH2, where X is Phe or Val (Harrison and Geppetti, 2001, Saria, 1999). This sequence is essential for their biological activity and thus there is a certain amount of cross reactivity amongst the tachykinin receptors and their ligands (Gerard, et al., 1991, Khawaja and Rogers, 1996). Each tachykinin has varying affinities for the tachykinin receptors, with SP having the greatest affinity for the tachykinin NK1 receptor (NK_1), NKA to NK_2 and NKB to NK_3 tachykinin receptors.

Tachykinin receptors have a rhodopsin-like membrane structure comprising of 7 hydrophobic transmembrane domains connected by extra- and intracellular loops and coupled to G-proteins (Harrison and Geppetti, 2001). NK_1 and NK_3 receptors are mainly found in the CNS, but are also present in peripheral tissues (Otsuka and Yoshioka, 1993). Throughout the brain, greatest NK_1 receptor immunoreactivity is found in the striatum, nucleus accumbens, hippocampus, hypothalamus and the raphe nuclei (Harrison and Geppetti, 2001), whereas NK_3 receptors are most abundant in the cortex and on glial cells (Yip and Chahl, 2000). In contrast, NK_2 receptors are widely distributed in the peripheral nervous system (PNS) especially in the smooth muscle of the respiratory, gastrointestinal and urinary tracts (Maggi, 1995).

SP binds to the hydrophobic ligand-binding pocket within the extracellular loops of the NK_1 receptor causing rapid internalisation of the ligand and its receptor (Harrison and Geppetti, 2001). Ligand binding stimulates the activity of adenylate cyclase and the conversion of adenosine triphosphate (ATP) to adenosine monophosphate, which inturn activates phospholipase C_B (PLC_B) (Saria, 1999). Activation of PLC_B results in an increased turnover of intracellular inositol 1,4,5-triphosphate and a subsequent elevation of intracellular calcium (Ca^{2+}) (Gerard, et al., 1991). The NK_1 receptor has a 5' untranslated region containing a cyclic AMP (cAMP) binding protein that responds to elevated levels of cAMP and Ca^{2+} by increasing gene transcription of SP (Saria, 1999). This creates a positive feedback loop for SP production and release. Conversely, SP may also block potassium channels causing membrane depolarisation and/or activate NK_1 autoreceptors to inhibit its own release (Harrison and Geppetti, 2001).

SP is synthesized from the preprotachykinin (PPT)-A gene, which also encodes NKA, neuropeptide K (NPK) and neuropeptide Y (NPY), the latter two being elongated versions of NKA (Hokfelt, et al., 2001). Alternative splicing of the PPT-A gene results in 3 distinct mRNAs: α-PPT-A, β-PPT-A and γ-PPT-A. Although all 3 PPT-A mRNAs encode for SP (Harrison and Geppetti, 2001), α-PPT-A mRNA is the main isoform of mRNA in the brain, whereas α- and γ-PPT-A mRNA are primarily expressed within the periphery (Severini, et al., 2002). NKB is encoded by the PPT-B gene and like PPT-A gene is conserved amongst species (Hoyle, 1998).

Synthesis of SP occurs within ribosomes in cell bodies of the dorsal root ganglia before it is packaged into large dense core vesicles with processing enzymes called convertases, which cleave at Lys-Arg, Arg-Arg or Arg-Lys bonds to release the active form of SP (Severini, et al., 2002). When stimulated, SP-containing vesicles undergo retrograde axonal transport to the terminal endings in both the CNS and PNS, where they undergo final enzymatic processing and post-translational enzymatic modifications such as C-terminal amidation (Hokfelt, et al., 2000). As previously mentioned, SP release is triggered by a small rise in intracellular Ca^{2+}, which will increase the pH within the vesicle resulting in alkinisation and release of SP by exocytosis (Otsuka and Yoshioka, 1993). NK_1 receptors are also synthesized and then anterogradely transported along axons to peripheral and perhaps central terminals. Thus, upon release SP can activate the postsynaptic NK_1 receptors (Malcangio and Bowery, 1999).

3.1 Substance P regulation of basal ganglia function

Substance P is important in regulating the function of the SN and BG (Bell, et al., 1998, Maubach, et al., 2001) where it acts as an excitatory neurotransmitter (Napier, et al., 1995). Like in other areas of the brain, SP is released in the BG due to an elevation in Ca^{2+} (Otsuka and Yoshioka, 1993). Once released, it may bind to NK_1 receptors located on striatal interneurons to increase the firing rate and depolarise membrane potentials causing the release of other BG neurotransmitters such as GABA, glutamate and acetylcholine (Aosaki and Kawaguchi, 1996, Bailey, et al., 2004, Kemel, et al., 2002).

It is now known that NK_1 receptors are also located on 90% of DA neurons in the SNc (L-W. Chen, et al., 2004). However, earlier studies reported that there was an absence of NK_1 receptors in the SN and a mismatch between SP and NK_1 in this region (Humpel and Saria, 1993). This mismatch in the expression and binding of SP in the SN was subsequently thought to be due to the rapid internalisation of the SP/NK_1 complex following SP binding resulting in NK_1 being mainly located intracellularly (Levesque, et al., 2007). Accordingly, through binding to NK_1 receptors on dopaminergic neurons, SP can directly cause the release of DA within the striatum (Galarraga, et al., 1999, Orosz and Bennett, 1990, Reid, et al., 1990a, Reid, et al., 1990b). Moreover, as DA receptors are located on SP-containing striatal projection neurons, DA or DA agonists can potentiate SP release within the SN (Humpel and Saria, 1993). Therefore, SP and DA within the BG are modulated through a positive feedback mechanism. Accordingly, an injection of SP into the BG induces behavioural effects such as sniffing, rearing, grooming and increased motor activity in rats by promoting striatal DA release (Saria, 1999). However in PD, the loss of striatal DA interrupts this positive feedback mechanism and therefore a reduction in striatal SP gene transcription and SP protein content within the SN has been observed.

3.2 Substance P expression in Parkinson's disease

Post-mortem immunohistochemical studies have shown that there is a loss of SP content in the striatum and SN in PD brains (De Ceballos and Lopez-Lozano, 1999, Mauborgne, et al., 1983, Nisbet, et al., 1995, Sivam, 1991, Tenovuo, et al., 1984). Along with this loss of SP, there is also a significant deficit of NK_1 receptors in the putamen and GP of PD patients compared to aged matched controls (Fernandez, et al., 1994). Moreover, in a case of idiopathic PD, where the person died shortly after diagnosis from an unrelated cause, LBs were observed in surviving SP-containing neurons of the pedunculopontine tegmental nucleus, suggesting that these SP neurons were affected early in PD (Gai, et al., 1991).

Decrease in SP has also been extensively studied in the 6-OHDA rodent and MPTP non-human primate models of PD. Like in human PD, there is a decrease in SP content in the SN and striatum in these animal models (Bannon, et al., 1995, Schwarting and Huston, 1996). However, in a study by Orosz and Bennet in 1990 using the 6-OHDA rat model of PD, it was shown that although there was a decline in SP-immunoreactivity and SP mRNA in tissue levels of the SN, there was a rise in SP-immunoreactivity in the extracellular space of the SN. Subsequently, it was suggested that this rise was a compensatory mechanisms for the loss of intracellular SP (Orosz and Bennett, 1990). This was the first study to show an increase in extracellular SP during PD. Due to the tissue loss of SP, 6-OHDA animals were given replacement SP treatment into either the lateral ventricle or directly into the SN restoring striatal DA content (Krasnova, et al., 2000). Additionally, pre-treatment with SP assisted the recovery from a 6-OHDA lesion. The authors suggested that this was due to prolonged changes in SP release that helped to negate the tissue loss of SP caused by 6-OHDA (Nikolaus, et al., 1997). Thus basal levels of SP are fundamental for proper function.

In the non-human primate MPTP model of PD, which represents the model most similar to human PD, it was shown that there was a reduction in striatal SP gene expression and that this deficiency in SP correlated with the degree of motor symptoms present (Wade and Schneider, 2001). However when primates were treated with L-DOPA the decrease in SP gene expression was reversed (Herrero, et al., 1995).

It is important to note that these studies have all been undertaken in post-mortem tissue or in models that replicate the end stage of the disease. Therefore, the SP changes observed may be a secondary effect due to the loss of DA input into the striatum and the activation of the direct pathway. Indeed, research in our laboratory has shown that SP may actually be increased in the early stages of PD. In nigrostriatal organotypic cell culture, 6-OHDA treatment caused an immediate and prolonged elevation in SP content that was significantly correlated with lactate dehydrogenase content, a marker of cell death. Furthermore, the 6-OHDA induced cell death was prevented by treatment with an NK_1 receptor antagonist (Thornton, et al., 2010).

Subsequent *in vivo* studies using the rodent striatal 6-OHDA model also measured SP content in the striatum and SN at days 3 and 7 following lesioning using an enzyme-linked immunosorbent assay (ELISA) method, which determines SP content from a standardized amount of protein (Figure 1). Despite the difference in SP content between the hemispheres in sham (control) animals, there was an apparent increase in SP content in the contralateral (left) and ipsilateral (right) striatum at both 3 and 7 days following 6-OHDA administration. However, SP content was not elevated within the SN until day 7 following 6-OHDA striatal lesions. Dopaminergic neuronal loss as assessed by tyrosine hydroxylase immunoreactivity was also not apparent at day 3 but had begun by day 7 and was significant by day 14 post-lesion. Nonetheless, a small loss of striatal DA terminals was observed by day 3. These results suggest that increased SP expression may contribute to the loss of dopaminergic terminals and neurons, however dopaminergic cell loss must also have initiated an increase in SP content within the SN. Furthermore, as the majority of dopaminergic degeneration occurs from day 7 to 14, the rise in SP content may act to potentiate this cell loss.

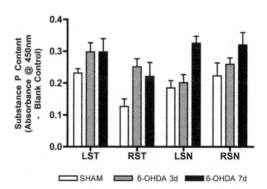

Fig. 1. Using an ELISA method, substance P content was semi-quantified within the striatum and substantia nigra following 6-OHDA intrastriatal injections. Results are displayed as mean+SEM (n=5/group).

Substance P has been associated with cell loss and functional deficits in other brain pathologies such as traumatic brain injury and stroke (Donkin, et al., 2009, R. J. Turner, et al., 2006). This detrimental effect of SP was credited to its ability to induce BBB breakdown and the subsequent genesis of cerebral oedema (R. Turner and Vink, 2007). Although cerebral oedema does not occur in PD, a decrease in BBB integrity has recently been linked to dopaminergic cell loss and the progression of PD (Bartels, et al., 2008, Kortekaas, et al., 2005). Moreover, SP has been shown to play an integral role in the inflammatory response within both the peripheral and central nervous systems (R.V. Alves, et al., 1999). Recently, neuroinflammation has also received much interest for its potential role in DA degeneration and disease progression. We therefore hypothesize that SP may be involved in dopaminergic cell death in early PD by promoting neuroinflammation and BBB dysfunction.

4. Potential role for substance P in dopaminergic degeneration in PD

4.1 Inflammatory processes

Two of the main inflammatory cells within the brain are microglia and astrocytes. Resting microglia are important for maintaining cellular homeostasis, and once activated are involved in the removal of cellular debris (Mosley, et al., 2006, Rock and Peterson, 2006). However, activated microglia produce proinflammatory trophic factors and cytokines such as interleukin-1 (IL-1), IL-2, IL-6 and tumour necrosis factor-α (TNF-α), all of which are potentially cytotoxic (Blum, et al., 2001). Chronic activation of microglia and therefore prolonged expression of cytokines can be especially damaging to neurons. Indeed, activated microglia have been observed in post-mortem PD tissue and in experimental models long after the induction of PD (Depino, et al., 2003, Marinova-Mutafchieva, et al., 2009, McGeer and McGeer, 2008). Moreover, in human cases and animal models of PD a rise in these proinflammatory factors and cytokines has been demonstrated in the SN, striatum and cerebrospinal fluid (CSF) (Jenner and Olanow, 1998, Liu and Hong, 2003).

Activated microglia can also generate reactive oxygen species (ROS) such as hydrogen peroxide and superoxide (O_2^-) through activation of NADPH oxidase (Wu, et al., 2003). Under normal conditions this is important for the microglial role in brain immune surveillance and ability to kill foreign organisms that enter the brain. However, excessive production of ROS can result in oxidative damage to proteins, lipids and DNA, resulting in dopaminergic cell death (reviewed by (Mosley, et al., 2006)). In addition, microglia contain inducible NOS (iNOS), enabling the secretion of nitric oxide (NO). NO can react with ROS to form reactive nitrogen species (RNS) such as peroxynitrite (ONOO-), which is more stable than O^{2-} and can cross cell membranes and thus can be more damaging to cells than ROS. Indeed, by-products of oxidative damage are found in the SN of PD brains at post-mortem (Marsden and Olanow, 1998).

Usually, the SN contains large numbers of microglia compared to other areas of the brain. This is consistent with dopaminergic neurons already being in a state of oxidative stress due to the production of ROS during normal DA metabolism, making these neurons particularly vulnerable to insults (Berretta, et al., 2005, Liu and Hong, 2003, Olanow, et al., 2004). Moreover, oxidative damage by ROS and RNS is exacerbated in PD due to a deficiency of glutathione and superoxide dismutase, two of the main antioxidant enzymes that scavenge ROS, RNS and reduce H_2O_2 to its non-reactive state (Canals, et al., 2001).

Apart from causing damage to cellular structures, RNS and ROS may also cause mitochondrial dysfunction. In PD, a 30 to 40% decrease in complex I (NADH dehydrogenase) activity of the electron transport chain (ETC) is observed in mitochondria within the SN (Blum, et al., 2001, Squire, et al., 2003). The ETC, through oxidative phosphorylation, produces ATP, an important energy source for cell organelles, enzymes and transport systems. Thus, mitochondrial dysfunction causes a bioenergetic deficit that leads to membrane depolarisation, disruption of Ca^{2+} homeostasis and further production of free radicals and ROS (Shults, 2004). Specifically, a reduction in ATP causes impairment of the mitochondrial membrane potential, and subsequent opening of the mitochondrial permeability transition pore. Pore opening stimulates the release of mitochondrial proteins, such as cytochrome c and apoptosis-inducing factor, that trigger apoptosis (Rego and Oliveira, 2003). Consistent with this, DA neurons are thought to die via apoptotic cell death cascades in PD (Olanow and Tatton, 1999).

With the loss of ATP production, there is also a consequential loss of the magnesium blockade of N-methyl-D-aspartate (NMDA) receptors, resulting in elevated levels of glutamate and NO (Q. Chen, et al., 1996). Dopaminergic neurons in the SN are rich in functional NMDA glutamate receptors and therefore affected by any change in glutamate levels (Olanow and Tatton, 1999). Glutamate, an excitatory amino acid, causes an increase in intracellular Ca^{2+} resulting in FR production, mitochondrial damage and activation of degradative enzymes. These enzymes, including proteases, endonucleases and phospholipases, result in degradation of plasma membranes, the cytoskeleton and nuclear material and subsequent cell death. This deleterious cascade of events, known as glutamate excitotoxicity, is also a major contributor to cell loss in PD (Beal, 1992).

Notably, production of ROS and RNS during inflammation and mitochondrial dysfunction are critically linked since activation of microglia can lead to mitochondrial dysfunction, and vice versa (Di Filippo, et al., 2010). The combined effects of these disease mechanisms in dopaminergic degeneration are further reinforced in experimental models of PD as the complex 1 inhibitor rotenone causes DA degeneration and microglial activation following either systemic or intracerebral administration (Gao, et al., 2003). Additionally, MPTP and 6-OHDA models also demonstrate both mitochondrial dysfunction and an exacerbated inflammatory response (Blum, et al., 2001, Chung, et al., 2010a).

Activation of microglia is not only a vicious cycle whereby the degeneration of neurons stimulates further microglial activation (Raivich, et al., 1999), it may also precede DA degeneration (Wojtera, et al., 2005). Activated microglia may prematurely phagocytose damaged DA neurons that may not have gone on to degenerate as evidence by the fact that phagocytotic CD68 positive microglia are observed prior to caspase-3 positive apoptotic DA neurons in the 6-OHDA model of PD (Marinova-Mutafchieva, et al., 2009).

The astrocytic response in PD has received less attention than microglia for its potential role in the pathogenesis of PD. Nevertheless, in all animal models of PD, there is an increase in glial fibrillary acidic protein immunoreactivity in both the striatum and SN, with the presence of reactive, hypertrophic astrocytes (Depino, et al., 2003, Takagi, et al., 2007). Furthermore, a 30% increase in these reactive astrocytes within the SN was seen in PD tissue at post-mortem (Wu, et al., 2003). However, activation of astrocytes may be both beneficial, through secretion of neurotrophic substances such as glial derived nerve factor and brain derived nerve factor, and detrimental through secretion of pro-inflammatory cytokines (Brahmachari, et al., 2006, Hirsch, 2000). These cytokines stimulate the activation of additional microglia or astrocytes, thereby further exacerbating the inflammatory response and tissue damage previously described for microglia (Chauhan, et al., 2008, Raivich, et al., 1999). In reactive astrocytes, myeloperoxidase produces RNS and damage to DA neurons (Choi, et al., 2005). However, the presence of astrocytes may be also beneficial as the density of astrocytes is low in the SNc compared to the ventral tegmental area, an area much less susceptible to DA damage in clinical and experimental models of PD. Nonetheless, reactive astrocytes are thought to contribute to disease progression, although their exact role remains controversial (Chung, et al., 2010b).

The CNS immune response in PD can result in apoptosis of neurons by causing mitochondrial dysfunction and production of cytokines. An increase in cytokines, especially TNFα, can initiate apoptosis through binding at the tumour necrosis factor-α receptor 1 (TNFαR1), a known cell death receptor located on dopaminergic cell bodies in the SN (Mladenovic, et al., 2004).

4.1.1 Substance P and inflammation

Substance P and its NK_1 receptor have long been known to be important mediators of CNS inflammation (Harrison and Geppetti, 2001, Martin, et al., 1992). SP binding at NK_1 receptors expressed on microglia and astrocytes may directly result in the activation of these glial cells in the CNS (Mantyh, et al., 1989, Marriott, 2004). SP can also cause the indirect activation of astrocytes and microglia through its ability to promote cytokine and NO production, as they are able to modulate the activation of each other during the inflammatory response (Brahmachari, et al., 2006, Rodrigues, et al., 2001). Furthermore, pro-inflammatory cytokine production, for example, Il-1β can upregulate the expression of NK_1 receptors on glial cells (Guo, et al., 2004). Due to its ability to modulate the inflammatory response, SP may play a critical role in inflammation-induced damage. Indeed, in bacterial diseases of the CNS, SP/NK_1 interactions exacerbate the glial immune responses through both initiating and progressing the subsequent inflammation (Chauhan, et al., 2008).

In vitro studies also have increased our understanding of the signal transduction pathways induced by SP in microglia and astrocytes and resulting in pro-inflammatory cytokine production. SP can stimulate the secretion of TNF-α from microglia and astrocytes following treatment with the endotoxin lipopolysaccharide (LPS) (Luber-Narod, et al., 1994). The presence of NK_1 receptors could not be demonstrated on microglia, therefore suggesting that this effect was mediated via the SP induced release of IL-1 from astrocytes, causing TNF-α release from both glial cell populations. However, the authors concede that their methods may have not have detected NK_1 receptors. Subsequent studies have shown functional NK_1 receptors expressed on murine microglia *in vitro* (Rasley, et al., 2002). The production of pro-inflammatory cytokines from glial cells has been shown to occur following the translocation of NF-κβ. SP by binding to NK_1 activated the NF-κβ pathway stimulating cytokine production (Lieb, et al., 1997). Moreover, SP has also been shown to induce IL-6 production by activating p39 MAPK pathway (Fiebich, et al., 2000).

The role of inflammation in dopaminergic cell loss is further confirmed by the efficacy of anti-inflammatory agents in PD as they have been shown to slow down disease progression (Qian, et al., 2010). A meta-analysis of peer reviewed data between 1966 and 2008 indicated NSAIDs may be slightly protective in PD through their ability to halt the pro-inflammatory response, prevent cyclooxygenase activity and scavenge ROS and RNS (Samii, et al., 2009). Furthermore, Minocycline, a microglial inhibitor, has advanced to phase III clinical trials (Tansey and Goldberg, 2010). These promising results suggest that inhibiting SP signalling through antagonism of the NK_1 receptor may reduce the inflammatory response in PD, thus offering a novel therapeutic target to slow the progression of PD.

4.2 Blood brain barrier dysfunction

Recently, BBB dysfunction has been implicated in the pathophysiology of PD. In clinical PD, p-glycoprotein function, a marker of BBB integrity, was reduced suggesting a loss of barrier integrity (Bartels, 2008; Kortekaas 2005). The authors suggested that this loss of barrier function may contribute to the progression of PD. In the SN the BBB is known to be weaker than in other brain regions and consequently is easily disrupted (Ionov, 2008). Notably, dopaminergic neurons demonstrate a greater vulnerability to barrier breakdown. In a study by Rite and colleagues (2007), intracerebral injection of vascular endothelium growth factor (VEGF) into the SN and striatum caused BBB breakdown as assessed by fluorescently tagged FITC-albumin infiltration. This resulted in dopaminergic terminal degeneration and apoptotic markers, caspase-3 and TUNEL expression in DA neurons. In contrast, injection of VEGF into the hippocampus caused no apparent apoptosis of hippocampal neurons (Rite, et al., 2007).

A correlation between BBB breakdown, the astrocytic and microglial response and dopaminergic degeneration has been previously described (Tomas-Camardiel, et al., 2004). In experimental models of PD, barrier dysfunction has been reported in MPTP, 6-OHDA and rotenone models of PD (Carvey, et al., 2005, Chao, et al., 2009, Ravenstijn, et al., 2008) and has also been observed in our own studies (unpublished). Further evidence for the BBB and CNS inflammation contributing to dopaminergic cell death is that mesenchymal stem cell (MSC) transplantation was found to be protective to DA neurons in the MPTP model of PD (Chao, et al., 2009). MSC transplantation reduced microglial activation and restored BBB function as reflected in reduced FITC-labelled albumin leakage, and returned expression of tight junction proteins, claudin 1 and 5 expression back to basal levels. The authors attributed this beneficial effect of MSCs expression of TGF-β1, which has an anti-inflammatory effect.

BBB dysfunction may also result in damage to DA neurons by allowing the influx of peripheral immune cells, such as blood borne macrophages, T-lymphocytes and leukocytes into the brain (Hunot, et al., 1999, Kortekaas, et al., 2005). Similar to CNS immune cells, peripheral immune cells secrete cytokines following the translocation of transcription factor NF-κβ. Accordingly, PD patients challenged with LPS had significantly exacerbated release of cytokines / chemokines from peripheral borne macrophage cells as compared to healthy controls (Reale, et al., 2009). Blood inflammatory cells such as neutrophils may also infiltrate through the disrupted BBB and activate microglia. Indeed, increased neutrophil infiltration, greater BBB permeability and decreased astrocyte numbers in SNc are thought to contribute to selective DA degeneration (Ji, et al., 2008). Furthermore, a study by Brochard and colleagues has shown that peripheral immune cells such as CD4+ T leukocytes are involved in MPTP induced cell death in mice while CD4+ null mice have reduced DA degeneration (Brochard, et al., 2009).

Thus, the infiltration and production of pro-inflammatory cytokines by peripheral cells can activate resident brain immune cells such as microglia. Therefore, not only do peripheral immune cells directly injure dopaminergic neurons, they can also indirectly activate microglia and astrocytes to further exacerbate inflammatory and cell death cascades. These results suggest that peripheral cytokine production and infiltration across the BBB may contribute to PD pathogenesis.

4.2.1 Substance P and blood brain barrier dysfunction

Along with its known role in modulating the peripheral immune response, SP is an important regulator of BBB integrity and can potentiate barrier breakdown through neurogenic inflammation. Neurogenic inflammation is a neurally elicited local inflammatory response characterised by vasodilation, protein extravasation and tissue swelling, which can be induced by certain types of injury or infection (Vink, et al., 2003). It is caused by a release of calcitonin-gene related peptide (CGRP) and SP from primary sensory nerve fibers surrounding blood vessels with subsequent activation of NK_1 receptors on endothelial cells (Lever, et al., 2003). CGRP, the most potent vasodilator, increases blood flow, bringing cytokines and inflammatory mediators to the area (Woie, et al., 1993), whereas SP binding to NK_1 receptors increases vessel permeability, leading to plasma extravasation and BBB breakdown (Hokfelt, et al., 2001). Neurogenic inflammation has been well described in the periphery but has also recently been reported to occur in the CNS (Nimmo, et al., 2004, R. Turner and Vink, 2007).

Another mechanism whereby SP may affect BBB permeability is through histamine. SP instigates the release of histamine from mast cells, to further increase vessel permeability and extravasation (R.V. Alves, et al., 1999). Thus, SP plays a central role in mediating extravascular migration of inflammatory cells into inflamed tissue (Harrison and Geppetti, 2001). Interestingly in PD, patients demonstrate elevated plasma histamine levels (Coelho, et al., 1991) and intranigral injection of histamine results in DA cell death and glial cell activation (Vizuete, et al., 2000).

5. Conclusion

We conclude that SP may be involved in the pathogenesis of PD, particularly in relation to inflammation and BBB breakdown. We suggest that the reported loss of SP expression in PD may be a secondary effect due to the decrease in striatal dopamine and therefore the loss of the SP/dopaminergic positive feedback mechanism. In contrast, SP may actually be increased within the BG *early* in PD and induce nigral BBB breakdown through neurogenic inflammation, as well as contribute to local inflammatory responses. Therefore, treatment with a NK_1 receptor antagonist may be a novel neuroprotective agent to slow the progression of PD.

6. References

Aizman, O., Brismar, H., Uhlen, P., Zettergren, E., Levey, A. I., Forssberg, H., Greengard, P.&Aperia, A., (2000). Anatomical and physiological evidence for D1 and D2 dopamine receptor colocalization in neostriatal neurons. *Nat Neurosci*. Vol. 3, No. 3, (Mar, 2000), pp. (226-30).

Alves, G., Forsaa, E. B., Pedersen, K. F., Dreetz Gjerstad, M.&Larsen, J. P., (2008). Epidemiology of Parkinson's disease. *J Neurol*. Vol. 255 Suppl 5, No., (Sep, 2008), pp. (18-32).

Alves, R. V., Campos, M. M., Santos, A. R. S.&Calixto, J. B., (1999). Receptor subtypes involved in tachykinin-mediated edema formation. *Peptides*. Vol. 20, No., 1999), pp. (921-927).

Aosaki, T.&Kawaguchi, Y., (1996). Actions of substance P on rat neostriatal neurons in vitro. *J Neurosci*. Vol. 16, No. 16, (Aug 15, 1996), pp. (5141-53).

Bailey, C. P., Maubach, K. A.&Jones, R. S., (2004). Neurokinin-1 receptors in the rat nucleus tractus solitarius: pre- and postsynaptic modulation of glutamate and GABA release. *Neuroscience*. Vol. 127, No. 2, 2004), pp. (467-79).

Bannon, M. J., Brownschidle, L. A., Tian, Y., Whitty, C. J., Poosch, M. S., D'sa, C.&Moody, C. A., (1995). Neurokinin-3 receptors modulate dopamine cell function and alter the effects of 6-hydroxydopamine. *Brain Res.* Vol. 695, No., 1995), pp. (19-24).

Bartels, A. L., Willemsen, A. T., Kortekaas, R., de Jong, B. M., de Vries, R., de Klerk, O., van Oostrom, J. C., Portman, A.&Leenders, K. L., (2008). Decreased blood-brain barrier P-glycoprotein function in the progression of Parkinson's disease, PSP and MSA. *J Neural Transm.* Vol. 115, No. 7, (Jul, 2008), pp. (1001-9).

Beal, M. F., (1992). Mechanisms of excitotoxicity in neurologic diseases. *Faseb J.* Vol. 6, No. 15, (Dec, 1992), pp. (3338-44).

Bell, M. I., Richardson, P. J.&Lee, K., (1998). Characterization of the mechanism of action of tachykinins in rat striatal cholinergic interneurons. *Neuroscience.* Vol. 87, No. 3, (Dec, 1998), pp. (649-58).

Bennett, M. C., (2005). The role of alpha-synuclein in neurodegenerative diseases. *Pharmacol Ther.* Vol. 105, No. 3, (Mar, 2005), pp. (311-31).

Berretta, N., Freestone, P. S., Guatteo, E., Castro, D. D., Geracitano, R., Bernardi, G., Mercuri, N. B.&Lipski, J., (2005). Acute Effects of 6-Hydroxydopamine on Dopaminergic Neurons of the Rat Substantia Nigra Pars Compacta In Vitro. *Neurotoxicology.* Vol., No., (May 9, 2005), pp.).

Blum, D., Torch, S., Lambeng, N., Nissou, M., Benabid, A. L., Sadoul, R.&Verna, J. M., (2001). Molecular pathways involved in the neurotoxicity of 6-OHDA, dopamine and MPTP: contribution to the apoptotic theory in Parkinson's disease. *Prog Neurobiol.* Vol. 65, No. 2, (Oct, 2001), pp. (135-72).

Brahmachari, S., Fung, Y. K.&Pahan, K., (2006). Induction of glial fibrillary acidic protein expression in astrocytes by nitric oxide. *J Neurosci.* Vol. 26, No. 18, (May 3, 2006), pp. (4930-9).

Brochard, V., Combadiere, B., Prigent, A., Laouar, Y., Perrin, A., Beray-Berthat, V., Bonduelle, O., Alvarez-Fischer, D., Callebert, J., Launay, J. M., Duyckaerts, C., Flavell, R. A., Hirsch, E. C.&Hunot, S., (2009). Infiltration of CD4+ lymphocytes into the brain contributes to neurodegeneration in a mouse model of Parkinson disease. *J Clin Invest.* Vol. 119, No. 1, (Jan, 2009), pp. (182-92).

Canals, S., Casarejos, M. J., de Bernardo, S., Rodriguez-Martin, E.&Mena, M. A., (2001). Glutathione depletion switches nitric oxide neurotrophic effects to cell death in midbrain cultures: implications for Parkinson's disease. *J Neurochem.* Vol. 79, No. 6, (Dec, 2001), pp. (1183-95).

Carvey, P. M., Zhao, C. H., Hendey, B., Lum, H., Trachtenberg, J., Desai, B. S., Synder, J., Zhu, Y. G.&Ling, Z. D., (2005). 6-hydroxydopamine-induced alteration in blood-brain barrier permeability. *Eur J Neurosci.* Vol. 22, No., 2005), pp. (1158-1168.).

Chao, Y. X., He, B. P.&Tay, S. S., (2009). Mesenchymal stem cell transplantation attenuates blood brain barrier damage and neuroinflammation and protects dopaminergic neurons against MPTP toxicity in the substantia nigra in a model of Parkinson's disease. *J Neuroimmunol.* Vol. 216, No. 1-2, (Nov 30, 2009), pp. (39-50).

Chauhan, V. S., Sterka, D. G., Jr., Gray, D. L., Bost, K. L.&Marriott, I., (2008). Neurogenic exacerbation of microglial and astrocyte responses to Neisseria meningitidis and Borrelia burgdorferi. *J Immunol.* Vol. 180, No. 12, (Jun 15, 2008), pp. (8241-9).

Chen, L.-W., Yung, K. K. L.&Chan, Y. S., (2004). Neurokinin peptides and neurokinin receptors as potential therapeutic intervention targets of basal ganglia in the prevention and treatment of Parkinson's disease. *Current Drug Targets*. Vol. 5, No., 2004), pp. (1-10).

Chen, Q., Veenman, C. L.&Reiner, A., (1996). Cellular expression of ionotropic glutamate receptor subunits on specific striatal neuron types and its implication for striatal vulnerability in glutamate receptor-mediated excitotoxicity. *Neuroscience*. Vol. 73, No. 3, (Aug, 1996), pp. (715-31).

Choi, D. K., Pennathur, S., Perier, C., Tieu, K., Teismann, P., Wu, D. C., Jackson-Lewis, V., Vila, M., Vonsattel, J. P., Heinecke, J. W.&Przedborski, S., (2005). Ablation of the inflammatory enzyme myeloperoxidase mitigates features of Parkinson's disease in mice. *J Neurosci*. Vol. 25, No. 28, (Jul 13, 2005), pp. (6594-600).

Chung, Y. C., Kim, S. R.&Jin, B. K., (2010a). Paroxetine prevents loss of nigrostriatal dopaminergic neurons by inhibiting brain inflammation and oxidative stress in an experimental model of Parkinson's disease. *J Immunol*. Vol. 185, No. 2, (Jul 15, 2010a), pp. (1230-7).

Chung, Y. C., Ko, H. W., Bok, E., Park, E. S., Huh, S. H., Nam, J. H.&Jin, B. K., (2010b). The role of neuroinflammation on the pathogenesis of Parkinson's disease. *BMB Rep*. Vol. 43, No. 4, (Apr, 2010b), pp. (225-32).

Coelho, M. H., Silva, I. J., Azevedo, M. S.&Manso, C. F., (1991). Decrease in blood histamine in drug-treated parkinsonian patients. *Mol Chem Neuropathol*. Vol. 14, No. 2, (Apr, 1991), pp. (77-85).

Contreras-Vidal, J. L.&Stelmach, G. E., (1996). Mini Review: Effects of Parkinsonism on motor control. *Life Sciences*. Vol. 58, No. 3, 1996), pp. (165-176).

De Ceballos, M. L.&Lopez-Lozano, J. J., (1999). Subgroups of parkinsonian patients differentiated by pertidergic immunostaining of caudate nuclues biopsies. *Peptides*. Vol. 20, No., 1999), pp. (249-257).

Depino, A. M., Earl, C., Kaczmarczyk, E., Ferrari, C., Besedovsky, H., del Rey, A., Pitossi, F. J.&Oertel, W. H., (2003). Microglial activation with atypical proinflammatory cytokine expression in a rat model of Parkinson's disease. *Eur J Neurosci*. Vol. 18, No. 10, (Nov, 2003), pp. (2731-42).

Deumens, R., Blokland, A.&Prickaerts, J., (2002). Modeling Parkinson's disease in rats: an evaluation of 6-OHDA lesions of the nigrostriatal pathway. *Exp Neurol*. Vol. 175, No. 2, (Jun, 2002), pp. (303-17).

Di Filippo, M., Chiasserini, D., Tozzi, A., Picconi, B.&Calabresi, P., (2010). Mitochondria and the link between neuroinflammation and neurodegeneration. *J Alzheimers Dis*. Vol. 20 Suppl 2, No., 2010), pp. (S369-79).

Donkin, J. J., Nimmo, A. J., Cernak, I., Blumbergs, P. C.&Vink, R., (2009). Substance P is associated with the development of brain edema and functional deficits after traumatic brain injury. *J Cereb Blood Flow Metab*. Vol. In press, No., 2009), pp.).

Fernandez, A., de Ceballos, M. L., Jenner, P.&Marsden, C. D., (1994). Neurotensin, substance P, delta and mu opioid receptors are decreased in basal ganglia of Parkinson's disease patients. *Neuroscience*. Vol. 61, No. 1, (Jul, 1994), pp. (73-9).

Fiebich, B. L., Schleicher, S., Butcher, R. D., Craig, A.&Lieb, K., (2000). The neuropeptide substance P activates p38 mitogen-activated protein kinase resulting in IL-6 expression independently from NF-kappa B. *J Immunol*. Vol. 165, No. 10, (Nov 15, 2000), pp. (5606-11).

Gai, W. P., Halliday, G. M., Blumbergs, P. C., Geffen, L. B.&Blessing, W. W., (1991). Substance P-containing neurons in the mesopontine tegmentum are severely affected in Parkinson's disease. *Brain*. Vol. 114 (Pt 5), No., (Oct, 1991), pp. (2253-67).

Galarraga, E., Hernandez-Lopez, S., Tapia, D., Reyes, A.&Bargas, J., (1999). Action of substance P (neurokinin-1) receptor activation on rat neostriatal projection neurons. *Synapse*. Vol. 33, No. 1, (Jul, 1999), pp. (26-35).

Gao, H. M., Liu, B.&Hong, J. S., (2003). Critical role for microglial NADPH oxidase in rotenone-induced degeneration of dopaminergic neurons. *J Neurosci*. Vol. 23, No. 15, (Jul 16, 2003), pp. (6181-7).

Gerard, N. P., Garraway, L. A., Eddy, J., R.L., Shows, T. B., Iijima, H., Paquet, J.-L.&Gerard, C., (1991). Human substance P receptor(NK-1): Organisation of the gene, chromosome localization, and functional expression of cDNA clones. *Biochemistry*. Vol. 30, No. 44, 1991), pp. (10640-10646).

Graybiel, A. M., (1990). Neurotransmitters and neuromodulators in the basal ganglia. *TINS*. Vol. 13, No. 7, 1990), pp. (244-254).

Guo, C. J., Douglas, S. D., Gao, Z., Wolf, B. A., Grinspan, J., Lai, J. P., Riedel, E.&Ho, W. Z., (2004). Interleukin-1beta upregulates functional expression of neurokinin-1 receptor (NK-1R) via NF-kappaB in astrocytes. *Glia*. Vol. 48, No. 3, (Nov 15, 2004), pp. (259-66).

Harrison, S.&Geppetti, P., (2001). Review: Substance P. *The International Journal of Biochemistry & Cell Biology*. Vol. 33, No., 2001), pp. (555-576).

Hauber, W., (1998). Involvement of basal ganglia transmitter systems in movement initiation. *Prog Neurobiol*. Vol. 56, No. 5, (Dec, 1998), pp. (507-40).

Herrero, M.-T., Augood, S. J., Hirsch, E. C., Javoy-Agid, F., Luquin, M. R., Agid, Y., Obeso, J. A.&Emson, P. C., (1995). Effects of L-DOPA on preproenkephalin and preprotachykinin gene expression in the MPTP-treated monkey striatum. *Neurosci*. Vol. 68, No. 4, 1995), pp. (1189-1198).

Hirsch, E. C., (2000). Glial cells and Parkinson's disease. *J Neurol*. Vol. 247 Suppl 2, No., (Apr, 2000), pp. (II58-62).

Hokfelt, T., Broberger, C., Xu, Z.-Q. D., Sergeyev, V., Ubink, R.&Diez, M., (2000). Neuropeptides- an overview. *Neuropharmacology*. Vol. 39, No., 2000), pp. (1337-1356).

Hokfelt, T., Pernow, B.&Wahren, J., (2001). Substance P: a pioneer amongst neuropeptides. *J of Internal Medicine*. Vol. 249, No., 2001), pp. (27-40).

Hoyle, C. H., (1998). Neuropeptide families: evolutionary perspectives. *Regul Pept*. Vol. 73, No. 1, (Jan 2, 1998), pp. (1-33).

Humpel, C.&Saria, A., (1993). Intranigral injection of selective neurokinin-1 and neurokinin-3 but not neurokinin-2 receptor agonists biphasically modulate striatal dopamine metabolism but not striatal preprotachykinin-A mRNA in the rat. *Neurosci Lett*. Vol. 157, No. 2, (Jul 23, 1993), pp. (223-6).

Hunot, S., Dugas, N., Faucheux, B., Hartmann, A., Tardieu, M., Debre, P., Agid, Y., Dugas, B.&Hirsch, E. C., (1999). FcepsilonRII/CD23 is expressed in Parkinson's disease and induces, in vitro, production of nitric oxide and tumor necrosis factor-alpha in glial cells. *J Neurosci*. Vol. 19, No. 9, (May 1, 1999), pp. (3440-7).

Ionov, I. D., (2008). Self-amplification of nigral degeneration in Parkinson's disease: a hypothesis. *Int J Neurosci*. Vol. 118, No. 12, (Dec, 2008), pp. (1763-80).

Jenner, P.&Olanow, C. W., (1998). Understanding cell death in Parkinson's disease. *Ann Neurol.* Vol. 44, No. 3 Suppl 1, (Sep, 1998), pp. (S72-84).

Ji, K. A., Eu, M. Y., Kang, S. H., Gwag, B. J., Jou, I.&Joe, E. H., (2008). Differential neutrophil infiltration contributes to regional differences in brain inflammation in the substantia nigra pars compacta and cortex. *Glia.* Vol. 56, No. 10, (Aug 1, 2008), pp. (1039-47).

Kemel, M. L., Perez, S., Godeheu, G., Soubrie, P.&Glowinski, J., (2002). Facilitation by endogenous tachykinins of the NMDA-evoked release of acetylcholine after acute and chronic suppression of dopaminergic transmission in the matrix of the rat striatum. *J Neurosci.* Vol. 22, No. 5, (Mar 1, 2002), pp. (1929-36).

Khawaja, A. M.&Rogers, D. F., (1996). Tachykinins: receptor to effector. *Int J Biochem Cell Biol.* Vol. 28, No. 7, 1996), pp. (721-738).

Kortekaas, R., Leenders, K. L., van Oostrom, J. C., Vaalburg, W., Bart, J., Willemsen, A. T.&Hendrikse, N. H., (2005). Blood-brain barrier dysfunction in parkinsonian midbrain in vivo. *Ann Neurol.* Vol. 57, No. 2, (Feb, 2005), pp. (176-9).

Krasnova, I. N., Bychkov, E. R., Lioudyno, V. I., Zubareva, O. E.&Dambinova, S. A., (2000). Intracerebroventricular administration of Substance P increases dopamine content in the brain of 6-hydroxydopamine-lesioned rats. *Neurosci.* Vol. 95, No. 1, 2000), pp. (113-117).

Leeman, S. E.&Ferguson, S. L., (2000). Substance P: an historical perspective. *Neuropeptides.* Vol. 34, No. 5, 2000), pp. (249-254).

Lever, I. J., Grant, A. D., Pezet, S., Gerard, N. P., Brain, S. D.&Malcangio, M., (2003). Basal and activity-induced release of substance P from primary afferent fibers in NK$_1$ receptor knockout mice: evidence for negative feedback. *Neuropharmacology.* Vol. 45, No. 8, 2003), pp. (1101-1110).

Levesque, M., Wallman, M. J., Parent, R., Sik, A.&Parent, A., (2007). Neurokinin-1 and neurokinin-3 receptors in primate substantia nigra. *Neurosci Res.* Vol. 57, No. 3, (Mar, 2007), pp. (362-71).

Lieb, K., Fiebich, B. L., Berger, M., Bauer, J.&Schulze-Osthoff, K., (1997). The neuropeptide substance P activates transcription factor NF-kappa B and kappa B-dependent gene expression in human astrocytoma cells. *J Immunol.* Vol. 159, No. 10, (Nov 15, 1997), pp. (4952-8).

Liu, B.&Hong, J. S., (2003). Role of microglia in inflammation-mediated neurodegenerative diseases: mechanisms and strategies for therapeutic intervention. *J Pharmacol Exp Ther.* Vol. 304, No. 1, (Jan, 2003), pp. (1-7).

Luber-Narod, J., Kage, R.&Leeman, S. E., (1994). Substance P enhances the secretion of tumor necrosis factor-alpha from neuroglial cells stimulated with lipopolysaccharide. *J Immunol.* Vol. 152, No. 2, (Jan 15, 1994), pp. (819-24).

Maggi, C. A., (1995). The mammalian tachykinin receptors. *Gen Pharmac.* Vol. 26, No. 5, 1995), pp. (911-944).

Malcangio, M.&Bowery, N. G., (1999). Peptide autoreceptors: does an autoreceptor exist for substance P. *TiPS.* Vol. 20, No., 1999), pp. (405-407).

Mantyh, P. W., Johnson, D. J., Boehmer, C. G., Catton, M. D., Vinters, H. V., Maggio, J. E., Too, H. P.&Vigna, S. R., (1989). Substance P receptor binding sites are expressed by glia in vivo after neuronal injury. *Proc Natl Acad Sci U S A.* Vol. 86, No. 13, (Jul, 1989), pp. (5193-7).

Marey-Semper, I., Gelman, M.&Levi-Strauss, M., (1995). A selective toxicity toward cultured mesencephalic dopaminergic neurons is induced by the synergistic effects of energetic metabolism impairment and NMDA receptor activation. *J Neurosci*. Vol. 15, No. 9, 1995), pp. (5912-5918).

Marinova-Mutafchieva, L., Sadeghian, M., Broom, L., Davis, J. B., Medhurst, A. D.&Dexter, D. T., (2009). Relationship between microglial activation and dopaminergic neuronal loss in the substantia nigra: a time course study in a 6-hydroxydopamine model of Parkinson's disease. *J Neurochem*. Vol. 110, No. 3, (Aug, 2009), pp. (966-75).

Marriott, I., (2004). The role of tachykinins in central nervous system inflammatory responses. *Front Biosci*. Vol. 9, No., (Sep 1, 2004), pp. (2153-65).

Marsden, C. D.&Olanow, C. W., (1998). The causes of Parkinson's disease are being unraveled and rational neuroprotective therapy is close to reality. *Ann Neurol*. Vol. 44, No. 3 Suppl 1, (Sep, 1998), pp. (S189-96).

Martin, F. C., Charles, A. C., Sanderson, M. J.&Merrill, J. E., (1992). Substance P stimulates IL-1 production by astrocytes via intracellular calcium. *Brain Res*. Vol. 599, No. 1, (Dec 18, 1992), pp. (13-8).

Maubach, K. A., Martin, K., Smith, D. W., Hewson, L., Frankshun, R. A., Harrison, T.&Seabrook, G. R., (2001). Substance P stimulates inhibitory synaptic transmission in the guinea pig basolateral amygdala in vitro. *Neuropharmacology*. Vol. 40, No. 6, (May, 2001), pp. (806-17).

Mauborgne, A., Javoy-Agid, F., Legrand, J. C., Agid, Y.&Cesselin, F., (1983). Decrease of substance P-like immunoreactivity in the substantia nigra and pallidum of parkinsonian brains. *Brain Res*. Vol. 268, No. 1, (May 23, 1983), pp. (167-70).

McGeer, P. L.&McGeer, E. G., (2008). Glial reactions in Parkinson's disease. *Mov Disord*. Vol. 23, No. 4, (Mar 15, 2008), pp. (474-83).

Mladenovic, A., Perovic, M., Raicevic, N., Kanazir, S., Rakic, L.&Ruzdijic, S., (2004). 6-Hydroxydopamine increases the level of TNFalpha and bax mRNA in the striatum and induces apoptosis of dopaminergic neurons in hemiparkinsonian rats. *Brain Res*. Vol. 996, No. 2, (Jan 23, 2004), pp. (237-45).

Mosley, R. L., Benner, E. J., Kadiu, I., Thomas, M., Boska, M. D., Hasan, K., Laurie, C.&Gendelman, H. E., (2006). Neuroinflammation, Oxidative Stress and the Pathogenesis of Parkinson's Disease. *Clin Neurosci Res*. Vol. 6, No. 5, (Dec 6, 2006), pp. (261-281).

Napier, T. C., Mitrovic, I., Churchill, L., Klitenick, M. A., Lu, X. Y.&Kalivas, P. W., (1995). Substance P in the ventral pallidum: projection from the ventral striatum, and electrophysiological and behavioral consequences of pallidal substance P. *Neuroscience*. Vol. 69, No. 1, (Nov, 1995), pp. (59-70).

Nikolaus, S., Huston, J. P., Korber, B., Thiel, C.&Schwarting, R. K. W., (1997). Pretreatment with neurokinin substance P but not with cholecystokinin-8S can alleviate functional deficits of partial nigrostriatal 6-hydoxydopamine lesion. *Peptides*. Vol. 18, No. 8, 1997), pp. (1161-1168).

Nimmo, A. J., Cernak, I., Heath, D. L., Hu, X., Bennett, C. J.&Vink, R., (2004). Neurogenic inflammation is associated with development of edema and functional deficits following traumatic brain injury in rats. *Neuropeptides*. Vol. 38, No. 1, (Feb, 2004), pp. (40-7).

Nisbet, A. P., Foster, O. J., Kingsbury, A., Eve, D. J., Daniel, S. E., Marsden, C. D.&Lees, A. J., (1995). Preproenkephalin and preprotachykinin messenger RNA expression in normal human basal ganglia and in Parkinson's disease. *Neuroscience*. Vol. 66, No. 2, (May, 1995), pp. (361-76).

Olanow, C. W.&Tatton, W. G., (1999). Etiology and pathogenesis of Parkinson's disease. *Annu Rev Neurosci*. Vol. 22, No., 1999), pp. (123-144).

Olanow, C. W., Agid, Y., Mizuno, Y., Albanese, A., Bonucelli, U., Damier, P., De Yebenes, J., Gershanik, O., Guttman, M., Grandas, F., Hallet, M., Hornykiewicz, O., Jenner, P., Katzenschlager, R., Langston, W. J., LeWitt, P., Melamed, E., Mena, M. A., Michel, P. P., Mytilineou, C., Obeso, J. A., Poewe, W., Quinn, N., Raisman-Vozari, R., Rajput, A. H., Rascol, O., Sampaio, C.&Stocchi, F., (2004). Levodopa in the treatment of Parkinson's disease: current controversies. *Movement Disorders*. Vol. 19, No. 9, 2004), pp. (997-1005).

Orosz, D.&Bennett, J. P., Jr., (1990). Baseline and apomorphine-induced extracellular levels of nigral substance P are increased in an animal model of Parkinson's disease. *Eur J Pharmacol*. Vol. 182, No. 3, (Jul 17, 1990), pp. (509-14).

Otsuka, M.&Yoshioka, K., (1993). Neurotransmitter functions of mammalian tachykinins. *Physiol Rev*. Vol. 73, No. 2, (Apr, 1993), pp. (229-308).

Qian, L., Flood, P. M.&Hong, J. S., (2010). Neuroinflammation is a key player in Parkinson's disease and a prime target for therapy. *J Neural Transm*. Vol. 117, No. 8, (Aug, 2010), pp. (971-9).

Raivich, G., Bohatschek, M., Kloss, C. U., Werner, A., Jones, L. L.&Kreutzberg, G. W., (1999). Neuroglial activation repertoire in the injured brain: graded response, molecular mechanisms and cues to physiological function. *Brain Res Brain Res Rev*. Vol. 30, No. 1, (Jul, 1999), pp. (77-105).

Rasley, A., Bost, K. L., Olson, J. K., Miller, S. D.&Marriott, I., (2002). Expression of functional NK-1 receptors in murine microglia. *Glia*. Vol. 37, No. 3, (Mar 1, 2002), pp. (258-67).

Ravenstijn, P. G., Merlini, M., Hameetman, M., Murray, T. K., Ward, M. A., Lewis, H., Ball, G., Mottart, C., de Ville de Goyet, C., Lemarchand, T., van Belle, K., O'Neill, M. J., Danhof, M.&de Lange, E. C., (2008). The exploration of rotenone as a toxin for inducing Parkinson's disease in rats, for application in BBB transport and PK-PD experiments. *J Pharmacol Toxicol Methods*. Vol. 57, No. 2, (Mar-Apr, 2008), pp. (114-30).

Reale, M., Iarlori, C., Thomas, A., Gambi, D., Perfetti, B., Di Nicola, M.&Onofrj, M., (2009). Peripheral cytokines profile in Parkinson's disease. *Brain Behav Immun*. Vol. 23, No. 1, (Jan, 2009), pp. (55-63).

Rego, A. C.&Oliveira, C. R., (2003). Mitochondrial dysfunction and reactive oxygen species in excitotoxicity and apoptosis: implications for the pathogenesis of neurodegenerative diseases. *Neurochem Res*. Vol. 28, No. 10, (Oct, 2003), pp. (1563-74).

Reid, M. S., Herrera-Marschitz, M., Hokfelt, T., Lindefors, N., Persson, H.&Ungerstedt, U., (1990a). Striatonigral GABA, dynorphin, substance P and neurokinin A modulation of nigrostriatal dopamine release: evidence for direct regulatory mechanisms. *Exp Brain Res*. Vol. 82, No. 2, 1990a), pp. (293-303).

Reid, M. S., Herrera-Marschitz, M., Hokfelt, T., Ohlin, M., Valentino, K. L.&Ungerstedt, U., (1990b). Effects of intranigral substance P and neurokinin A on striatal dopamine release--I. Interactions with substance P antagonists. *Neuroscience.* Vol. 36, No. 3, 1990b), pp. (643-58).

Ribeiro-da-Silva, A.&Hokfelt, T., (2000). Neuroanatomical localisation of Substance P in the CNS and sensory neurons. *Neuropeptides.* Vol. 34, No. 5, 2000), pp. (256-271).

Rite, I., Machado, A., Cano, J.&Venero, J. L., (2007). Blood-brain barrier disruption induces in vivo degeneration of nigral dopaminergic neurons. *J Neurochem.* Vol. 101, No. 6, (Jun, 2007), pp. (1567-82).

Rock, R. B.&Peterson, P. K., (2006). Microglia as a pharmacological target in infectious and inflammatory diseases of the brain. *J Neuroimmune Pharmacol.* Vol. 1, No. 2, (Jun, 2006), pp. (117-26).

Rodrigues, R. W. P., Gomide, V. C.&Chadi, G., (2001). Astroglial and microglial reaction after partial nigrostriatal degeneration induced by the striatal injection of different doses of 6-hydroxydopamine. *International Journal of Neuroscience.* Vol. 109, No., 2001), pp. (91-126).

Samii, A., Etminan, M., Wiens, M. O.&Jafari, S., (2009). NSAID use and the risk of Parkinson's disease: systematic review and meta-analysis of observational studies. *Drugs Aging.* Vol. 26, No. 9, 2009), pp. (769-79).

Saria, A., (1999). The tachykinin NK_1 receptor in the brain: pharmacology and putative functions. *Eur J of Pharmacol.* Vol. 375, No., 1999), pp. (51-60).

Schwarting, R. K.&Huston, J. P., (1996). Unilateral 6-hydroxydopamine lesions of meso-striatal dopamine neurons and their physiological sequelae. *Prog Neurobiol.* Vol. 49, No. 3, (Jun, 1996), pp. (215-66).

Severini, C., Improta, G., Falconieri-Erspamer, G., Salvadori, S.&Erspamer, V., (2002). The tachykinin peptide family. *Pharmacol Rev.* Vol. 54, No., 2002), pp. (385-322).

Shults, C. W., (2004). Mitochondrial dysfunction and possible treatments in Parkinson's disease-a review. *Mitochondrion.* Vol. 4, No. 5-6, (Sep, 2004), pp. (641-8).

Sil'kis, I. G., (2002). A possible mechanism for the dopamine-evoked synergistic disinhibition of thalamic neurons via the "direct" and "indirect" pathways in the basal ganglia. *Neurosci Behav Physiol.* Vol. 32, No. 3, (May-Jun, 2002), pp. (205-12).

Silkis, I., (2001). The cortico-basal ganglia-thalamocortical circuit with synaptic plasticity. II. Mechanism of synergistic modulation of thalamic activity via the direct and indirect pathways through the basal ganglia. *Biosystems.* Vol. 59, No. 1, (Jan, 2001), pp. (7-14).

Sivam, S. P., (1991). Dopamine dependent decrease in enkephalin and substance P levels in basal ganglia regions of postmortem Parkinsonian brains. *Neuropeptides.* Vol. 18, No., 1991), pp. (201-207).

Sutoo, D., Yabe, K.&Akiyama, K., (1999). Quantitative imaging of substance P in the human brain using a brain mapping analyzer. *Neurosci Res.* Vol. 35, No., 1999), pp. (339-346).

Takagi, S., Hayakawa, N., Kimoto, H., Kato, H.&Araki, T., (2007). Damage to oligodendrocytes in the striatum after MPTP neurotoxicity in mice. *J Neural Transm.* Vol. 114, No. 12, 2007), pp. (1553-7).

Tansey, M. G.&Goldberg, M. S., (2010). Neuroinflammation in Parkinson's disease: its role in neuronal death and implications for therapeutic intervention. *Neurobiol Dis.* Vol. 37, No. 3, (Mar, 2010), pp. (510-8).

Tenovuo, O., Rinne, U. K.&Viljanen, M. K., (1984). Substance P immunoreactivity in the post-mortem parkinsonian brain. *Brain Res*. Vol. 303, No. 1, (Jun 11, 1984), pp. (113-6).

Thornton, E., Tran, T. T.&Vink, R., (2010). A substance P mediated pathway contributes to 6-hydroxydopamine induced cell death. *Neurosci Lett*. Vol. 481, No. 1, (Aug 30, 2010), pp. (64-7).

Tomas-Camardiel, M., Rite, I., Herrera, A. J., de Pablos, R. M., Cano, J., Machado, A.&Venero, J. L., (2004). Minocycline reduces the lipopolysaccharide-induced inflammatory reaction, peroxynitrite-mediated nitration of proteins, disruption of the blood-brain barrier, and damage in the nigral dopaminergic system. *Neurobiol Dis*. Vol. 16, No. 1, (Jun, 2004), pp. (190-201).

Turner, R.&Vink, R., (2007). Inhibition of neurogenic inflammation as a novel treatment for ischemic stroke. *Drug News Perspect*. Vol. 20, No. 4, (May, 2007), pp. (221-6).

Turner, R. J., Blumbergs, P. C., Sims, N. R., Helps, S. C., Rodgers, K. M.&Vink, R., (2006). Increased substance P immunoreactivity and edema formation following reversible ischemic stroke. *Acta Neurochir Suppl*. Vol. 96, No., 2006), pp. (263-6).

van der Stelt, M.&Di Marzo, V., (2003). The endocannabinoid system in the basal ganglia and in the mesolimbic reward system: implications for neurological and psychiatric disorders. *Eur J Pharmacol*. Vol. 480, No. 1-3, (Nov 7, 2003), pp. (133-50).

Vink, R., Young, A., Bennett, C. J., Hu, X., Connor, C. O., Cernak, I.&Nimmo, A. J., (2003). Neuropeptide release influences brain edema formation after diffuse traumatic brain injury. *Acta Neurochir Suppl*. Vol. 86, No., 2003), pp. (257-60).

Vizuete, M. L., Merino, M., Venero, J. L., Santiago, M., Cano, J.&Machado, A., (2000). Histamine infusion induces a selective dopaminergic neuronal death along with an inflammatory reaction in rat substantia nigra. *J Neurochem*. Vol. 75, No. 2, (Aug, 2000), pp. (540-52).

Wade, T. V.&Schneider, J. S., (2001). Expression of striatal preprotachykinin mRNA in symptomatic and asymptomatic 1-methyl-4-phenyl-1,2,3,6-tetrahydropyridine-exposed monkeys is related to parkinsonian motor signs. *J Neurosci*. Vol. 21, No. 13, (Jul 1, 2001), pp. (4901-7).

Wardas, J., Peitraszek, M., Wolfarth, S.&Ossowska, K., (2003). The role of metabotropic glutamate receptors in regulation of striatal proenkephalin expression: Implications for the therapy of Parkinson's disease. *Neurosci*. Vol. 122, No., 2003), pp. (747-756).

Woie, K., Koller, M. E., Heyeraas, K. J.&Reed, R. K., (1993). Neurogenic inflammation in rat trachea is accompanied by increased negativity of interstitial fluid pressure. *Circ Res*. Vol. 73, No. 5, (Nov, 1993), pp. (839-45).

Wojtera, M., Sikorska, B., Sobow, T.&Liberski, P. P., (2005). Microglial cells in neurodegenerative disorders. *Folia Neuropathol*. Vol. 43, No. 4, 2005), pp. (311-21).

Wu, D. C., Teismann, P., Tieu, K., Vila, M., Jackson-Lewis, V., Ischiropoulos, H.&Przedborski, S., (2003). NADPH oxidase mediates oxidative stress in the 1-methyl-4-phenyl-1,2,3,6-tetrahydropyridine model of Parkinson's disease. *Proc Natl Acad Sci U S A*. Vol. 100, No. 10, (May 13, 2003), pp. (6145-50).

Yelnik, J., (2002). Functional anatomy of the basal ganglia. *Mov Disord*. Vol. 17 Suppl 3, No., 2002), pp. (S15-21).

Yip, J.&Chahl, L. A., (2000). Localization of tachykinin receptors and fos-like immunoreactivity induced by substance P in guinea pig brain. *Clinical and Experimental Pharmacology and Physiology.* Vol. 27, No., 2000), pp. (943-946).

6

Mitochondrial Haplogroups Associated with Japanese Parkinson's Patients

Shigeru Takasaki
Toyo University, Izumino 1-1-1, Ora-gun Itakuracho, Gunma,
Japan

1. Introduction

Mitochondria are essential cytoplasmic organelles generating cellular energy in the form of adenosine triphosphate by oxidative phosphorylation. Most cells contain hundreds of mitochondria, each of which has several mitochondrial DNA (mtDNA) copies, so each cell contains thousands of mtDNA copies. mtDNA has a very high mutation rate, and when a mutation occurs the cell initially contains a mixture of wild-type and mutant mtDNAs, a situation known as heteroplasmy. If the percentage of mutant mtDNA increases enough that the cell's ATP production falls below the level needed for normal cell function, disease symptoms appear and become progressively worse. A wide variety of diseases — such as Parkinson's disease (PD), Alzheimer's disease (AD), and cancer — are reportedly linked to mitochondrial dysfunction, and it is clear that mitochondrial diseases encompass an extraordinary assemblage of clinical problems (Wallace 1999; Vila and Przedborski 2003; Taylor and Turnbull 2005).

Although mtDNA mutations have been reported to be related both to a wide variety of diseases and aging (Lin *et al.* 1992; Schoffner *et al.* 1993; Kosel *et al.* 1994; Mayr-Wohlfart *et al.* 1996; Schnopp *et al.* 1996; Simon *et al.* 2000; Tanaka *et al.* 2002; Dawson and Dawson 2003; Ross *et al.* 2003; Lustbader *et al.* 2004; Niemi *et al.* 2005; Alexe *et al.* 2007; Fuku *et al.* 2007; Chinnery *et al.* 2008; Kim *et al.* 2008; Maruszak *et al.* 2008; Feder *et al.* 2008), there are few reports regarding the relations between all mtDNA mutations and either disease patients or centenarians. The previous reports have also focused on mutations causing amino acid replacements in mitochondrial proteins and, although mitochondrial functions can of course be affected directly by amino acid replacements, they can also be affected indirectly by mutations in mtDNA control regions. It is therefore important to examine the relations between all mtDNA mutations and disease patients or centenarians.

In the article reported here the relations between Japanese PD patients and their mitochondrial single nucleotide polymorphism (mtSNP) frequencies were analyzed using a method based on radial basis function (RBF) networks (Poggio and Girosi 1990; Wu and McLarty 2000) and a modified method based on RBF network predictions (Takasaki 2009). In addition, the relations between the haplogroups of the PD patients and those of the other four classes of people (centenarians, AD patients, T2D patients, and healthy non-obese young males) are also described using the same analysis method. The results described here are quite different from those reported previously (Saxena *et al.* 2006; Alexe *et al.* 2007; Fuku *et al.* 2007; Bilal *et al.* 2008).

2. Materials and methods

2.1 mtSNPs

We used complete mtDNA sequences available in GiiB Human Mitochondrial Genome Polymorphism Database (http://mtsnp.tmig.or.jp/mtsnp). The mtSNPs used were those in 96 Japanese PD patients (43 males and 53 females), 96 Japanese centenarians (30 males and 66 females), 96 Japanese AD patients (20 males and 76 females), 96 Japanese type 2 diabetes (T2D) patients (54 males and 42 females), and 96 Japanese healthy non-obese young males (Tanaka *et al.* 2004).

2.2 RBF-based method of mtSNP classification

A RBF network is an artificial network used in supervised learning problems such as regression, classification, and time series prediction. In supervised learning a function is inferred from examples (training set) that a teacher supplies. The elements in the training set are paired values of the independent (input) variable and dependent (output) variable.

The RBF network shown in Fig. 1 was learned from the training set as the mtSNPs of the PD patients were regarded as correct and the mtSNPs of other four classes of people (centenarians, AD patients, T2D patients, and healthy non-obese young males) were regarded as incorrect. Similarly, in the mtSNP classification for the centenarians the mtSNPs of the centenarians are regarded as correct and those of the other four classes are regarded as incorrect. The mtSNPs of the AD patients, T2D patients, and healthy non-obese young males were also classified this way.

The mitochondrial genome sequences of the PD patients were partitioned into two sets: training data comprising the sequences of 64 of the PD patients, and validation data comprising the sequences of the other 32 PD patients. The training and validation steps are described in detail elsewhere (Takasaki *et al.* 2006).

2.3 Modified classification method based on probabilities predicted by the RBF network

Since a RBF network can predict the probabilities that persons with certain mtSNPs belong to certain classes (e.g., PD patients, centenarians, AD patients, T2D patients, or healthy non-obese young males), these predicted probabilities are used to identify mtSNP features. By examining the relations between individual mtSNPs and the persons with high predicted probabilities of belonging to one of these classes, we are able to identify other mtSNPs useful for distinguishing between the members in different classes. A modified classification method based on the probabilities predicted by the RBF network was thus carried out in the following way (Takasaki 2009).

1. Select the analysis target class (i.e., PD patients, centenarians, AD patients, T2D patients, or healthy non-obese young males).
2. Rank individuals according to their predicted probabilities of belonging to the target class.
3. Either select individuals whose probabilities are greater than a certain value or select the desired number of individuals from the top, and set them as a modified cluster.

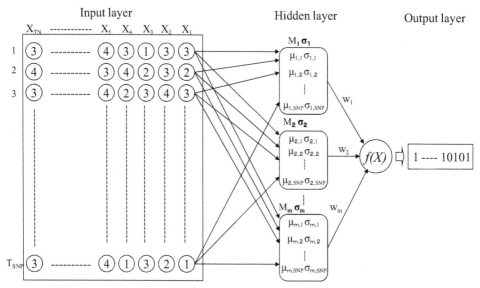

Fig. 1. RBF network representation of the relations between individual mtSNPs and the PD patients. The input layer is the set of mtSNP sequences represented numerically (A, G, C, and T are converted to 1, 2, 3, and 4). The hidden layer classifies the input vectors into several clusters depending on the similarities of individual input vectors. The output layer is determined depending on which analysis is carried out. In the case of PD patients, 1 corresponds to PD patients and 0 corresponds to other four classes of people. In the case of centenarians, 1 corresponds to centenarians and 0 corresponds to other four classes of people. The AD patients, T2D patients, and healthy non-obese young males are also carried out in similar way. X_i : i-th input vector, TN : maximum number of vectors (in this example, TN=320 (64x5)), T_{SNP} : maximum number of mtSNPs (in this example, T_{SNP} =562), M_m: the location vector, m: the number of basis functions, μ: basis function, σ: standard deviation, w_i: i-th weighting variable, $f(X)$: weighted sum function.

3. Results and discussion

3.1 Associations between haplogroups and the mtSNPs of the PD patients

When the mtSNPs of the PD patients were classified by the RBF-based method described above, ten mtSNP clusters were obtained. The average predicted probabilities of these clusters for becoming the PD patients were respectively 63%, 62.5%, 52.9%, 30%, 29.4%, 15.4%, 7.7%, 4.3%, 3.4% and 0%. Then the 15 individuals with the highest probabilities of becoming PD patients were selected using the modified classification method, and their nucleotide distributions at individual mtDNA positions were examined. After that, the relations between Asian/Japanese haplogroups and the mtSNPs for the PD patients were examined (Herrnstadt et al. 2002; Kong et al. 2003; Tanaka et al. 2004). The associations between the haplogroups and mtSNPs for the PD patients are shown in Fig. 2. The features of associations for the PD patients were L3-M-M7b2 (33%), L3-M-G2a (27%), L3-N-B4e (13%), B5b (13%), and N9a (7%).

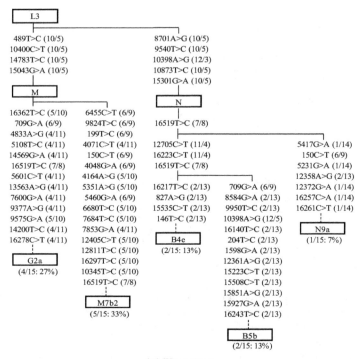

(A) PD patients

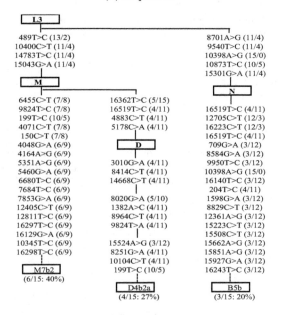

(B) Centenarians

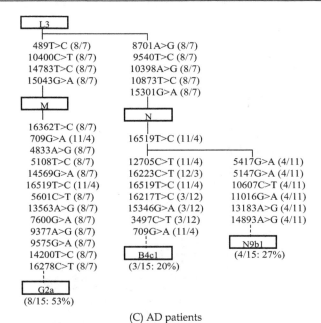

(C) AD patients

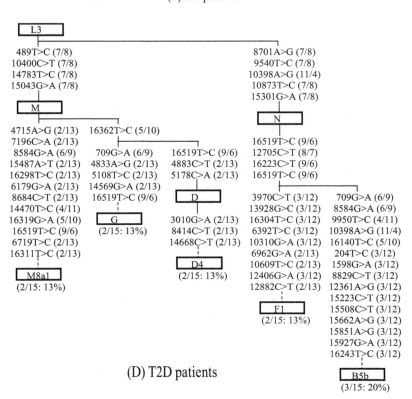

(D) T2D patients

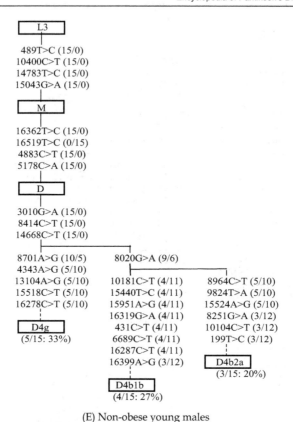

(E) Non-obese young males

Fig. 2. Associations between haplogroups and the mtSNPs of the 15 persons with the highest probabilities of becoming PD patients. This description of associations is based on the phylogenetic tree for macrohaplogroups M and N described in Tanaka *et al.* [26]. The locus of mtDNA polymorphism (mmm), the normal nucleotide (rCRS) at the position mmm (N_N), the mtDNA mutation at that position (N_M), the number of the mtDNA mutations at mmm in individual clusters (Y), and the number of the normal nucleotides at mmm in individual clusters (X) are expressed as $mmmN_N{>}N_M$ (Y/X). For example, 489T>C (10/5) indicates the mtDNA locus (489), the normal nucleotide at that position (T), the mutation at that position (C), the number of mutations (10), and the number of the normal nucleotides in the cluster (5). (B) Centenarians, (C) AD patients, (D) T2D patients, (E) Non-obese young males.

To compare the mitochondrial haplogroups of the PD patients with those of other classes of people, we used the same modified method to examine the relations between the other four classes (i.e., centenarians, AD patients, T2D patients, and non-obese young males) and their mtSNPs. The associations between the haplogroups and mtSNPs for four classes of Japanese people are shown in Fig. 2 B to E. The centenarians were associated haplogroups L3-M-M7b2 (40%), L3-M-D-D4b2a (27%), and L3-N-B5b (20%); the AD patients were associated haplogroups L3-M-G2a (53%), L3-N-B4c1 (20%), and N9b1 (27%); the T2D patients were associated haplogroups L3-M-D-D4 (13%), L3-M-M8a1 (13%), G (13%), L3-N-B5b (20%), and F1 (13%); and the healthy non-obese young males were associated haplogroups L3-M-D-D4g

(33%), D4b2a (20%), and D4b1b (27%). The relations among the haplogroups for these five classes of people are listed in Table 1.

Classification consideration	PD patients	Centenarians	AD patients	T2D patients	Non-obese males
15 persons from the top				M8a1 (13%)	
	M7b2 (33%)	M7b2 (40%)			
				G (13%)	
	G2a (27%)		G2a (53%)		
				D4 (13%)	
					D4b1b (27%)
					D4b2a (20%)
		D4b2a (27%)			
					D4g (33%)
	B4e (13%)				
	B5b (13%)	B5b (20%)		B5b (20%)	
			B4c1 (20%)		
	N9a (7%)				
			N9b1 (27%)		
				F1 (13%)	
Persons whose probabilities are greater than 50%				M8a1 (4%)	
	M7a1a (19%)				
	M7b2 (14%)	M7b2 (13%)			
				G (11%)	
			G1 (9%)		
	G1a (14%)				
	G2a (11%)		G2a (17%)		
			D4 (19%)	D4 (47%)	
		D4a (15%)			
					D4b1b (24%)
					D4b2 (35%)
		D4b2a (9%)			
		D4b2b (16%)			
					D4g (29%)
				D5a (6%)	
	B4e (5%)				
			B4c1 (11%)		
	B5b (5%)	B5b (7%)		B5b (6%)	
	N9a (16%)		N9a (4%)		
			N9b1 (9%)	N9b1 (6%)	
			F1 (11%)	F1 (6%)	

Table 1. The relations among the haplogroups for five classes of people

In Table 1 we see that the haplogroup Mb2 was common in PD patients and centenarians, G2a was common in PD patients and AD patients; and B5b was common in PD patients, centenarians, and T2D patients. The haplogroups of the PD patients are therefore different from those of the other four classes of people. The results are therefore considered new findings.

Then individuals whose probabilities of becoming PD patients were greater than 50% were selected, and the nucleotide distributions of those 37 persons were examined. The associations between haplogroups and the mtSNPs of those PD patients are shown in Fig. 3. Individuals whose probabilities of becoming PD patients were greater than 50% were classified into more haplogroups than were the 15 persons most likely to become PD patients. The ratios of the haplogroups M7b2, G2a, B4e, B5b and N9a for the 15 persons most likely to become PD patients were respectively changed from 33% to 14%, 27% to 11%, 13%

to 5%, 13% to 5%, and 7% to 16%, and new haplogroups M7a1a (19%) and G1a (14%) were classified for the persons whose probabilities were greater than 50%. The other four classes of people were also examined for the persons whose probabilities were greater than 50%. The selected numbers of the four classes were 55 for centenarians, 47 for AD patients, 47 for T2D patients, and 17 for healthy non-obese young males. The associations between the haplogroups and mtSNPs for four classes of people are shown in Fig. 3 B to E. The centenarians were associated haplogroups L3-M-M7b2 (13%), L3-M-D-D4a (15%), D4b2a (9%), D4b2b (16%), and L3-N-B5b (7%); the AD patients were associated haplogroups L3-M-G1 (9%), G2a (17%), L3-M-D-D4 (19%), L3-N-F1 (11%), B4c1 (11%), N9a (4%), and N9b1 (9%); the T2D patients were associated haplogroups L3-M-M8a1 (4%), G (11%), L3-M-D-D4 (47%), D5a (6%), L3-N-F1 (6%), B5b (6%), and N9b1 (6%); and the healthy non-obese young males were associated haplogorups L3-M-D-D4g (29%), D4b1b (24%), and D4b2 (35%). The relations among the haplogroups of the selected persons for the five classes of people are also listed in Table 1, where one sees that the individual classes of people were classified into more haplogroups when the mtSNP analysis was based on the persons whose probabilities were greater than 50% than they were when the analysis was based on the highest 15 persons from the top.

3.2 Comparison with previous works for T2D patients and Centenarians
Although there is no report regarding the relations between mtSNP haplogroups and PD patients but there were a few studies concerning the relations between mtSNP haplogroups and T2D patients or centenarians, the differences between previous works and the work reported here are discussed based on the mtSNP haplogroups obtained.

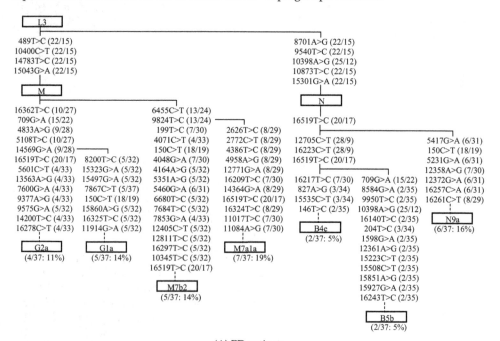

(A) PD patients

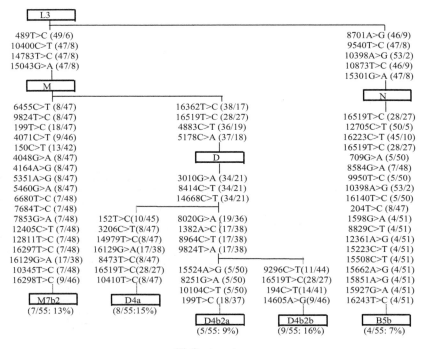

(B) Centenarians

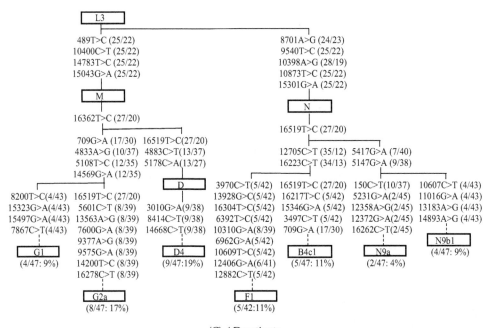

(C) AD patients

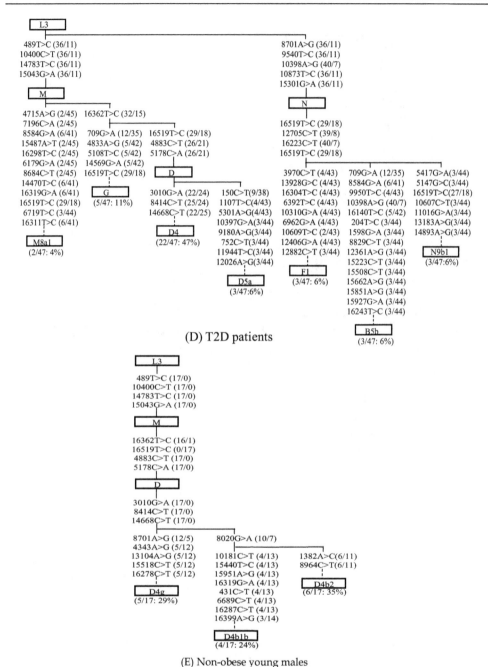

(D) T2D patients

(E) Non-obese young males

Fig. 3. Associations between haplogroups and the mtSNPs of the persons whose probabilities of becoming PD patients are greater than 50%. (B) Centenarians, (C) AD patients, (D) T2D patients, (E) Non-obese young males.

Fuku et al. (2007) reported that the mitochondrial haplogroup F in Japanese individuals had a significantly increased risk of type 2 diabetes mellitus (T2DM) (odds ratio 1.53, P=0.0032) using hospital based sampling data for large-scale association study (Fuku et al., 2007). They indicated that there were three mtSNPs in the haplogroup F – 3970C>T, 13928G>C, and 10310G>A. In the present analysis, the risk of T2D patients for the haplogroup F1 was approximately 13% (Fig. 2D). Other haplogroups related to the risk of T2D patients were B5b (20%), M8a1 (13%), D4 (13%) and G (13%) (Fig. 2D and Table 2). There were therefore big differences between the analyses of Fuku et al. (2007) and the results reported here. The significantly increased risk of T2DM was the haplogroup F in Fuku et al. (2007), whereas that of the results obtained was the haplogroup B5b. Although Fuku et al. (2007) indicated that the haplogroup F was the increased risk of T2DM, the F has four sub-haplogroups F1, F2, F3, and F4. In the work reported here, the only haplogroup F1 was obtained by the modified clustering method. The haplogroup F by Fuku et al. (2007) was characterized by three mtSNPs – 3970C>T, 13928G>C, and 10310G>A, whereas the haplogroup F1 by the proposed method was featured by many mtSNPs – 3970C>T, 13928G>C, 16304T>C, 6392T>C, 10310G>A, 6962G>A, 10609T>C, 12406G>A, and 12882C>T (Tanaka et al., 2004) (Fig. 2D). Furthermore, as Saxena et al. (2006) reported that there was no evidence of association between common mtDNA polymorphism and type 2 diabetes mellitus, the results obtained may indicate new findings for T2D patients (Saxena et al., 2006).

In addition, Alexe et al. (2007) reported the associations between Asian haplogroups and the longevity of Japanese people using the same GiiB data (Alexe et al., 2007). They showed the enrichment of longevity phenotype in mtDNA haplogroups D4b2b, D4a, and D5 in the Japanese population using statistical techniques (t-test and P-value). However, the results here showed that the haplogroups M7b2, D4b2a, and B5b were associated with Japanese centenarians. There is therefore no common haplogroup in both methods. Alexe et al. (2007) showed that the haplogroup D5 was characterized by mtSNPs 11944T>C, 12026A>G, 1107T>C, 5301A>G, 10397A>G, and 752C>T, whereas there was no frequency in the corresponding mtSNPs in the present analysis. Although they reported that the centenarian enrichment was not found in the haplogroup D4b2a, the present results showed that the corresponding D4b2a was characterized by many mtSNPs with a frequency of 27% (Fig. 2B). Although Alexe et al. (2007) described that there was no haplogroup having mtSNPs significantly enriched in centenarians other than D mega-group in M macrohaplogroup, the present analysis indicated that the haplogroup M7b2 was characterized by many mtSNPs (Fig. 2B and 3B). They also reported that there was no enrichment haplogroup for centenarians in macrohaplogroup N, whereas the haplogroup B5b obtained by the proposed method also had many mtSNPs enriched in centenarians (Figs. 2B and 3B).

Bilal et al. (2008) reported the haplogroup D4a was a marker for extreme longevity in Japan by analyzing the complete mtDNA sequences from 112 Japanese semi-supercentenarians (aged over 105 years old) combined with previously published data (Bilal et al., 2008). These semi-supercentenarians were also examined using the proposed method. Since the predicted probabilities of individual clusters for the semi-supercentenarians were lower than those of the centenarians, 43 individuals with predicted probabilities over 46% (the average is 54%) were selected. The obtained results were the haplogroups D4a (30%), B4c1a (14%), M7b2 (12%), F1 (9%), M1 (7%) and B5b (2%) shown in Fig. 4. As the highest haplogroup was D4a, this was the same as the marker described by Bilal et al. (2008). However, there are other haplogroups indicating the characteristics of semi-supercentenarians. This means that other haplogroups also have the possibilities of becoming semi-supercentenarians. The common haplogroups between the centenarians and semi-supercentenarians were M7b2 and B5b.

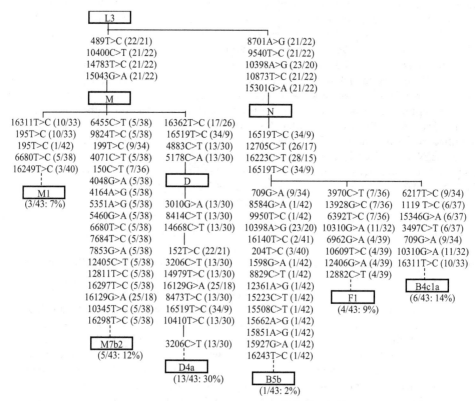

Fig. 4. Associations between Asian/Japanese haplogroups and mtSNPs of semi-supercentenarians.

3.3 Differences between statistical technique and the modified RBF method

Although the haplogroups of the PD patients were obtained by the modified RBF method, there are clear differences between the previously reported statistical technique and the method described here. As the previously reported methods analyzed the relations between mtSNPs and Japanese PD patients, centenarians, AD patients, T2D patients, or semi-supercentenarians using standard statistical techniques (Alexe et al., 2007; Fuku et al., 2007; Bilal et al., 2008), they could not indicate mutual relations among the other classes of people — centenarians, AD patients, T2D patients and healthy non-obese young males. On the other hand, the proposed method was able to show differences and mutual relations among these classes of people. In addition, the prediction probabilities of associations between mtSNPs and these classes of people cannot be obtained by the statistical techniques used in the previous methods, whereas the method proposed is able to compute them based on learning mtSNPs of individual classes.

It is considered that the relations among individual mtSNPs for these classes of people should be analyzed as mutual mtSNP connections in the entire mtSNPs. A learning method, a RBF network, was therefore adopted for extracting individual characteristics from the entire mtSNPs, although the previous methods used standard statistical techniques.

	Statistical technique	Proposed method
Technique	Relative relations between target and normal data	Supervised learning (RBF) by using correct and incorrect data
Analysis position	Each locus of mtDNA polymorphisms (independent position)	Entire loci of mtDNA polymorphisms (succesive positions)
Input (required data)	Target (individual cases) and control (normal data)	Correct (individual cases) and incorrect (others except correct)
Output (results)	Odds ratio or relative risk	Clusters with predictions
Analysis	Check odds ratio or relative risk at each position	Check individuals in clusters based on prediction probabilities

Table 2. Differences between the statistical technique and the proposed (modified RBF) method

The differences between standard statistical technique and the proposed method are listed in Table 2. In the statistical technique, the analysis of odds ratios or relative risks is based on the relative relations between target and control data at each polymorphic mtDNA locus. In the modified RBF method, on the other hand, clusters indicating predicted probabilities are examined on the basis of the RBF using correct and incorrect data for the entire polymorphic mtDNA loci. The statistical technique determines characteristics of haplogroups using independent mtDNA polymorphisms that indicate high odds ratios, whereas the modified RBF method determines them by checking individuals with high predicted probabilities. This means that the statistical technique uses the results of independent mutation positions, whereas the modified RBF method uses the results of entire mutation positions. As there are the differences between the two methods, which method is better depends on future research. Furthermore, the method described here may have possibilities for use in the initial diagnosis of various diseases or longevity on the basis of the individual predicted probabilities.

4. Acknowledgement

I thank Dr. Y. Kawamura for his encouragement and technical support.

5. References

Alexe, G., Fuku, N., Bilal, E., Ueno, H., Nishigaki, Y., Fujita, Y., Ito, M., Arai, Y., Hirose, N., Bhanot, G., and Tanaka, M. (2007). Enrichment of longevity phenotype in mtDNA haplogroups D4b2b, D4a, and D4 in the Japanese population, Hum. Genet. 121: 347 – 356.

Bilal, E., Rabadan, R., Alexe, G., Fuku, N., Ueno, H., Nishigaki, Y., Fujita, Y., Ito, M., Arai, Y., Hirose, N., Ruckenstein, A., Bhanot, G., and Tanaka, M. (2008). Mitochondrial DNA Haplogroup D4a Is a Marker for Extreme Longevity in Japan, PLoS ONE 3(6): e2421.

Chinnery, P.F., Mowbray, C., Patel, S.K., Elson, J.L., Sampson, M., Hitman, G.A., McCarthy, M.I., Hattersley,A.T., and Walker, M. (2008). Mitochondrial DNA haplogroups and type 2 diabetes: a study of 897 cases and 1010 controls, J Med Genet. 44: e80.

Dawson, T.M., and Dawson, V.L. (2003). Molecular Pathway of Neurodegeneration in Parkinson's Disease, Science 302: 819 – 822.

Fuku, N., Park, K.S., Yamada, Y., Nishigaki, Y., Cho, Y.M., Matsuo, H., Segawa, T., Watanabe, S., Kato, K., Yokoi, K., Nozawa, Y., Lee, K.H., and Tanaka M. (2007). Mitochondrial Haplogroup N9a Confers Resistance against Type 2 diabetes in Asians, Am J Hum Genet. 80: 407 – 415.

Feder, J., Blech, I., Ovadia, O., Amar, S., Wainstein, J., Raz, I., Dadon, S., Arking, D.E., Glaser, B., and Mishmar, D. (2008). Differences in mtDNA haplogroup distribution among 3 Jewish populations alter susceptibility to T2DM complications, BMC Genomics 9: 198.

Herrnstad, C., Elson, J.L., Fahy, E., Preston, G., Turnbull, D.M., Anderson, C., Ghosh, S.S., Olefsky, J.M., Beal, M.F., Davis, R.E., and Howell, N. (2002). Reduced-median-network Analysis of complete mitochondrial DNA coding-region sequences for major African, Asian and European haplogroups, Am J Hum Genet. 70: 1152 – 1171.

Kim, W., Yoo, T.K., Shin, D.J., Rho, H.W., Jin, H.J., Kim, E.T., and Bae, Y.S. (2008). Mitochondrial haplogroup analysis reveals no association between the common genetic lineages and prostate cancer in the Korean population, PLoS ONE 3: e2211.

Kosel, S., Egensperger, R., Mehraein, P., and Graeber, M.B. (1994). No association of mutations at nucleotide 5460 of mitochondrial NADH dehydrogenase with Alzheimer's disease, Biochem. Biophy. Res. Comm. 203: 745 – 749.

Kong, Q.P., Yao, Y.G., Sun, C., Bandelt, H.J., Zhu, C.L., and Zhang, Y.P. (2003). Phylogeny of East Asian mitochondrial DNA lineages inferred from complete sequences, Am J Hum Genet. 73: 671 – 676.

Lin, F., Lin, R., Wisniewski, H.M., Hwang, Y., Grundke-Iqbal, I., Healy-Louie, G., and Iqbal, K. (1992). Detection of point mutations in codon 331 of mitochondrial NADH dehydrogenase subunit 2 in Alzheimer's brains, Biochem. Biophy. Res. Comm. 182: 238 – 246.

Lustbader, J.W., Cirilli, M., Lin, C., Xu, H.W., Takuma, K., Wang, N., Caspersen, C., Chen, X., Pollak, S., Chaney, M., Trinchese, F., Liu, S., Gunn-Moore, F., Lue, L.F., Walker, D.G., Kuppusamy, P., Zewier, Z.L., Arancio, O., Stern, D., Yan, S.S., and Wu, H. (2004). ABAB DirectlyLinks Aβ to Mitochondrial Toxicity in Alzheimer's Disease, Science 304: 448 – 452.

Mayr-Wohlfart, U., Paulus, C., and Rodel, G. (1996). Mitochondrial DNA mutations in multiple sclerosis patients with severe optic involvement, Acta Neurol. Scand. 94: 167 – 171.

Maruszak, A., Canter, J.A., Styczynska, M., Zekanowski, C., and Barcikowska, M. (2008). Mitochondrial haplogroup H and Alzheimer's disease – Is there a connection?, Neurobiol Aging, doi: 10.1016.

Niemi, A.K., Moilanen, J.S., Tanaka M., Hervonen, A., Hurme, M., Lehtimaki, T., Arai, Y., Hirose, N., and Majamaa, K. A. (2005). A combination of three common inherited mitochondrial DNA polymorphisms promotes longevity in Finnish and Japanese subjects, Eur. J Hum. Genet. 13: 166 – 170.

Poggio, T., and Girosi, F. (1990). Networks for approximation and learning, Proc. of IEEE 78: 1481–1497.

Ross, O.A., MaCormack, R., Maxwell, L.D., Duguid, R.A., Quinn, D.J., Barnett, Y.A., Rea, I.M., El-Agnaf, O.M., Gibson, J.M., Wallace, A., Middleton, D., and Curran, M.D. (2003). mt4216C variant in linkage with the mtDNA TJ cluster may confer a susceptibility to mitochondrial dysfunction resulting in an increased risk of Parkinson's disease in Irish, Exp Gerontol. 38: 397 – 405.

Saxena, R., de Bakker, PIW., Singer, K., Mootha, V., Burtt, N., Hirschhorn, J.N., Gaudet, D., Isomaa, B., Daly, M.J., Groop, L., Ardlie, K.G., and Altshuler, D. (2006). Comprehensive Association Testing of Common Mitochondrial DNA Variation in Metabolic Disease, Am J Hum Genet. 79: 54 – 61.

Schoffner, J.M., Brown, M.D., Torroni, A., Lott, M.T., Cabell, M.F., Miorra, S.S., Beal, M.F., Yang, C.C., Gearing, M., Salvo, R., Watts, R.L., Juncos, J.L., Hansen, L.A., Crain, B.J., Fayad, M., Reckord, C.L., and Wallace, D.C. (1993). Mitochondrial DNA variants observed in Alzheimer disease and Parkinson disease Patients, Genomics 17: 171 – 184.

Schnopp, N.M., Kosel, S., Egensperger, R., and Graeber, M.B. (1996). Regional heterogeneity of mtDNA hetroplasmy in parkinsonian brain, Clin Neuropathol. 15: 348 – 352.

Simon, D.K., Mayeux, R., Marder, K., Kowall, N.W., Beal, M.F., and Jons, D.R. (2000). Mitochondrial DNA mutations in complex I and tRNA genes in Parkinson's disease, Neurology 54: 703 – 709.

Tanaka, M., Fuku, N., Takeyasu, T Guo, L.J., Hirose, R., Kurata, M., Borgeld, H.J., Yamada, Y., Maruyama, W., Arai, Y., Hirose, N., Oshida, Y., Sato, Y., Hattori, N., Mizuno, Y., Iwata, S., and Yagi, K. (2002). Golden Mean to Longevity: Rareness of Mitochondrial Cytochrome b Varianats in Centenarians But Not in Patients With Parkinson's Disease, J. Neuro. Res. 70: 347 – 355.

Tanaka, M., Cabrera, V.M., Gonzalez, A.M., Larruga, J.M., Takeyasu, T., Fuku, N., Guo, L.J., Hirose, R., Fujita, Y., Kurata, M., Shinoda, K., Umetsu, K., Yamada, Y., Oshida, Y., Sato, Y., Hattori, N., Mizuno, Y., Arai, Y., Hirose, N., Ohta, S., Ogawa, O., Tanaka, Y., Kawamori, R., Shamoto-Nagai, M., Maruyama, W., Shimokata, H., Suzuki, R., and Shimodaira, H. (2004). Mitochondrial genome variation in Eastern Asia and the peopling of Japan, Genome Research 14: 1832 – 1850.

Takasaki, S., Kawamura, Y., and Konagaya, A. (2006). Selecting effective siRNA sequences by using radial basis function network and decision tree learning, BMC Bioinformatics 7: s5-s22, doi: 10.1186/147-2105-7-s5-s22.

Takasaki S (2009) Mitochondrial haplogroups associated with Japanese centenarians, Alzheimer's patients, Parkinson's patients, type 2 diabetic patients and healthy non-obese young males. J. Genetics and Genomics. 36: 425–434.

Taylor, R.W., and Turnbull, D.M. (2005). Mitochondrial DNA Mutations in Human Disease, Nature Rev. Genetics 6: 389 – 402.

Vila, M., and Przedborski, S. (2003). Targeting Programmed Cell Death Neurodegenerative Diseases, Nature Rev. Neuro. 4: 1 – 11.

Wallace, D.C. (1999). Mitochondrial Diseases in Man and Mouse, Science 283: 1482 – 1488.

Wu. C.H., and McLarty, J.W. (2000). Neural Networks and Genome Informatics. Elsevier Science Ltd., NY.

7

Noradrenergic Mechanisms in Parkinson's Disease and L-DOPA-Induced Dyskinesia: Hypothesis and Evidences from Behavioural and Biochemical Studies

Amal Alachkar
University of Aleppo
Syria

1. Introduction

The key pathological characteristic of Parkinson's disease PD is the degeneration of dopaminergic neurons in the substantia nigra pars compacta SNc that project to the striatum (Barolin and Horykiewicz 1967). The depletion of dopamine leads to abnormalities of the transmission in striatal projections to the lateral or medial segments of the globus pallidus, or to the substantia nigra reticulata SNr (Brotchie et al, 1993; Albin et al., 1989). It is well known, however, that in PD, besides dopaminergic degeneration, a considerable loss of noradrenergic neurons, as well as, a decrease of noradrenaline levels in several brain regions occurs (Hornykiewicz & Kish 1987).

Interestingly, the neural loss in PD in Locus coreleus is greater than that of dopamine in the substantia nigra (Zarow et al., 2003).

The influence of noradrenergic neurotransmission on dopamine-mediated behaviour has been the focus of several studies over the last four decades, and has confirmed the importance of the relationship between dopaminergic and noradrenergic pathways in the control of locomotor activity. The progressive neurodegeneration of the main noradrenergic nucleus – the locus coeruleus LC – might influence not only the progression of Parkinson's disease but also the response to dopaminergic replacement. Furthermore, additional evidences support the notion that noradrenaline deficit might be relevant for the pathogenesis of long-term complications of L-DOPA treatment such as the wearing-off phenomenon and dyskinesias (Bezard et al., 2001; Obeso et al., 2000; Marsden and Parkes, 1976).

However, in spite of the bulk of data on the influence of the alterations of noradrenergic transmission on locomotor behaviour, much of these data is conflicting and not conclusive. Therefore, definitive conclusions, as to the specific role of the noradrenergic system in the generation of symptoms of Parkinson's disease and L-DOPA-induced dyskinesia LID, cannot yet be drawn.

Based on a number of behavioural studies, demonstrating the alleviation of dyskinesia by α_2 adrenergic receptor antagonists, in addition to other biochemical studies, this chapter aims to test the hypothesis that the noradrenergic system plays a role in the neural mechanisms underlying Parkinson's disease and L-DOPA-induced dyskinesia.

The model presented here suggests that the degeneration of noradrenergic neurons contributes to the pathophysiology and symptomatology of PD, and that the remaining intact noradrenergic neurons exert a compensatory mechanism in PD. Furthermore, we suggest a role for L-DOPA metabolites in the mechanism of LID; this role might be mediated through the activation of α_2 adrenoceptors.

Our data and other studies presented in this chapter demonstrate a potential role for noradrenergic system in Parkinson's disease and LID.

2. Parkinson's disease and L-DOPA-induced dyskinesia

Parkinson's disease is a progressive hypokinetic neurodegenerative disorder, characterised by bradykinesia, rigidity, tremor, akinesia, and abnormal posture. Non-motor symptoms such as cognitive decline, depression, sleep disturbances and autonomic and sensorimotor dysfunction also occur (Marsden, 1990, Remy et al., 2005; Schapira, 2008). The key pathological characteristic of Parkinson's disease is the degeneration of dopaminergic neurons in the substantia nigra that project to the striatum (Barolin and Horykiewicz 1967).

Dopamine neurons degenerate with advancing age more than other neuronal systems in the brain (Fearnley & Lees, 1991). Neurons in the SNc and VTA are lost at a rate of 1% per year in parkinsonian patients compared to 0.5% per year in non-parkinsonian subjects (Scherman et al, 1989). Parkinsonian symptoms become apparent when striatal dopamine levels fall by about 70% (Altar and Marien, 1989). Post-mortem studies show substantial depletion of dopamine in the putamen. In caudal parts of the putamen, dopamine content is less than 1% of control levels, whereas the dopamine content of the caudate nucleus is relatively well preserved i.e. 40% of control levels (Hornykiewicz, 1973; Kish et al, 1988). The degeneration of cells in the SNc is accompanied by the presence of eosinophilic intraneuronal, cytoplasmic inclusions called Lewy bodies, which are characterised by a central core and peripheral halo (McGeer et al, 1988; Quinn et al, 1989). Lewy bodies show immunoreactivity for tubulin and ubiquitin (Jellinger, 1990).

The loss of dopaminergic neurons in the substantia nigra pars compacta, which results in a reduction in the level of dopamine in the striatum, leads to alterations in the activity of striatal output nuclei. This results in changes in the other nuclei basal ganglia, which can be summarized as following: (a) Degeneration of the nigrostriatal pathway, (b) the underactivity of the GABA/dynorphin striato-medial pallidal/SNr nigral pathway, (c) the overactivity of the GABA/enkephalin striato-lateral-pallidal pathway, (d) the overactivity of the subthalamic nucleus, (e) the overactivity of the GABA medial pallidal/SNr (output regions of the basal ganglia) -thalamic projection (Brotchie et al, 1993). The overactivity of basal ganglia output results in increased inhibition of excitatory glutamatergic projections from the thalamus to the cortex. Cortical motor outputs are, thus, underactive leading to the movement paucity in Parkinson's disease (Albin et al., 1989).

Although the predominant pathology of PD is the loss of dopaminergic cells in the substantia nigra, however, there is also degeneration of other neurotransmission systems, such as cholinergic, noradrenergic, serotoninergic and peptidergic brainstem nuclei (Jellinger, 1991).

Some of these alterations in neurotransmitters occur before the appearance of parkinsonian symptoms (Bezard et al, 2001). Noradrenaline (NA) is particularly implicated in certain symptoms of Parkinson's disease. Biochemical analysis revealed that 40-80% of the brain's content of NA is depleted in PD (Agid, et al., 1987; Gerlach et al, 1994).

Current strategies for the treatment of PD still depend largely on the replacement of lost dopamine. Levodopa, a precursor of dopamine, has proved very successful as an antiparkinsonian agent (Cotzias et al 1967). L-DOPA can cross the blood-brain barrier and is converted to dopamine by aromatic amino acid decarboxylase, presumably in the striatum at the synaptic sites of surviving nigrostriatal cells (Melamed et al 1984). However, due to the massive degeneration of nigrostriatal terminals, it is unlikely that the majority of dopamine synthesis occurs in nigrostriatal terminals (Snyder & Zigmond, 1990). Within the striatum, 5-HT terminals, striatal interneurons and glial cells also contain aromatic amino acid decarboxylase, and these sites may play a role in the conversion of L-DOPA to dopamine in the degenerated striatum (Opacka-Juffry, 1995; Mura et al, 1995).

Initially, L-DOPA is successful in reversing parkinsonian symptoms, akinesia, rigidity and tremor. However, as treatment progresses, the effectiveness of L-DOPA treatment decreases and dyskinesia, fluctuations in mobility and freezing episodes, occur (Marsden & Parkes, 1976; Mouradian et al, 1991). With the progress of treatment, the dose of L-DOPA required to induce dyskinesia gradually decreases and the dose of L-DOPA required to alleviate parkinsonian symptoms is increased, thereby, resulting in the development of a narrow therapeutic window (Mouradian et al, 1988).

The mechanism, underlying L-DOPA-induced dyskinesia, is still far from being fully understood. The fact, that dyskinesia results from prolonged replacement of dopamine, suggests that it arises through the overactivity of dopaminergic mechanisms. Similarities in the choreic dyskinesia seen among various brain disorders, i.e. L-DOPA-induced dyskinesia, tardive dyskinesia and hemiballism, has led to the suggestion of a common mechanism for all dyskinesia (Crossman (review) 1990).

According to the most acceptable model, L-DOPA-induced dyskinesia is associated with an imbalance of basal ganglia circuitry in favour of the direct pathway. Data obtained from animal models of PD have implicated a relative underactivity of the indirect pathway, and overactivity of the direct pathway. The net effect of the overactive GABAergic projection in the direct and indirect pathways and the underactive glutamatergic projection of the STN, will lead to the cumulative inhibitory effects on the output nuclei of the basal ganglia. This, in turn, leads to the decrease of the inhibition of thalamocortical neurons and overactivation of cortical motor areas.

- PD.: Decreased activity in the dopaminergic nigrostriatal pathway, Overactivity of the GABA striato-lateral-pallidal pathway, Overactivity of the subthalamic nucleus, Overactivity of the regions of the basal ganglia that project to non-basal ganglia motor regions, i.e., the medial pallidal segment and the SNr (Blandini et al, 2000).

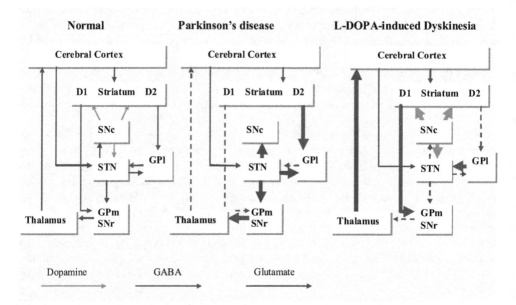

Fig. 1. Diagram illustrating the changes in the organisation of the basal ganglia in Parkinson's disease and L-DOPA-induced Dyskinesia.

- LID: Increased activity in the dopaminergic nigrostriatal pathway, Underactivity of the GABA striato-lateral-pallidal pathway, Underactivity of the subthalamic nucleus, Underactivity of the regions of the basal ganglia that project to non-basal ganglia motor regions, i.e., the medial pallidal segment and the SNr.

3. Noradrenergic system

The main noradrenergic system is the locus coeruleus LC (A6-cell group), in which about 45% of brain noradrenergic cells are present.

The total estimated number of noradrenergic neurons in the LC of the normal young adult human brain ranges from 45,000 to 60,000 (Baker et al, 1989; , German et al., 1988). The vast majority (90%) of LC efferent projections remain ipsilateral (Ader et al., 1980; Mason & Fibiger, 1979; Room et al., 1981). There are two types of LC axonal terminals: regular synaptic terminals, and varicosities that are believed to cause an extra-synaptic release of noradrenaline, which then may diffuse over a distance (Aoki, 1992; Beaudet & Descarries, 1978; Koda et al., 1978; Parnavelas & Papadopoulos, 1989).

The main projections of the LC are to the neocortex, where LC neurons project to all layers of the neocortex, although the density of fibres varies according to the cortical regions and the species (Morrison et al, 1979; Morrison et al, 1982). The LC also sends efferents to the hippocampus, amygdala, septum, thalamus and hypothalamus. Morphologically different types of neurons in the locus coeruleus project to different regions of the CNS (Loughlin, et al, 1986), and the axons of LC neurons are extensively ramified, as one axon may branch up to 100,000 times (Moore & Bloom, 1979). Noradrenaline may co-exist with other neurotransmitters and modulators, and the type of modulators co-existing with NA depends, in part, on species. For instance, noradrenergic neurons have been reported to have immunoreactive staining for enkephalin in cats, vasopressin in rats, and neuropeptide Y (NPY) in rats and humans (Caffe et al, 1985).

The firing activity of noradrenergic neurons in the LC is regulated by somatodendritic autoreceptors of the α_2- adrenergic subtype. These receptors are believed to decrease the firing rate of NA neurons primarily through an increase in potassium conductance.

The firing rate of LC cells is influenced by behavioural activity and sensory input and seems to relate closely to arousal and sleep-waking cycles (Astone –Jones et al, 1991). The LC cells are completely inactive during rapid-eye-movement (REM) sleep (Aston-Jones & Bloom, 1981). The changes in cell firing in sleep-waking cycles suggest a contribution of LC to the mechanisms controlling sleep-waking states (Foote et al, 1980; Mallick, 2002).

Numbers of LC cells and the concentration of brain noradrenaline decline with age in normal brain respectively by 25% and 50% between the fourth and ninth decades of life (Mann, 1983; Mann et al, 1983).

4. Noradrenaline functions

Electrophysiological and behavioural studies have revealed an important role for noradrenaline in attention, arousal and waking (Grant and Redmond 1984; Kumar, 2003). There is an increase in the activity of the LC in rats and primates during high awareness, whereas the activity is decreased during grooming, feeding and sleeping (Grant and Redmond 1984). Furthermore, the α_2 adrenoceptor agonist clonidine increases the total duration of sleep and significantly reduces the duration of REM sleep. In contrast, yohimbine, an α_2 adrenoceptor antagonist, reverses the effects of clonidine (Autret et al, 1977).

Noradrenaline has also been implicated in controlling feeding behaviour (Goldman et al, 1985). Injection of noradrenaline or the α_2 receptor agonist clonidine into the area of the paraventricular nucleus (PVN), caused a potent feeding response in satiated animals, an effect probably mediated via α_2 adrenoceptors located postsynaptically (Weiss &Leibowitz, 1985; Goldman et al, 1985). Further studies have suggested that feeding behaviour is stimulated by low levels of clonidine, and decreased by further production of noradrenaline (Bungo et al, 1999).

The noradrenaline system has also been implicated in anxiety-related behaviours since α_2 agonists are of clinical benefit in treating some types of anxiety (Hoehen-Saric et al, 1981; Crespi, 2009), while α_2 antagonists elicit intense anxiety (Charney et al, 1983; Graeff, 1994). However, it is not clear whether these effects are mediated through pre-or postsynaptic adrenoceptors. A study by Tanak et al., has suggested that the increased release of noradrenaline in the locus coeruleus is, in part, involved in the frustration of anxiety and/or fear in animals exposed to stress (Tanaka et al, 2000). On the other hand, genetic studies on α_{2a} adrenoceptor knock-out mice suggest that α_{2a} may play a protective role in some types of depression and anxiety (Schramm et al, 2001).

Noradrenaline is also involved in cognitive processes such as memory, learning and selective attention (Franowicz, & Arnsten, 1998; Franowicz et al, 2002; Gibbs & Summers, 2002; Marrs et al, 2005; Timofeeva & Levin, 2008). In Alzheimer Type Dementia (ATD), both the concentration of noradrenaline and the noradrenaline transporters sites are significantly decreased in a number of brain regions including the Locus coeruleus, cingulate gyrus, putamen, hypothalamus, medial thalamic nucleus, and raphe area (Arai et al, 1984; Tejani et al, 1993).

Evidence has accumulated suggesting that noradrenaline is also involved in controlling body temperature (Lin et al, 1981, Sallinen et al, 1997), endocrine secretion (Endroczi et al, 1978; Valet et al, 1989; Ruffolo et al, 1991), and sexual behaviour (Morales et al, 1987; Guiliano & Rampin, 1997).

5. Noradrenaline in the basal ganglia

The synthesis of noradrenaline (Glowinski & Iverson, 1966) and its release (Coyle & Henry, 1973) was initially demonstrated in the striatum. Later studies revealed that the striatum receives little noradrenergic projection from the locus coeruleus and has low levels of dopamine β-hydroxylase (Swanson & Hartman, 1975). Nevertheless, the striatum shows high levels of α_2 adrenoceptor gene expression (mRNA) (Scheinin et al, 1994) and high radioligand binding to α_{2C} adrenoceptors (Uhlen et al, 1997). Noradrenergic terminals and uptake sites have also been demonstrated in the SNc (Fuxe, 1965), subthalamic nucleus (Carpenter et al, 1981b; Parent & Hazrati, 1995; Belujon et al, 2007) and the SNr (Gehlert et al, 1993).

The precise role of noradrenaline in the basal ganglia is not yet clear. However, the noradrenergic inputs to the basal ganglia appear to have a modulatory effect on other neurotransmitters in different structures of the basal ganglia.

Noradrenaline derived from the LC may induce an inhibition of striatal neurons trans-synaptically activated by nigral stimulation (Fujimoto et al, 1981). It has been shown that the α_2 antagonist yohimbine increases the synthesis and release of dopamine in the striatum, while the agonist clonidine can reverse this effect (Anden and Grabowska, 1976). α_2 presynaptic heteroreceptors also seem to regulate the release of amino acid neurotransmitters such as glutamic acid, aspartic acid, GABA as evaluated with synaptosoms (Bristow and Bennett, 1988, Kamisaki, et al, 1992, Bickler and Hansen, 1996, Pralong and Magistretti, 1995). Immunocytochemical studies reveal that 94% of spiny GABAergic neurons in the striatum contain α_{2C} adrenergic receptors (Holmberg et al, 1999), which are negatively coupled to adenylyl cyclase (Zhang et al, 1999). These α_{2C} receptors are thought to play a regulatory role on the direct and indirect pathways of the basal ganglia by modulating GABA transmission. Recent studies on α_2 receptor knock-out mice indicate that α_{2a} and α_{2C} adrenoceptors are located on different neurons in the striatum, and that striatal GABA release is mediated by the activation of α_{2C} but not α_{2a} adrenoceptor (Zhang & Ordway, 2003). These authors suggest that the effect of α_{2C} on GABA release might be mediated by dopamine.

In the basal ganglia, α adrenoceptors are mainly found in the striatum, globus pallodus, substantia nigra pars compacta SNc and substantia nigra pars reticulata SNr (Unnerstall et al, 1984; Boyajian et al, 1987; Uhlen et al, 1997; Winzer-Srhan et al, 1997).

Noradrenergic pathways might have a significant role in regulating basal ganglia function and thus motor activity by modulating the spontaneous activity of the STN neurons. Accordingly, noradrenaline has been reported to induce stimulation of the firing rate of a neuronal subpopulation of the subthalamic nucleus, and this stimulation was suggested to be mediated through the activation of α_1 adrenoceptors (Arcos et al, 2003).

The modulation of dopamine neurone firing by the noradrenergic system of the locus coeruleus in the rat has provided further evidence for the role of noradrenaline in regulating the activity of the basal ganglia. Interestingly, noradrenaline has been reported to evoke excitation followed by inhibition of the electrical activity of dopaminergic cells (Grenhoff et al, 1993; Grenhoff et al, 1995).

The SNr represents, with medial segment of globus pallidus, the main output regions of the basal ganglia and therefore, plays a crucial role in movement initiation. The GABAergic neurons in the substantia nigra are spontaneously active and the modulation of their activity would significantly influence the basal ganglia functions. Indeed, there is evidence supporting the regulatory action of noradrenaline upon the neurons of the SNr. Noradrenaline has been demonstrated to increase the tonic firing of principal cells in the SNr (Berretta et al, 2000). On the other hand, we demonstrated the stimulatory effects of both the activation and blockade of α_2 adrenergic receptors on the release of GABA from slices of the SNr. (Alachkar et al, 2006).

6. Noradrenaline- dopamine interaction

The interaction between dopamine and noradrenaline systems has been demonstrated, previously, in the brain. Dopamine, for instance, has long been demonstrated to have stimulatory actions upon noradrenergic neurons in the locus coeruleus (Persson and Waldeck, 1970). On the other hand, noradrenaline has been shown to reduce the spontaneous firing of dopaminergic neurons in the SNc (White & Wang, 1984), although, other workers have reported excitatory responses of the SNc to the stimulation of the locus coeruleus (Grenhoff, 1993). Other studies have provided evidences for the mutual inhibition of dopaminergic and noradrenergic systems (Persson & Waldeck, 1970; Guiard et al, 2008). A number of studies indicate, interestingly, that dopamine is co-released with noradrenaline from noradrenergic neurons in the locus coeruleus (Anden et al, 1973; Devoto et al, 2001).

On the other hand, dopamine may activate α_2 adrenoceptors in more than a region in the brain (Segawa et al, 1998; Cornil et al, 2002; Alachkar et al, 2010a). It is well documented that a molecular relationship exists, at the level of the amino acid sequence, between α_2 and dopamine D2 receptors, in that D2 dopamine receptors are more closely related to α_2 adrenoceptors than to D1 dopaminergic receptors (Harrison et al, 1991).

NA was found to act as a D1 dopaminergic agonist (Kubrusly et al., 2007), and mimic the effect of DA on the DA D2 receptor (Onali et al., 1985). Furthermore, it was demonstrated that NA binds to the human DA D4 receptor with high affinity (Lanau et al., 1997; Newman-Tancredi et al., 1997) and 10% of total D2-like receptors are of the DA D4 receptor located in the caudate putamen (Tarazi et al., 1997).

α_2 adrenoceptor mRNA, type A and C, is present in high levels in the striatum and locus coeruleus (Nicholas et al, 1993; Scheinin et al, 1994, our unpublished results), with receptors binding located in the striatum, and SNr (Rosin et al, 1996; Lee et al, 1998a,b).

The presence of noradrenaline uptake sites in the SNr (Gehlert et al, 1995; Strazielle et al, 1999) indicates noradrenaline release in this nucleus.

The NA could affect the activity of the SNr through their direct noradrenergic projections and their indirect influence by the action of SNc and other parts of basal ganglia.

7. Noradrenaline in Parkinson's disease

In Parkinson's disease, a significant loss of noradrenergic cells of the locus coeruleus and the noradrenergic pathways occurs, in addition to the degeneration of the nigrostriatal dopaminergic pathway, (Hornykiewicz & Kish 1987; Zarow et al., 2003). Moreover, there is a considerable decrease in NA levels in a number of brain structures including the hypothalamus, cerebral cortex, substantia nigra and caudate nucleus in patients with this disease (Fahn et al, 1971; Rinne & Sonninen, 1973; Kish et al, 1984). The significance of the loss of LC cells to Parkinson's disease is still largley unknown. It is possible that noradrenergic depletion contributes to the degeneration of other brain nuclei. Postmortem studies have revealed that the symptoms of depression and dementia in PD were associated with a significant loss of noradrenergic neurons in the LC and NA depletion in the cortex (Zweig et al., 1993; Bosboom et al., 2004; Remy et al., 2005; Ridderinkhof et al., 2004; Ramos and Arnsten, 2007). LC-noradrenergic neurotransmitter system may be involved in the pathogenesis of non-motor symptoms in PD. A decrease in α_2 receptor density in the prefrontal cortex has also been shown in animal models of Parkinson's disease (Mavridis et al, 1991). Administration of α_2-adrenergic agonist was demonstrated to improve the cognitive impairments in PD patients (Remy et al., 2005; Riekkinen and Riekkinen, 1999).

The great extent to which LC cell loss occurs in PD is emphasized by the study by Zarow et al. who, interestingly, demonstrated that the greatest loss of neurons in PD was found in the LC (83.2%). The degree of cell loss in the LC seemed to be even more extensive than that observed in the substantia nigra (77.8% loss) (Zarow et al. 2003). Significant depletions (>80%) of noradrenaline in the substantia nigra pars compacta and reticulata, of postmortem PD brains have also been described (Taquet et al., 1982).

The NA depletion in the LC was proved to decrease DA release in the striatum (Lategan et al., 1990; Lategan et al., 1992). Furthermore, clinical studies have indicated that some motor symptoms of PD are likely to result from noradrenergic lesions (Grimbergen et al., 2009). These findings suggest the implication of the LC-noradrenergic system in the pathophysiology of PD.

Experimental data suggest that the LC noradrenaline system may have a neuroprotective role on dopaminergic SN neurons (Gesi et al, 2000). For instance, noradrenaline depletion significantly increased MPTP- as well as methylamphetamine-induced striatal dopamine depletion in mice and monkeys (Forani et al, 1995, Marien et al 1993; Archer and Fredriksson, 2006; Nishi et al., 1991). Furthermore, lesions of LC by 6-OHDA in MPTP treated monkeys produced a more significant depletion and greater loss of substantia nigra cell compared to normal controls, and impaired the recovery which usually occurs from the parkinsonian manifestations induced by MPTP (Mavridis et al, 1991; Bing et al, 1994). A potentiation of parkinsonian symptoms following locus coeruleus noradrenaline depletion has been reported in 6-OHDA-lesioned rats (Srinivasan & Schmidt, 2003).

The mechanism by which the locus coeruleus may protect dopaminergic neurons is still unknown. The activation of α_2 adrenoceptors by clonidine, α_2 agonist, has been demonstrated to suppress MPTP-induced reduction of striatal dopamine and tyrosine hydroxylase activity in mice (Bristow and Bennett, 1988; Fornai et al, 1995).

Noradrenaline may exert its neuroprotective effects by facilitating the release of trophic factors, such as the nerve growth factor NGF; this was suggested to occur through an action on β-adrenoceptors on the glial cells (Mochetti et al, 1989). Noradrenaline may suppress the formation of toxic MPP^+ from MPTP by inhibiting the production of glial monoamine oxidase B in the substantia nigra (Stone and Ariano, 1989). Interestingly, the administration of L-threo-3, 4 dihydroxyphenylserine (L-threo-DOPS) an immediate precursor of noradrenaline, seems to alleviate parkinsonian symptoms (Narabayashi et al, 1984). Although L-threo DOPS causes an increase in dopamine as well as noradrenaline levels, its anti-parkinsonian action was inhibited by adrenoceptor antagonists and dopamine β-hydroxylase inhibitors. The α_2 adrenoceptor antagonist R47 243 has been found to reverse some parkinsonian signs in a monkey in which MPTP's effects had been progressive, by a mechanism that is still unknown (Colpaert et al, 1991). On the other hand, blockade of α_2 adrenoceptors counteracted to some extent the development of parkinsonian symptoms and neurochemical alterations in the rotenone model of Parkinson's disease (Alam et al, 2009). In addition Belujon et al have provided behavioral and electrophysiological evidence for the noradrenergic modulation of subthalamic nucleus activity in intact and 6-hydroxydopamine-lesioned rats. The authors have shown that the firing of STN neurons is controlled by noradrenergic system through the activation of α_1- and α_2 adrenergic receptors (Belujon et al, 2007).

Firing activity of LC-noradrenergic neurons was demonstrated to increase in rats after the SNc lesion (Guiard et al, 2008; Wang et al., 2009), which may imply an overactivity of LC-noradrenergic neurons and enhanced influence of LC in rats with SNc lesion.

On the other hand, lesions of the LC in rat models of PD caused further hyperactivity of SNr neurons implying that LC-noradrenergic system may play a role in decreasing the activity of the output regions of the basal ganglia (wang et al, 2010). Intact noradrenergic neurons of the LC were believed to play a crucial role in the compensational mechanism after the dopaminergic depletion in the SNc (Gesi et al., 2000; Rommelfanger and Weinshenker, 2007).

8. Noradrenaline and L-DOPA-induced dyskinesia

Progressive neurodegeneration of the noradrenergic neurons in the locus coeruleus was suggested to influence the response to dopaminergic replacement (Cotzias et al., 1967), and the pathogenesis of long-term complications of L-DOPA treatment (Bezard et al., 2001; Marsden and Parkes, 1976; Obeso et al., 2000).

The involvement of noradrenergic transmission in L-DOPA-induced dyskinesia has been the focus of several investigations. This was based on the well documented interaction between dopaminergic and noradrenergic system. Early studies on reserpine-treated rats revealed that the hyperkinesia induced by L-DOPA was mediated via activation of the noradrenergic system (Anden et al, 1969; Stromber & Svensson, 1971). A number of studies substantiated evidence that the noradrenergic system may have a modulatory effect on L-DOPA-induced dyskinesia. Gomez-Mancilla and Bedard (1993) investigated the effects of several agents acting on the noradrenergic system in the brain on L-DOPA-induced dyskinesia. They reported that the α_2 adrenergic receptor antagonist, yohimbine, decreased L-DOPA-induced dyskinesia without reducing the anti-parkinsonian action of L-DOPA, in MPTP-treated monkeys. Further studies have reported that the reduction of dyskinesia can be mediated by blocking the actions of α_2 adrenergic receptors, shown using a number of α_2 antagonists (Henry et al 1999, Fox et al 2001; Grondin et al, 2000; Rascol, 2001; Savola et al, 2003; Dekundy et al, 2007). The mechanism by which α_2 antagonists can alleviate L-DOPA-induced dyskinesia is unknown; however, activation of α_2 adrenoceptors on the striatal output neuron terminals has been suggested to reduce GABA release and inhibition of the lateral segment of the globus pallidus (GPl) in the indirect pathway (Henry et al, 1999). Therefore, blockade at these sites may up-regulate the inhibitory striatopallidal connections and reduce STN inhibition and dyskinesia. The other explanation for the effect of α_2 adrenoceptor antagonists in reducing L-DOPA-induced dyskinesia may be the blockade of the action of noradrenaline synthesised from levodopa on α_{2c} receptors in the basal ganglia (Fox et al, 2001). There is evidence that local administration of NA into the lesioned striatum can induce dyskinetic movements in rats in a similar manner to intrastriatal L-DOPA treatment (Buck & Ferger, 2009).

On the other hand, noradrenaline synthesized from exogenous L-DOPA administered in Parkinson's disease therapy may, in part, be involved in the locomotor activity produced by L-DOPA (Dolphin et al, 1976). This implies that at least some symptoms of LID are mediated through the activation of the noradrenergic system. Therefore, the therapeutic actions of α_2 antagonists may be correlated with this noradrenergic disruption in Parkinson's disease and LID.

Fox et al., have reported that α_2 antagonism reduces L-DOPA-induced dyskinesia but did not affect apomorphine-induced dyskinesia suggesting that L-DOPA-induced dyskinesia but not dopamine agonist-induced dyskinesia, involves activation of adrenoceptors (Fox et al, 2001). The authors suggested that the pharmacological characteristics of the neural mechanisms underlying levodopa-induced dyskinesia and dopamine agonist-induced dyskinesia in parkinsonism are distinct, at least with respect to the involvement of α_2 adrenoceptors.

9. Noradrenergic mechanisms in PD and LID: A theory

9.1 Parkinson's disease PD

We present here a model to explain the mechanism by which noradrenergic system may modulate the activity of the basal ganglia in PD.This model attempts to answer the question of whether noradrenergic abnormalities reflect a response to, or the cause of, the PD. Our scenario is based on the discussion above and most importantly the following three observations:

- Certain evidences support the belief that LC lesion may exacerbate the abnormal activity of basal ganglia in PD, resulting in a further overactivity of the SNr neurons. This implies that LC-noradrenergic system may play a role in decreasing the activity of the output regions of the basal ganglia in PD (wang et al, 2010).
- Further evidence indicates that the firing activity of LC-noradrenergic neurons increases after the SNc lesion (Guiard et al, 2008; Wang et al., 2009), which may imply an overactivity of LC-noradrenergic neurons; and enhanced influence of LC in PD.
- Several studies have described the anti-parkinsonian effects of the blockade of α_2 inhibitory receptors. Although the site of action of these receptors is not known for certain, the data of other several studies conform to a model where alpha-2 antagonists produce their effects in the SNr by interacting with GABAergic transmission.

According to our model, changes in Parkinson's disease that occur in noradrenergic transmission contribute to the mechanism of PD, and partially compensate for the degeneration of the dopaminergic system.

Based on the discussion above, we propose that in Parkinson's disease, the degeneration of 83% of LC neurons and depletion of noradrenaline exacerbate the Parkinsonian symptoms through increasing the overactivity of the substantia nigra pars reticulata. On the other hand, the destruction of the dopamine-containing cells in the SNc results in a decrease in the inhibition, by dopamine, on the firing of the locus coeruleus and therefore, the remaining intact noradrenergic neurons of the LC are deemed to play a crucial role in the compensational mechanism after the dopaminergic depletion in the SNc (Gesi et al., 2000; Rommelfanger and Weinshenker, 2007). Noradrenaline released from overactive remaining LC neurons is thought to act as an inhibitory transmitter on α_2 adrenoceptors located on the GABAergic striatal projecting neurons, and on the neurons of SNr. This would decrease the firing rate and the activity of the inhibitory GABAergic projection of SNr (which is overactive in PD) to the motor regions of the thalamus, and hence alleviate Parkinsonian symptoms. Accordingly, noradrenaline may contribute to the pathological and the compensational mechanisms in Parkinson's disease. The prevalence of one of these two contradictory effects of noradrenergic system depends mainly on the extent of the degeneration of LC cells. The greater degeneration of LC noradrenergic neurons indicates more extensive abnormalities of the basal ganglia and overactivity of SNr, and thus further potentiation of the Parkinsonian symptoms.

9.2 L-DOPA-induced dyskinesia LID
Administration of L-DOPA with an AADC inhibitor, NSD1015, produced hyperlocomotor activity in reserpine-treated rats (Alachkar et al, 2010b). It seems likely that L-DOPA, or one or more of its metabolites not formed via routes involving direct decarboxylation of L-DOPA, are responsible for the generation of hyperkinesia. Significantly, α_2 receptor antagonist, rauwolscine, reduced centre vertical movement induced by L-DOPA and NSD1015 and shifted the time-course response curve to the left, (i.e. it caused earlier onset of L-DOPA and NSD1015 action). Thus, the behavioural effect of L-DOPA and NSD1015 given together is exerted, at least, in part, by the noradrenergic system.

The prediction, arising from studies on the behavioural effects of L-DOPA, is that manipulation of α_2 or/and dopamine receptors by L-DOPA or its metabolites may result in hyperlocomotor activity. This prediction was tested in a study by radioligand binding in membranes prepared from cell lines expressing α_2 and dopaminergic receptors (Alachkar et al, 2010a). We reported that 3-MT bound to α_{2a} receptors with high affinity compared to α_{2C} adrenoceptors and dopaminergic receptors. The finding in the same study that dopamine bound to α_2 adrenoceptors with relatively high affinities, provides evidence confirming previous reports on the direct activation of α_2 adrenoceptors by dopamine (Cornil et al, 2002; Zhang et al, 1999).

A mechanism underlying the hyperkinesia induced by L-DOPA following the inhibition of central decarboxylase was suggested. According to these results, L-DOPA is metabolised in two steps leading to the formation of 3-MT, which will cause hyperkinesia (Nakazato & Akiyama, 2002; Nakazato, 2002), possibly through interaction with D1, or α_{2a} adrenoceptors (Alachkar et al, 2010a). The reduction of vertical hyperlocomotor activity by rauwolscine supports that 3-MT interacts with α_2 adrenoceptors (Alachkar et al, 2010b).

In Parkinson's disease, there is a decrease in the activity (Gjedde et al., 1993; Kuwabara et al., 1995) and expression (Ichinose et al., 1994) of the enzyme aromatic amino acid decarboxylase AADC. Interestingly, treatment with L-DOPA produces a further decrease in AADC (Tanaka et al., 1973; Fisher et al, 2000) and an increase of COMT (Liu et al, 2000; Zhao et al, 2001). In view of these observations, we propose that following long-term treatment with L-DOPA, the major portion of exogenous L-DOPA will not be metabolised to dopamine, instead a large portion of L-DOPA will be methylated to 3,O, methyldopa. 3-O-methyldopa has a longer half-life than L-DOPA itself (15 hours vs ½ hour) (Kuruma et al, 1971; Cedarbaum, 1987) and, consequently, 3,O,methyldopa formed from exogenous L-DOPA accumulates in the plasma and the brain to be subsequently metabolised slowly (Kuruma et al, 1971). The decarboxylation of 3,O,methyldopa leads to the formation of 3-MT. The significance of methoxy groups in the production of abnormal induced movements was the focus of very early studies (Ericsson et al, 1971). A number of early studies suggested that the occupation of the meta position by a OCH_3 group in the absence of similar groups at the para position caused hyperkinesias in rats (Hornykiewicz, 1966) and induced abnormal movements (Huntington chorea) in humans (Ericsson & Wertman, 1971). More recent studies have confirmed these early finding, as 3-MT was demonstrated to induce hyperactivity in rats (Nakazato & Akiyama, 2002; Nakazato, 2002). As a result, 3-MT seems to be the candidate metabolite to induce dyskinesia following long term treatment with L-DOPA in Parkinson's disease.

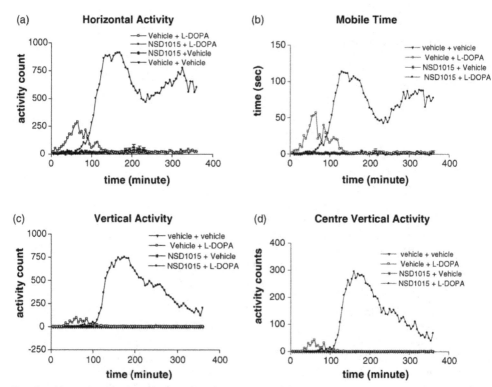

Fig. 2. **Effect of NSD1015 on the stimulant action of L-DOPA on locomotor activity.**

3-MT was found to bind to α_{2a} adrenoceptors with relatively high affinity (Alachkar et al, 2010a). The pharmacological experiments to determine whether 3-MT acts as an agonist or antagonist at α_{2a} adrenoceptors have not yet been undertaken. However, the similarities in the chemical structures between 3-MT and other catecholamines such as α-methylnoradrenaline and epinephrine, which are known to activate α_2 adrenoceptors, suggest that 3-MT may act as an agonist at these receptors. According to the present scenario, a high concentration of 3,O,methyldopa, and hence 3-MT will occur in Parkinson's disease and following long-term treatment with L-DOPA. The 3-MT will then bind to α_{2a} receptors located presynaptically on the locus coeruleus terminals in the SNr. This hypothesis is supported by the finding of Mela et al. (2007) who demonstrated an increase in extracellular GABA release after administration of L-DOPA in dyskinetic rats in the substantia nigra pars reticulata (Mela et al., 2007).

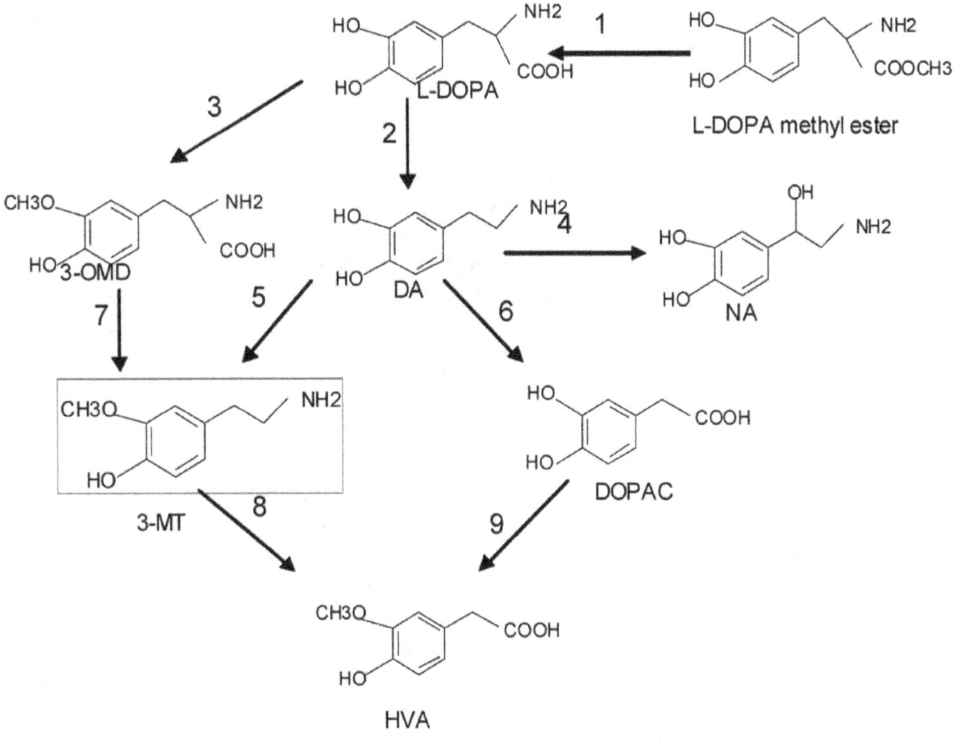

Fig. 3. l-DOPA and dopamine metabolic pathways. Abbreviations: l-DOPA, l-3,4-dihydroxyphenylalanine; DA dopamine; NA noradrenaline; 3-OMD 3-O-methyldopa; 3-MT 3-methoxytyramine; DOPAC dihydroxyphenylacetic acid; HVA homovanilic acid. (1) Esterase or hydrolase; (2) aromatic amino acid decarboxylase AADC; (3) catechol O-methyl transferase COMT; (4) dopamine _-hydroxylase BDH; (5) COMT; (6) monoamine oxidase MAO; (7) unknown; (8) MAO; (9) COMT (Alachkar et al, 2010a).

The activation of α_2 inhibitory autoreceptors would result in an inhibition of noradrenaline release from these terminals and, therefore, a decrease in the inhibitory tone on GABA release from striato-nigral projection to the SNr. This leads to the increase of the activity of the GABAergic direct pathway, resulting in an increase of the inhibition of the output regions of the basal ganglia, counteracting the underactivity of this structure, which is the key pathological mechanism of LID. Thus, the abnormalities in noradrenergic transmission may contribute to, or facilitate, the development of LID.

Previous experimental studies have demonstrated that α_2 adrenoceptor antagonists such as yohimbine reduce L-DOPA-induced dyskinesia in rodent (Lundblad et al., 2002; Dekundy et al., 2007) as well as primate models (Gomez-Mancilla and Bedard, 1993). Moreover, some α_2 adrenoceptor antagonists like idazoxan and fipamezole have shown antidyskinetic efficacy without compromising the anti-parkinsonian action of L-DOPA in monkey studies (Grondin et al., 2000; Fox et al., 2001; Savola et al., 2003) and clinical trials.

A series of behavioural studies have demonstrated the therapeutic benefits of non-selective α_2 antagonists in reducing LID in animal models of Parkinson's disease (Henry et al, 1999; Gomez-mancilla & Bedard, 1993). The anti-dyskinetic effects of the α_{2a} selective antagonist fipamezole in non-human primate model of PD have been demonstrated (Savola et al, 2003). It was suggested in this study that in LID, the activation of α_2 adrenoceptors that regulate the activity of the direct pathway, by L-DOPA or its metabolites, may facilitate LID (Savola et al, 2003). Although the exact site of α_2 adrenoceptor antagonist was not determined in the study by Savola et al, the authors have reached a similar conclusion by suggesting the involvement of the direct pathway in the mechanism of α_2 adrenoceptor antagonists.

According to the previous discussion, the anti-dyskinetic effect of α_2 adrenoceptors can be simply explained by the blockade, by the antagonist, of the effect of 3-MT at the inhibitory presynaptic α_{2a} in the terminals of locus coeruleus projection to the substantia nigra, resulting in facilitation of noradrenaline release. Noradrenaline, subsequently, exerts an inhibitory action on the GABAergic projection in the direct pathway, counteracting the overactivity of this pathway.

10. Conclusion

In conclusion, the discussions presented in this review demonstrate a potential role for noradrenergic system in Parkinson's disease and LID. Several lines of evidence suggest that the noradrenergic system regulates the activity of the direct pathway of the basal ganglia, through presynaptic α_2 receptors located in the SNr, and the indirect pathway through pre- and postsynaptic α_2 in the striatum, and α_2 and α_2 in the subthalamic nucleus. The model presented here suggests that the degeneration of noradrenergic neurons contributes to the pathophysiology and symptomatology of PD, and that the remaining intact noradrenergic neurons exert a compensatory mechanism in PD. Furthermore, we suggest a role for L-DOPA metabolites in the mechanism of LID; this role might be mediated through the activation of α_2 adrenoceptors. According to this model, the anti-dyskinesic action of α_2 antagonists might be mediated by the blockade of α_{2a} adrenoceptors located in the terminals of locus coeruleus projection to the SNr.

11. References

Ader, J.P., P. Room, F. Postema, J. Korf, Bilaterally diverging axon collaterals and contralateral projections from rat locus coeruleus neurons, demonstrated by fluorescent retrograde double labeling and norepinephrine metabolism, J. Neural Transm. 49 (1980) 207-208. ISSN: 0300-9564

Agid, Y., F. Javoy-Agid, M. Ruberg (1987). "Biochemistry of neurotransmitters in Parkinson's disease In: Marsden CD, Fahn S, eds. Movement Disorders. New York: Butterworth & Co. 1987;166-230.

Noradrenergic Mechanisms in Parkinson's Disease and L-DOPA-Induced Dyskinesia: Hypothesis and Evidences
from Behavioural and Biochemical Studies

143

Alachkar, A., Brotchie, J. M., Jones, O. (2006). "alpha2-Adrenoceptor-mediated modulation of the release of GABA and noradrenaline in the rat substantia nigra pars reticulata." Neurosci Lett 395(2): 138-42. ISSN: 0304-3940

Alachkar, A., Brotchie, J. M., Jones, O. (2010a) "Binding of dopamine and 3-methoxytyramine as l-DOPA metabolites to human alpha(2)-adrenergic and dopaminergic receptors." Neurosci Res 67(3): 245-9. ISSN: 1872-8111

Alachkar, A., Brotchie, J. M., Jones, O. (2010b) "Locomotor response to L-DOPA in reserpine-treated rats following central inhibition of aromatic L-amino acid decarboxylase: further evidence for non-dopaminergic actions of L-DOPA and its metabolites." Neurosci Res 68(1): 44-50. ISSN: 1872-8111

Alam, M., W. Danysz, Schmidt, W. J. Dekundy, A. (2009). "Effects of glutamate and alpha2-noradrenergic receptor antagonists on the development of neurotoxicity produced by chronic rotenone in rats." Toxicol Appl Pharmacol 240(2): 198-207. ISSN: 1096-0333

Albin, R. L., J. W. Aldridge, A. B.Young, S.Gilman (1989). "Feline subthalamic nucleus neurons contain glutamate-like but not GABA-like or glycine-like immunoreactivity." Brain Res 491(1): 185-8. ISSN: 0006-8993

Altar, C. A. and M. R. Marien (1989). "Preservation of dopamine release in the denervated striatum." Neurosci Lett 96(3): 329-34. ISSN: 0304-3940

Anden, N. and M. Grabowska (1976). "Pharmacological evidence for a stimulation of dopamine neurons by noradrenaline neurons in the brain." Eur J Pharmacol 39(2): 275-82. ISSN: 0014-2999

Anden, N. E., A. Carlsson, J. Haggendal, (1969). "Adrenergic mechanisms." Annu Rev Pharmacol 9: 119-34. ISSN: 0066-4251

Anden, N. E., C. V. Atack, T. H. Svensson, (1973). "Release of dopamine from central noradrenaline and dopamine nerves induced by a dopamine-beta-hydroxylase inhibitor." J Neural Transm 34(2): 93-100. ISSN: 0300-9564

Aoki, C., Beta-adrenergic receptors: astrocytic localization in the adult visual cortex and their relation to catecholamine axon terminals as revealed by electron microscopic immunocytochemistry, J. Neurosci. 12 (1992) 781–792. ISSN: 0270-6474

Arai, H., K. Kosaka, R. izuka (1984). "Changes of biogenic amines and their metabolites in postmortem brains from patients with Alzheimer-type dementia." J Neurochem 43(2): 388-93. ISSN: 0022-3042

Archer, T., Fredriksson, A., 2006. Influence of noradrenaline denervation on MPTP-induced deficits in mice. J.Neural Transm. 113, 1119–1129. ISSN: 0300-9564

Arcos, D., A. Sierra, A. Nunez, G. Flores, J. Aceves, J. A. Arias-Montano (2003). "Noradrenaline increases the firing rate of a subpopulation of rat subthalamic neurons through the activation of alpha1-adrenoceptors." Neuropharmacology 45(8): 1070-9. ISSN: 0028-3908

Aston-Jones, G. and F. E. Bloom (1981). "Activity of norepinephrine-containing locus coeruleus neurons in behaving rats anticipates fluctuations in the sleep-waking cycle." J Neurosci 1(8): 876-86. ISSN: 0270-6474

Aston-Jones, G., C. Chiang, T. Alexinsky (1991). "Discharge of noradrenergic locus coeruleus neurons in behaving rats and monkeys suggests a role in vigilance." Prog Brain Res 88: 501-20. ISSN: 0079-6123

Autret, A., M. Minz, T. Beillevaire, H. P. Cathala, H. Schmitt (1977). "Effect of clonidine on sleep patterns in man." Eur J Clin Pharmacol 12(5): 319-22. ISSN: 0031-6970

Baker, K.G., I. Tork, J.P. Hornung, P. Halasz, The human locus coeruleus complex: an immunohistochemical and three dimensional reconstruction study, Exp. Brain Res. 77 (1989) 257– 270. ISSN: 0014-4819

Barolin, G. S. and O. Hornykiewicz (1967). "[On the diagnostic value of homovanillic acid in the cerebrospinal fluid]." Wien Klin Wochenschr 79(44): 815-8. ISSN: 0043-5325

Beaudet, A., L. Descarries, The monoamine innervation of rat cerebral cortex: synaptic and nonsynaptic axon terminals, Neuroscience 3 (1978) 851–860. ISSN: 0306-4522

Belujon, P., Bezard, E.,Taupignon,A., Bioulac, B., Benazzouz,A., 2007. Noradrenergic modulation of subthalamic nucleus activity: behavioral and electrophysiological evidence in intact and 6-hydroxydopamine-lesioned rats. J. Neurosci. 27, 9595–9606. ISSN: 1529-2401

Berretta, N., G. Bernardi, N. B. Mercuri (2000). "Alpha(1)-adrenoceptor-mediated excitation of substantia nigra pars reticulata neurons." Neuroscience 98(3): 599-604. ISSN: 0306-4522

Bezard, E., P. Ravenscroft, C. E. Gross, A. R. Crossman, J. M. Brotchie (2001). "Upregulation of striatal preproenkephalin gene expression occurs before the appearance of parkinsonian signs in 1-methyl-4-phenyl- 1,2,3,6-tetrahydropyridine monkeys." Neurobiol Dis 8(2): 343-50. ISSN: 0969-9961

Bickler, P. E. and B. M. Hansen (1996). "Alpha 2-adrenergic agonists reduce glutamate release and glutamate receptor-mediated calcium changes in hippocampal slices during hypoxia." Neuropharmacology 35(6): 679-87. ISSN: 0028-3908

Bing, G., Y. Zhang, Y. Watanabe, B. S. McEwen, E. A. Stone (1994). "Locus coeruleus lesions potentiate neurotoxic effects of MPTP in dopaminergic neurons of the substantia nigra." Brain Res 668(1-2): 261-5. ISSN: 0006-8993

Bosboom, J., Stoffers, D., Wolters, E., 2004. Cognitive dysfunction and dementia in Parkinson's disease. J. Neural Transm. 111, 1303–1315. ISSN: 0300-9564

Boyajian, C. L., S. E. Loughlin, F. M. Leslie (1987). "Anatomical evidence for alpha-2 adrenoceptor heterogeneity: differential autoradiographic distributions of [3H]rauwolscine and [3H]idazoxan in rat brain." J Pharmacol Exp Ther 241(3): 1079-91. ISSN: 0022-3565

Bristow, L. J. and G. W. Bennett (1988). "Biphasic effects of intra-accumbens histamine administration on spontaneous motor activity in the rat; a role for central histamine receptors." Br J Pharmacol 95(4): 1292-302. ISSN: 0007-1188

Brotchie, J., A. Crossman, I. Mitchell, S. Duty, C. Carroll, A. Cooper, B. Henry, N. Hughes, Y. Maneuf (1993). "Chemical signalling in the globus pallidus in parkinsonism." Prog Brain Res 99: 125-39. ISSN: 0079-6123

Buck, K. and B. Ferger (2009). "Comparison of intrastriatal administration of noradrenaline and l-DOPA on dyskinetic movements: a bilateral reverse in vivo microdialysis study in 6-hydroxydopamine-lesioned rats." Neuroscience 159(1): 16-20. ISSN: 0306-4522

Bungo, T., M. Shimojo, Y.Masuda, Y. H. Choi, D. M. Denbow, M. Furuse (1999). "Induction of food intake by a noradrenergic system using clonidine and fusaric acid in the neonatal chick." Brain Res 826(2): 313-6. ISSN: 0006-8993

Caffe, A. R., F. W. van Leeuwen, R. M. Buijs, G. J. de Vries, M. Geffard, (1985). "Coexistence
    of vasopressin, neurophysin and noradrenaline immunoreactivity in medium-sized
    cells of the locus coeruleus and subcoeruleus in the rat." Brain Res 338(1): 160-4.
    ISSN: 0006-8993
Carpenter, M. B., S. C. Carleton, J. T. Keller, P. Conte (1981). "Connections of the subthalamic
    nucleus in the monkey." Brain Res 224(1): 1-29. ISSN: 0006-8993
Cedarbaum, J. M. (1987). "Clinical pharmacokinetics of anti-parkinsonian drugs." Clin
    Pharmacokinet 13(3): 141-78. ISSN: 0312-5963
Charney, D. S., G. R. Heninger, D. E., Redmond, Jr. (1983). "Yohimbine induced anxiety and
    increased noradrenergic function in humans: effects of diazepam and clonidine."
    Life Sci 33(1): 19-29. ISSN: 0024-3205
Colpaert, F. C., A. D. Degryse, H. V. Van Craenendonck (1991). "Effects of an alpha 2
    antagonist in a 20-year-old Java monkey with MPTP-induced parkinsonian signs."
    Brain Res Bull 26(4): 627-31. ISSN: 0361-9230
Cornil, C. A., J. Balthazart, P.Motte, L. Massotte, V. Seutin, (2002). "Dopamine activates
    noradrenergic receptors in the preoptic area." J Neurosci 22(21): 9320-30. ISSN:
    1529-2401
Cotzias, G. C., M. H. Van Woert, L. M. Schiffer (1967). "Aromatic amino acids and
    modification of parkinsonism." N Engl J Med 276(7): 374-9. ISSN: 0028-4793
Coyle, J. T. and D. Henry (1973). "Catecholamines in fetal and newborn rat brain." J
    Neurochem 21(1): 61-7. ISSN: 0022-3042
Crespi, F. (2009). "Anxiolytics antagonize yohimbine-induced central noradrenergic activity:
    a concomitant in vivo voltammetry-electrophysiology model of anxiety." J Neurosci
    Methods 180(1): 97-105. ISSN: 1872-678X
Crossman, A. R. (1990). "A hypothesis on the pathophysiological mechanisms that underlie
    levodopa- or dopamine agonist-induced dyskinesia in Parkinson's disease:
    implications for future strategies in treatment." Mov Disord 5(2): 100-8. ISSN: 0885-
    3185
Dekundy A, Lundblad M, Danysz W, Cenci MA (2007) Modulation of L-DOPA-induced
    abnormal involuntary movements by clinically tested compounds: further
    validation of the rat dyskinesia model. Behav Brain Res 179(1):76–89. ISSN: 0166-
    4328
Devoto, P., G. Flore, L.Pira, M. Diana, L. Gessa, (2002). "Co-release of noradrenaline and
    dopamine in the prefrontal cortex after acute morphine and during morphine
    withdrawal." Psychopharmacology (Berl) 160(2): 220-4. ISSN: 0033-3158
Dolphin, A., P. Jenner, C. D. Marsden (1976). "Noradrenaline synthesis from L-DOPA in
    rodents and its relationship to motor activity." Pharmacol Biochem Behav 5(4): 431-
    9. ISSN: 0091-3057
Endroczi, E., I. Marton, Z. Radnai, J. Biro (1978). "Effect of the depletion on brain
    noradrenaline on the plasma FSH and growth hormone levels in ovariectomized
    rats." Acta Endocrinol (Copenh) 87(1): 55-60. ISSN: 0001-5598
Ericsson, A. D. and B. G. Wertman (1971). "Sensitivity studies of L-dopa metabolites in
    reserpinized rats and their clinical significance." Neurology 21(11): 1129-33. ISSN:
    0028-3878

Ericsson, A. D., B. G. Wertman, K. M. Duffy (1971). "Reversal of the reserpine syndrome with L-dopa metabolites in reserpinized rats." Neurology 21(10): 1023-9. ISSN: 0028-3878

Fahn, S., L. R. Libsch, R. W. Cutler (1971). "Monoamines in the human neostriatum: topographic distribution in normals and in Parkinson's disease and their role in akinesia, rigidity, chorea, and tremor." J Neurol Sci 14(4): 427-55. ISSN: 0022-510X

Fearnley JM, Lees AJ. 1991. Ageing and Parkinson's disease: Substantia nigra regional selectivity. Brain 114:2283–2301.

Fisher, A., C. S. Biggs, O. Eradiri, M. S. Starr (2000). "Dual effects of L-3,4-dihydroxyphenylalanine on aromatic L-amino acid decarboxylase, dopamine release and motor stimulation in the reserpine-treated rat: evidence that behaviour is dopamine independent." Neuroscience 95(1): 97-111. ISSN: 0306-4522

Foote, S. L., G. Aston-Jones, F. E. Bloom (1980). "Impulse activity of locus coeruleus neurons in awake rats and monkeys is a function of sensory stimulation and arousal." Proc Natl Acad Sci U S A 77(5): 3033-7. ISSN: 0027-8424

Fornai, F., L. Bassi, et al. (1995). "Norepinephrine loss exacerbates methamphetamine-induced striatal dopamine depletion in mice." Eur J Pharmacol 283(1-3): 99-102. ISSN: 0014-2999

Fox, S. H., B. Henry, M. P. Hill, D. Peggs, A. R. Crossman, J. M. Brotchie, (2001). "Neural mechanisms underlying peak-dose dyskinesia induced by levodopa and apomorphine are distinct: evidence from the effects of the alpha(2) adrenoceptor antagonist idazoxan." Mov Disord 16(4): 642-50. ISSN: 0885-3185

Franowicz, J. S. and A. F. Arnsten (1998). "The alpha-2a noradrenergic agonist, guanfacine, improves delayed response performance in young adult rhesus monkeys." Psychopharmacology (Berl) 136(1): 8-14. ISSN: 0033-3158

Franowicz, J. S., L. E. Kessler, C. M. Borja, B. K. Kobilka, L. E. Limbird, Arnsten, A. F. (2002). "Mutation of the alpha2A-adrenoceptor impairs working memory performance and annuls cognitive enhancement by guanfacine." J Neurosci 22(19): 8771-7. ISSN: 1529-2401

Fujimoto, S., M. Sasa, S. Takori (1981). "Inhibition from locus coeruleus of caudate neurons activated by nigral stimulation." Brain Res Bull 6(3): 267-74. ISSN: 0361-9230

Fuxe, K. (1965). "Evidence for the Existence of Monoamine Neurons in the Central Nervous System. Iv. Distribution of Monoamine Nerve Terminals in the Central Nervous System." Acta Physiol Scand 64: SUPPL 247:37+. ISSN: 0302-2994

Gehlert, D. R., S. L. Gackenheimer, D. W. Robertson (1993). "Localization of rat brain binding sites for [3H]tomoxetine, an enantiomerically pure ligand for norepinephrine reuptake sites." Neurosci Lett 157(2): 203-6. ISSN: 0304-3940

Gerlach, M., D. Ben-Shachar, P. Riederer, M. B. Youdim (1994). "Altered brain metabolism of iron as a cause of neurodegenerative diseases?" J Neurochem 63(3): 793-807. ISSN: 0022-3042

German, D.C., B.S. Walker, K. Manaye, W.K. Smith, D.J. Woodward, A.J. North, The human locus coeruleus: computer reconstruction of cellular distribution, J. Neurosci. 8 (1988) 1776–1788. ISSN: 0270-6474

Gesi M, Soldani P, Giorgi FS, Santinami A, Bonaccorsi I, Fornai F. The role of the locus coeruleus in the development of Parkinson's disease. Neurosci Biobehav Rev 2000;24:655–68. ISSN: 0149-7634

Gibbs, M. E. and R. J. Summers (2002). "Role of adrenoceptor subtypes in memory consolidation." Prog Neurobiol 67(5): 345-91. ISSN: 0301-0082

Gjedde, A., G. C. Leger, P. Cumming, Y. Yasuhara, A. C. Evans, M. Guttman, H. Kuwabara (1993). "Striatal L-dopa decarboxylase activity in Parkinson's disease in vivo: implications for the regulation of dopamine synthesis." J Neurochem 61(4): 1538-41. ISSN: 0022-3042

Glowinski, J. and L. Iversen (1966). "Regional studies of catecholamines in the rat brain. 3. Subcellullar distribution of endogenous and exogenous catecholamines in various brain regions." Biochem Pharmacol 15(7): 977-87. ISSN: 0006-2952

Goldman, C. K., L. Marino, S. F. Leibowitz (1985). "Postsynaptic alpha 2-noradrenergic receptors mediate feeding induced by paraventricular nucleus injection of norepinephrine and clonidine." Eur J Pharmacol 115(1): 11-9. ISSN: 0014-2999

Gomez-Mancilla, B. and P. J. Bedard (1993). "Effect of nondopaminergic drugs on L-dopa-induced dyskinesias in MPTP-treated monkeys." Clin Neuropharmacol 16(5): 418-27. ISSN: 0362-5664

Graeff, F. G. (1994). "Neuroanatomy and neurotransmitter regulation of defensive behaviors and related emotions in mammals." Braz J Med Biol Res 27(4): 811-29. ISSN: 0100-879X

Grant, S. J. and D. E. Redmond, Jr. (1984). "Neuronal activity of the locus ceruleus in awake Macaca arctoides." Exp Neurol 84(3): 701-8. ISSN: 0014-4886

Grenhoff, J., M. Nisell, S. Ferre, G. Aston-Jones, T. H. Svensson (1993). "Noradrenergic modulation of midbrain dopamine cell firing elicited by stimulation of the locus coeruleus in the rat." J Neural Transm Gen Sect 93(1): 11-25. ISSN: 0300-9564

Grenhoff, J., R. A. North, S. W. Johnson (1995). "Alpha 1-adrenergic effects on dopamine neurons recorded intracellularly in the rat midbrain slice." Eur J Neurosci 7(8): 1707-13. ISSN: 0953-816X

Grimbergen, Y., Langston, J., Roos, R., Bloem, B., 2009. Postural instability in Parkinson's disease: the adrenergic hypothesis and the locus coeruleus. Expert. Rev. Neurother. 9, 279-290. ISSN: 1744-8360

Grondin, R., A. Hadj Tahar, V. D. Doan, P. Ladure, P. J. Bedard (2000). "Noradrenoceptor antagonism with idazoxan improves L-dopa-induced dyskinesias in MPTP monkeys." Naunyn Schmiedebergs Arch Pharmacol 361(2): 181-6. ISSN: 0028-1298

Guiard, B. P., M. El Mansari, P. Blier (2008) "Cross-talk between dopaminergic and noradrenergic systems in the rat ventral tegmental area, locus ceruleus, and dorsal hippocampus." Mol Pharmacol 74(5): 1463-75. ISSN: 1521-0111

Guiard, B. P., M. El Mansari, Z. Merali, P. Blier (2008) "Functional interactions between dopamine, serotonin and norepinephrine neurons: an in-vivo electrophysiological study in rats with monoaminergic lesions." Int J Neuropsychopharmacol 11(5): 625-39. ISSN: 1461-1457

Guiliano, F., O. Rampin, G. Benoit, A. Jardin (1997). "[The peripheral pharmacology of erection]." Prog Urol 7(1): 24-33. ISSN: 1166-7087

Harrison, J. K., D. D. D'Angelo, D. D. D'Angelo, D. W. Zeng, K. R. Lynch, (1991). "Pharmacological characterization of rat alpha 2-adrenergic receptors." Mol Pharmacol 40(3): 407-12. ISSN: 0026-895X

Henry, B., S. H. Fox, D. Peggs, A. R. Crossman, J. M. Brotchie, (1999b). "The alpha2-adrenergic receptor antagonist idazoxan reduces dyskinesia and enhances anti-parkinsonian actions of L-dopa in the MPTP-lesioned primate model of Parkinson's disease." Mov Disord 14(5): 744-53. ISSN: 0885-3185

Hoehn-Saric, R., A. F. Merchant, M. L. Keyser, V. K. Smith (1981). "Effects of clonidine on anxiety disorders." Arch Gen Psychiatry 38(11): 1278-82. ISSN: 0003-990X

Holmberg, M., M. Scheinin, H. Kurose, R. Miettinen (1999). "Adrenergic alpha2C-receptors reside in rat striatal GABAergic projection neurons: comparison of radioligand binding and immunohistochemistry." Neuroscience 93(4): 1323-33. ISSN: 0306-4522

Hornykiewicz, O. (1966). "Dopamine (3-hydroxytyramine) and brain function." Pharmacol Rev 18(2): 925-64. ISSN: 0031-6997

Hornykiewicz, O. (1973). "Parkinson's disease: from brain homogenate to treatment." Fed Proc 32(2): 183-90. ISSN: 0014-9446

Hornykiewicz, O. and S. J. Kish (1987). "Biochemical pathophysiology of Parkinson's disease." Adv Neurol 45: 19-34. ISSN: 0091-3952

Ichinose, H., T. Ohye, K. Fujita, F. Pantucek, K.Lange, P. Riederer, T. Nagatsu, (1994). "Quantification of mRNA of tyrosine hydroxylase and aromatic L-amino acid decarboxylase in the substantia nigra in Parkinson's disease and schizophrenia." J Neural Transm Park Dis Dement Sect 8(1-2): 149-58. ISSN: 0936-3076

Jellinger, K. (1990). "New developments in the pathology of Parkinson's disease." Adv Neurol 53: 1-16. ISSN: 0091-3952

Jellinger, K. A. (1991). "Pathology of Parkinson's disease. Changes other than the nigrostriatal pathway." Mol Chem Neuropathol 14(3): 153-97. ISSN: 1044-7393

Kamisaki, Y., T. Hamada, K. Maeda, M. Ishimura, T. Itoh, (1993). "Presynaptic alpha 2 adrenoceptors inhibit glutamate release from rat spinal cord synaptosomes." J Neurochem 60(2): 522-6. ISSN: 0022-3042

Kish, S. J., K. S. Shannak, A. H. Rajput, J. J. Gilbert, O. Hornykiewicz (1984). "Cerebellar norepinephrine in patients with Parkinson's disease and control subjects." Arch Neurol 41(6): 612-4. ISSN: 0003-9942

Kish, S. J., K. Shannak, O. Hornykiewicz (1988). "Uneven pattern of dopamine loss in the striatum of patients with idiopathic Parkinson's disease. Pathophysiologic and clinical implications." N Engl J Med 318(14): 876-80. ISSN: 0028-4793

Koda, L.Y., J.A. Schulman, F.E. Bloom, Ultrastructural identification of noradrenergic terminals in rat hippocampus: unilateral destruction of the locus coeruleus with 6-hydroxydopamine, Brain Res. 145 (1978) 190–195. ISSN: 0006-8993

Kubrusly RC, Ventura AL, de Melo Reis RA, Serra GC, Yamasaki EN, Gardino PF, de Mello MC, de Mello FG (2007) Norepinephrine acts as D1-dopaminergic agonist in the embryonic avian retina: late expression of beta1-adrenergic receptor shifts norepinephrine specificity in the adult tissue. Neurochem Int 50(1):211–218. ISSN: 0197-0186

Kumar, V. M. (2003). "Role of noradrenergic fibers of the preoptic area in regulating sleep." J Chem Neuroanat 26(2): 87-93. ISSN: 0891-0618

Kuruma, I., G. Bartholini, R. Tissot, A. Pletscher (1971). "The metabolism of L-3-O-methyldopa, a precursor of dopa in man." Clin Pharmacol Ther 12(4): 678-82. ISSN: 0009-9236

Kuwabara, H., P. Cumming, Y. Yasuhara, G. C. Leger, M. Guttman, M. Diksic, A. C. Evans, A. Gjedde, (1995). "Regional striatal DOPA transport and decarboxylase activity in Parkinson's disease." J Nucl Med 36(7): 1226-31. ISSN: 0161-5505

Lanau F, Zenner MT, Civelli O, Hartman DS (1997) Epinephrine and norepinephrine act as potent agonists at the recombinant human dopamine D4 receptor. J Neurochem 68(2):804–812. ISSN: 0022-3042

Lategan, A., Marien, M., Colpaert, F., 1990. Effects of locus coeruleus lesions on the release of endogenous dopamine in the rat nucleus accumbens and caudate nucleus as determined by intracerebral microdialysis. Brain Res. 523, 134–138. ISSN: 0006-8993

Lategan, A., Marien, M., Colpaert, F., 1992. Suppression of nigrostriatal and mesolimbic dopamine release in vivo following noradrenaline depletion by DSP-4: a microdialysis study. Life Sci. 50, 995–999. ISSN: 0024-3205

Lee, A., A. E. Wissekerke, D. L. Rosin, K. R. Lynch (1998a). "Localization of alpha2C-adrenergic receptor immunoreactivity in catecholaminergic neurons in the rat central nervous system." Neuroscience 84(4): 1085-96. ISSN: 0306-4522

Lee, A., D. L. Rosin, E. J. Van Bockstaele (1998b). "alpha2A-adrenergic receptors in the rat nucleus locus coeruleus: subcellular localization in catecholaminergic dendrites, astrocytes, and presynaptic axon terminals." Brain Res 795(1-2): 157-69. ISSN: 0006-8993

Lin, M. T., J. J. Jou, W. C. Ko (1981). "Effects of intracerebroventricular injection of clonidine on metabolic, respiratory, vasomotor and temperature responses in the rabbit." Naunyn Schmiedebergs Arch Pharmacol 315(3): 195-201. ISSN: 0028-1298

Liu, X. X., K. Wilson, C. G. Charlton (2000). "Effects of L-dopa treatment on methylation in mouse brain: implications for the side effects of L-dopa." Life Sci 66(23): 2277-88. ISSN: 0024-3205

Loughlin, S. E., S. L. Foote, F. E. Bloom (1986). "Efferent projections of nucleus locus coeruleus: topographic organization of cells of origin demonstrated by three-dimensional reconstruction." Neuroscience 18(2): 291-306. ISSN: 0306-4522

Lundblad M, Andersson M, Winkler C, Kirik D, Wierup N, Cenci MA. Pharmacological validation of behavioural measures of akinesia and dyskinesia in a rat model of Parkinson's disease. Eur J Neurosci 2002;15:120–32. ISSN: 0953-816X

Mallick, B. N., S. Majumdar, M. Faisal, V. Yadav, V. Madan, D. Pal (2002). "Role of norepinephrine in the regulation of rapid eye movement sleep." J Biosci 27(5): 539-51. ISSN: 0250-5991

Mann, D., The locus coeruleus and its possible role in ageing and degenerative disease of the human central nervous system, Mech. Ageing Dev. 23 (1983) 73– 94. ISSN: 0047-6374

Mann, D.M., P.O. Yates, J. Hawkes, The pathology of the human locus ceruleus, Clin. Neuropathol. 2 (1983) 1 –7. ISSN: 0722-5091

Marien, M., M. Briley, F. Colpaert (1993). "Noradrenaline depletion exacerbates MPTP-induced striatal dopamine loss in mice." Eur J Pharmacol 236(3): 487-9. ISSN: 0014-2999

Marrs, W., Kuperman, J., Avedian, T., Roth, R. H., Jentsch, J. D. (2005). "Alpha-2 adrenoceptor activation inhibits phencyclidine-induced deficits of spatial working memory in rats." Neuropsychopharmacology 30(8): 1500-10. ISSN: 0893-133X

Marsden, C. D. (1990). "Parkinson's disease." Lancet 335(8695): 948-52. ISSN: 0140-6736

Marsden, C. D. and J. D. Parkes (1976). ""On-off" effects in patients with Parkinson's disease on chronic levodopa therapy." Lancet 1(7954): 292-6. ISSN: 0140-6736

Mason, S.T., H.C. Fibiger, Regional topography within noradrenergic locus coeruleus as revealed by retrograde transport of horseradish peroxidase, J. Comp. Neurol. 187 (1979) 703– 724. ISSN: 0021-9967

Mavridis, M., F.C. Colpaert, M.J. Millan, Differential modulation of (+)-amphetamine-induced rotation in unilateral substantia nigra-lesioned rats by alpha 1 as compared to alpha 2 agonists and antagonists, Brain Res. 562 (1991) 216–224. ISSN: 0006-8993

McGeer, P. L., S. Itagaki, B. E. Boyes, E. G. McGeer (1988). "Reactive microglia are positive for HLA-DR in the substantia nigra of Parkinson's and Alzheimer's disease brains." Neurology 38(8): 1285-91. ISSN: 0028-3878

Melamed, E., F. Hefti, V. Bitton, M. Globus (1984). "Suppression of L-dopa-induced circling in rats with nigral lesions by blockade of central dopa-decarboxylase: implications for mechanism of action of L-dopa in parkinsonism." Neurology 34(12): 1566-70. ISSN: 0028-3878

Mocchetti, I., M. A. De Bernardi, A. M. Szekely, H. Alho, G. Brooker, E. Costa, (1989). "Regulation of nerve growth factor biosynthesis by beta-adrenergic receptor activation in astrocytoma cells: a potential role of c-Fos protein." Proc Natl Acad Sci U S A 86(10): 3891-5. ISSN: 0027-8424

Moore, R. Y. and F. E. Bloom (1979). "Central catecholamine neuron systems: anatomy and physiology of the norepinephrine and epinephrine systems." Annu Rev Neurosci 2: 113-68. ISSN: 0147-006X

Morales, A., M. Condra, J. A. Owen, D. H. Surridge, J. Fenemore, C. Harris, (1987). "Is yohimbine effective in the treatment of organic impotence? Results of a controlled trial." J Urol 137(6): 1168-72. ISSN: 0022-5347

Morrison, J. H., M. E. Molliver, R. Grzanna, J. T. Coyle (1979). "Noradrenergic innervation patterns in three regions of medial cortex: an immunofluorescence characterization." Brain Res Bull 4(6): 849-57. ISSN: 0361-9230

Morrison, J. H., S. L. Foote, D. O'Connor, F. E. Bloom (1982). "Laminar, tangential and regional organization of the noradrenergic innervation of monkey cortex: dopamine-beta-hydroxylase immunohistochemistry." Brain Res Bull 9(1-6): 309-19. ISSN: 0361-9230

Mouradian, M. M., I. J. Heuser, F. Baronti, M. Giuffra, K. Conant, L. Davis, T. Chase, T. N. (1991). "Comparison of the clinical pharmacology of (-)NPA and levodopa in Parkinson's disease." J Neurol Neurosurg Psychiatry 54(5): 401-5. ISSN: 0022-3050

Mouradian, M. M., J. L. Juncos, G. Fabbrini, J. Schlegel, J. J. Bartko, T. N. Chase, (1988). "Motor fluctuations in Parkinson's disease: central pathophysiological mechanisms, Part II." Ann Neurol 24(3): 372-8. ISSN: 0364-5134

Mura, A., D. Jackson, M. S. Manley, S. J. Young, P. M. Groves (1995). "Aromatic L-amino acid decarboxylase immunoreactive cells in the rat striatum: a possible site for the conversion of exogenous L-DOPA to dopamine." Brain Res 704(1): 51-60. ISSN: 0006-8993

Nakazato, T. (2002). "The medial prefrontal cortex mediates 3-methoxytyramine-induced behavioural changes in rat." Eur J Pharmacol 442(1-2): 73-9. ISSN: 0014-2999

Nakazato, T. and A. Akiyama (2002). "Behavioral activity and stereotypy in rats induced by L-DOPA metabolites: a possible role in the adverse effects of chronic L-DOPA treatment of Parkinson's disease." Brain Res 930(1-2): 134-42. ISSN: 0006-8993

Narabayashi, H., T. Kondo, T. Nagatsu, A. Hayashi, T. Suzuki, (1984). "DL-threo-3,4-dihydroxyphenylserine for freezing symptom in parkinsonism." Adv Neurol 40: 497-502. ISSN: 0091-3952

Newman-Tancredi A, Audinot-Bouchez V, Gobert A, Millan MJ (1997) Noradrenaline and adrenaline are high affinity agonists at dopamine D4 receptors. Eur J Pharmacol 319(2–3):379–383. ISSN: 0014-2999

Nicholas, A. P., V. Pieribone, T. Hokfelt (1993). "Distributions of mRNAs for alpha-2 adrenergic receptor subtypes in rat brain: an in situ hybridization study." J Comp Neurol 328(4): 575-94. ISSN: 0021-9967

Nishi, K., Kondo, T., Narabayashi, H., 1991. Destruction of norepinephrine terminals in 1-methyl-4-phenyl-1236-tetrahydropyridine (MPTP)-treated mice reduces locomotor activity induced by L-DOPA. Neurosci. Lett. 123, 244–247. ISSN: 0304-3940

Obeso JA, Olanow CW, Nutt JG. Levodopa motor complications in Parkinson's disease. Trends Neurosci 2000; 23:S2-7. ISSN: 0166-2236

Onali P, Olianas MC, Gessa GL (1985) Characterization of dopamine receptors mediating inhibition of adenylate cyclase activity in rat striatum. Mol Pharmacol 28(2):138–145. ISSN: 0026-895X

Opacka-Juffry, J. and D. J. Brooks (1995). "L-dihydroxyphenylalanine and its decarboxylase: new ideas on their neuroregulatory roles." Mov Disord 10(3): 241-9. ISSN: 0885-3185

Parent, A. and L. N. Hazrati (1995). "Functional anatomy of the basal ganglia. II. The place of subthalamic nucleus and external pallidum in basal ganglia circuitry." Brain Res Brain Res Rev 20(1): 128-54. PMID: 7711765

Parnavelas, J.G., G.C. Papadopoulos, The monoaminergic innervations of the cerebral cortex is not diffuse and nonspecific, Trends Neurosci. 12 (1989) 315– 319. ISSN: 0166-2236

Persson, T. and B. Waldeck (1970). "Further studies on the possible interaction between dopamine and noradrenaline containing neurons in the brain." Eur J Pharmacol 11(3): 315-20. ISSN: 0014-2999

Pralong, E. and P. J. Magistretti (1995). "Noradrenaline increases K-conductance and reduces glutamatergic transmission in the mouse entorhinal cortex by activation of alpha 2-adrenoreceptors." Eur J Neurosci 7(12): 2370-8. ISSN: 0953-816X

Quinn, N. P., P. Luthert, M. Honavar, C. D. Marsden (1989). "Pure akinesia due to lewy body Parkinson's disease: a case with pathology." Mov Disord 4(1): 85-9. ISSN: 0885-3185

Ramos, B., Arnsten, A., 2007. Adrenergic pharmacology and cognition: focus on the prefrontal cortex. Pharmacol. Ther. 113, 523–536. ISSN: 0163-7258

Rascol, O., I. Arnulf, H. Peyro-Saint Paul, C. Brefel-Courbon, M. Vidailhet, C. Thalamas, A. M. Bonnet, S. Descombes, B. Bejjani, N. Fabre, J. L. Montastruc, Y. Agid (2001). "Idazoxan, an alpha-2 antagonist, and L-DOPA-induced dyskinesias in patients with Parkinson's disease." Mov Disord 16(4): 708-13. ISSN: 0885-3185

Remy, P., Doder, M., Lees, A., Turjanski, N., Brooks, D., 2005. Depression in Parkinson's disease: loss of dopamine and noradrenaline innervation in the limbic system. Brain 128, 1314–1322. ISSN: 1460-2156

Ridderinkhof, K., Ullsperger, M., Crone, E., Nieuwenhuis, S., 2004. The role of the medial frontal cortex in cognitive control. Science 306, 443–447. ISSN: 1095-9203

Riekkinen, M., Riekkinen, P.J., 1999. Alpha2-adrenergic agonist clonidine for improving spatial working memory in Parkinson's disease. J. Clin. Psychopharmacol. 19, 444–449. ISSN: 0271-0749

Rinne, U. K. and V. Sonninen (1973). "Brain catecholamines and their metabolites in Parkinsonian patients. Treatment with levodopa alone or combined with a decarboxylase inhibitor." Arch Neurol 28(2): 107-10. ISSN: 0003-9942

Rollema, H., (1992). "Indole-N-methylation of beta-carbolines: the brain's bioactivation route to toxins in Parkinson's disease?" Ann N Y Acad Sci 648: 263-5. ISSN: 0077-8923

Rommelfanger KS, Weinshenker D (2007) Norepinephrine: The redheaded stepchild of Parkinson's disease. Biochem Pharmacol 74(2):177–190. ISSN: 0006-2952

Room, P., F. Postema, J. Korf, Divergent axon collaterals of rat locus coeruleus neurons: demonstration by a fluorescent double labeling technique, Brain Res. 221 (1981) 219– 230. ISSN: 0006-8993

Rosin, D. L., E. M. Talley, A.Lee, R. L. Stornetta, B. D. Gaylinn, P. G. Guyenet, K. R. Lynch (1996). "Distribution of alpha 2C-adrenergic receptor-like immunoreactivity in the rat central nervous system." J Comp Neurol 372(1): 135-65. ISSN: 0021-9967

Ruffolo, R. R., Jr., A. J. Nichols, Hieble (1991). "Metabolic regulation by alpha 1- and alpha 2-adrenoceptors." Life Sci 49(3): 171-83. ISSN: 0024-3205

Sallinen, J., R. E. Link, A. Haapalinna, T. Viitamaa, M. Kulatunga, B. Sjoholm, E. Macdonald, M. Pelto-Huikko, T. Leino, G. S. Barsh, B. K. Kobilka, M. Scheinin (1997). "Genetic alteration of alpha 2C-adrenoceptor expression in mice: influence on locomotor, hypothermic, and neurochemical effects of dexmedetomidine, a subtype-nonselective alpha 2-adrenoceptor agonist." Mol Pharmacol 51(1): 36-46. ISSN: 0026-895X

Savola, J. M., M. Hill, M. Engstrom, H. Merivuori, S. Wurster, S. G. McGuire, S. H. Fox, A. R. Crossman, J. M. Brotchie (2003). "Fipamezole (JP-1730) is a potent alpha2 adrenergic receptor antagonist that reduces levodopa-induced dyskinesia in the MPTP-lesioned primate model of Parkinson's disease." Mov Disord 18(8): 872-83. ISSN: 0885-3185

Schapira, A., 2008. Progress in Parkinson's disease. Eur. J. Neurol. 15, 1. ISSN: 1468-1331

Scheinin, M., J. W. Lomasney, D. M. Hayden-Hixson, U. B. Schambra, M. G. Caron, R. J. Lefkowitz, R. T. Fremeau, Jr. (1994). "Distribution of alpha 2-adrenergic receptor subtype gene expression in rat brain." Brain Res Mol Brain Res 21(1-2): 133-49. ISSN: 0169-328X

Scherman, D., C. Desnos, F. Darchen, P. Pollak, F. Javoy-Agid, Y. Agid (1989). "Striatal dopamine deficiency in Parkinson's disease: role of aging." Ann Neurol 26(4): 551-7. ISSN: 0364-5134

Schramm, N. L., M. P. McDonald, L. E. Limbird (2001). "The alpha(2a)-adrenergic receptor plays a protective role in mouse behavioral models of depression and anxiety." J Neurosci 21(13): 4875-82. ISSN: 1529-2401

Segawa, T., H. Ito, Inoue, K. Wada, H. Minatoguchi, S.Fujiwara, H. (1998). "Dopamine releases endothelium-derived relaxing factor via alpha 2-adrenoceptors in canine vessels: comparisons between femoral arteries and veins." Clin Exp Pharmacol Physiol 25(9): 669-75. ISSN: 0305-1870

Snyder, G. L. and M. J. Zigmond (1990). "The effects of L-dopa on in vitro dopamine release from striatum." Brain Res 508(2): 181-7. ISSN: 0006-8993

Srinivasan, J. and W. J. Schmidt (2003). "Potentiation of parkinsonian symptoms by depletion of locus coeruleus noradrenaline in 6-hydroxydopamine-induced partial degeneration of substantia nigra in rats." Eur J Neurosci 17(12): 2586-92. ISSN: 0953-816X

Stone, E. A. and M. A. Ariano (1989). "Are glial cells targets of the central noradrenergic system? A review of the evidence." Brain Res Brain Res Rev 14(4): 297-309. PMID: 2560410

Strazielle, C., R. Lalonde, C. Hebert, T. A. Reader (1999). "Regional brain distribution of noradrenaline uptake sites, and of alpha1-alpha2- and beta-adrenergic receptors in PCD mutant mice: a quantitative autoradiographic study." Neuroscience 94(1): 287-304. ISSN: 0306-4522

Stromberg, U. and T. H. Svensson (1971). "L-DOPA induced effects on motor activity in mice after inhibition of dopamine-beta-hydroxylase." Psychopharmacologia 19(1): 53-60. ISSN: 0033-3158

Swanson, L. W. and B. K. Hartman (1975). "The central adrenergic system. An immunofluorescence study of the location of cell bodies and their efferent connections in the rat utilizing dopamine-beta-hydroxylase as a marker." J Comp Neurol 163(4): 467-505. ISSN: 0021-9967

Tanaka, M., M. Yoshida, H. Emoto, H. Ishii (2000). "Noradrenaline systems in the hypothalamus, amygdala and locus coeruleus are involved in the provocation of anxiety: basic studies." Eur J Pharmacol 405(1-3): 397-406. ISSN: 0014-2999

Tanaka, M., T. Oshima, S. Hayashi, C. Ishibashi, S. Kobayashi (1973). "Enhancement of the pharmacological action of 3,4-dihydroxy-L-phenylalanine(L-dopa) and reduction of dopa decarboxylase activity in rat liver after chronic treatment with L-dopa." Eur J Pharmacol 22(3): 360-2. ISSN: 0014-2999

Taquet, H., F. Javoy-Agid, F. Cesselin, M. Hamon, J.C. Legrand, Y. Agid, Microtopography of methionine-enkephalin, dopamine and noradrenaline in the ventral mesencephalon of human control and Parkinsonian brains, Brain Res. 235 (1982) 303–314. ISSN: 0006-8993

Tarazi FI, Kula NS, Baldessarini RJ (1997) Regional distribution of dopamine D4 receptors in rat forebrain. Neuroreport 8(16): 3423–3426. ISSN: 0959-4965

Tejani-Butt, S. M., Yang, J., Zaffar, H. (1993). "Norepinephrine transporter sites are decreased in the locus coeruleus in Alzheimer's disease." Brain Res 631(1): 147-50. ISSN: 0006-8993

Timofeeva, O. A. & Levin E. D. (2008). "Idazoxan blocks the nicotine-induced reversal of the memory impairment caused by the NMDA glutamate receptor antagonist dizocilpine." Pharmacol Biochem Behav 90(3): 372-81. ISSN: 0091-3057

Uhlen, S., J. Lindblom, A. Johnson, J. E. Wikberg (1997). "Autoradiographic studies of central alpha 2A- and alpha 2C-adrenoceptors in the rat using [3H]MK912 and subtype-selective drugs." Brain Res 770(1-2): 261-6. ISSN: 0006-8993

Unnerstall, J. R., T. A. Kopajtic, M. J. Kuhar (1984). "Distribution of alpha 2 agonist binding sites in the rat and human central nervous system: analysis of some functional, anatomic correlates of the pharmacologic effects of clonidine and related adrenergic agents." Brain Res 319(1): 69-101. ISSN: 0006-8993

Valet, P., M. Taouis, M. A. Tran, P. Montastruc, M. Lafontan, M. Berlan (1989). "Lipomobilizing effects of procaterol and yohimbine in the conscious dog:

comparison of endocrinological, metabolic and cardiovascular effects." Br J Pharmacol 97(1): 229-39. ISSN: 0007-1188

Wang, T., Zhang, Q.J., Liu, J., Wu, Z.H., Wang, S., 2009. Firing activity of locus coeruleus noradrenergic neurons increases in a rodent model of Parkinsonism. Neurosci. Bull. 25, 15–20. ISSN: 1673-7067

Wang, Y., Q. J. Zhang, Liu, J. Ali, U. Gui, Z. H. Hui, Y. P. Chen, L. Wu, Z. H. Li, Q. (2010). "Noradrenergic lesion of the locus coeruleus increases apomorphine-induced circling behavior and the firing activity of substantia nigra pars reticulata neurons in a rat model of Parkinson's disease." Brain Res 1310: 189-99. 1872-6240

Weiss, G. F. and S. F. Leibowitz (1985). "Efferent projections from the paraventricular nucleus mediating alpha 2-noradrenergic feeding." Brain Res 347(2): 225-38. ISSN: 0006-8993

White, F. J. and R. Y. Wang (1984). "A10 dopamine neurons: role of autoreceptors in determining firing rate and sensitivity to dopamine agonists." Life Sci 34(12): 1161-70. ISSN: 0024-3205

Winzer-Serhan, U. H., H. K. Raymon, R. S. Broide, Y. Chen, F. M. Leslie (1997). "Expression of alpha 2 adrenoceptors during rat brain development--I. Alpha 2A messenger RNA expression." Neuroscience 76(1): 241-60. ISSN: 0306-4522

Zarow, C., S.A. Lyness, J.A. Mortimer, H.C. Chui, Neuronal loss is greater in the locus coeruleus than nucleus basalis and substantia nigra in Alzheimer and Parkinson diseases, Arch. Neurol. 60 (2003) 337–341. ISSN: 0003-9942

Zhang, W. and G. A. Ordway (2003). "The alpha(2C)-adrenoceptor modulates GABA release in mouse striatum." Brain Res Mol Brain Res 112(1-2): 24-32. ISSN: 0169-328X

Zhang, W., V. Klimek, J. T. Farley, M. Y. Zhu, G. A. Ordway (1999). "alpha2C adrenoceptors inhibit adenylyl cyclase in mouse striatum: potential activation by dopamine." J Pharmacol Exp Ther 289(3): 1286-92. ISSN: 0022-3565

Zhao, W. Q., L. Latinwo, X. X. Liu, E. S. Lee, N. Lamango, C. G. Charlton (2001). "L-dopa upregulates the expression and activities of methionine adenosyl transferase and catechol-O-methyltransferase." Exp Neurol 171(1): 127-38. ISSN: 0014-4886

Zweig, R., Cardillo, J., Cohen, M., Giere, S., Hedreen, J., 1993. The locus ceruleus and dementia in Parkinson's disease. Neurology 43, 986–991. ISSN: 0028-3878

8

Neurotensin as Modulator of Basal Ganglia-Thalamocortical Motor Circuit – Emerging Evidence for Neurotensin NTS$_1$ Receptor as a Potential Target in Parkinson's Disease

Luca Ferraro[1], Tiziana Antonelli[1], Sarah Beggiato[1], Maria Cristina Tomasini[1], Antonio Steardo[1], Kjell Fuxe[2] and Sergio Tanganelli[1]
[1]*Department of Clinical and Experimental Medicine, Section of Pharmacology, University of Ferrara, Italy and IRET Foundation, Ozzano Emilia, Bologna*
[2]*Department of Neuroscience, Karolinska Institute, Stockholm*
[1]*Italy*
[2]*Sweden*

1. Introduction

This chapter is focused on the putative role of neurotensin in the development of Parkinson's disease, a neurodegenerative disorder mainly characterized by a progressive loss of nigrostriatal dopaminergic neurons (Schimpff et al., 2001). Although a direct causal role of neurotensin in Parkinson's disease has not yet clearly demonstrated, some convincing animal and human studies support the potential role of the peptide in the etiopathogenesis of this motor disorder. Special emphasis is placed on the significance that neurotensin plays on basal ganglia neuroplasticity and neurodegeneration. This is mainly supported by recent findings clearly demonstrating that neurotensin enhances glutamate excitotoxicity in mesencephalic dopamine neurons and that neurotensin receptors are involved in the modulation of NMDA-induced excitotoxicity (Antonelli et al., 2002; 2004). Through these mechanisms neurotensin could contribute to the development and/or the progression of neurodegenerative disorders. The possible use of neurotensin receptor antagonists, in combination with conventional therapy, in the treatment of Parkinson's disease, is also discussed.

2. Basal ganglia

In Parkinson's disease, the degeneration of dopaminergic neurons in the substantia nigra pars compacta and the consequent striatal dopamine deficiency lead to a cascade of functional modifications in the activity of the basal ganglia-thalamocortical motor circuit, responsible for the motor disturbances characteristic of the pathology (Silkis, 2001). The basal ganglia are a collective group of structures, which include the neostriatum (caudate nucleus and putamen), the external and internal parts of the globus pallidus, the subthalamic nucleus, the substantia nigra pars reticulata and the substantia nigra pars compacta.

From a simplistic point of view, motor information coming from glutamatergic neurons located in several areas of the cerebral cortex, reach the striatum, which represents the primary input nucleus of the basal ganglia. These information, processed in the striatum, are transmitted by the so called "direct" and "indirect" pathways, to the main output nuclei of the basal ganglia (substantia nigra pars reticulata and the internal part of the globus pallidus; Fig. 1). The "indirect pathway" encompasses a trisynaptic link including *i)* GABAergic/enkephalinergic neurons, which connect the striatum to the external part of the globus pallidus; *ii)* the external part of the globus pallidus GABAergic neurons projecting to subthalamic nucleus and *iii)* glutamatergic subthalamic nucleus neurons, which project to the basal ganglia output structures (internal part of the globus pallidus/substantia nigra pars reticulata) and send collaterals to external part of the globus pallidus (Gerfen, 1992). On the other hand, the "direct" monosynaptic pathway consists of GABAergic neurons which directly connect the striatum to the main basal ganglia output structures (substantia nigra pars reticulata and the internal part of the globus pallidus). Outputs from these nuclei consist of inhibitory GABAergic neurons projecting to the ventral-anterior and ventrolateral nuclei of the thalamus which, through excitatory glutamatergic fibers, project back to the prefrontal and motor cortices. The differences in neuronal connectivity between the "direct" and "indirect" pathways show dissimilar functional consequences: the stimulation of the "direct pathway" inhibits substantia nigra pars reticulata and the internal part of the globus pallidus activity, thus leading to a disinhibition of thalamocortical neurons and a consequent facilitation of motor initiation. On the contrary, the stimulation of the "indirect pathway" produces motor inhibition. In spite of the model of the "direct" and "indirect" pathways is an oversimplification of the basal ganglia organization, it still represents the cornerstone for modern research on the basal ganglia functions (for review, Smith and Villalba, 2008).

Dopamine released by terminals of neurons located in substantia nigra pars compacta markedly affects the functional activity of the striatum. In the striatum dopamine D_1 and D_2 receptor subtypes are respectively expressed on the "direct" and "indirect" striatonigral pathways and modulate motor information (Gerfen, 2003). Although the degree of this anatomical separation of D_1 and D_2 receptors has been for a time a controversial topic, recent studies, using transgenic mice have confirmed that dopamine receptor subtypes have mainly a different expression on separate populations of GABAergic medium-spiny projection neurons (Wang et al., 2006; Galvan and Wichmann, 2008). Due to the different location of its receptor subtypes, striatal dopamine physiologically activates the "direct pathway" (D_1 receptors) and inhibits the "indirect pathway" (D_2), leading to an increase of thalamocortical motor drive (*see* above). In addition, striatal glutamate release from corticostriatal glutamatergic terminals is tonically inhibited by dopaminergic input coming from the substantia nigra pars compacta and activating dopamine D_2 heteroreceptors (Bamford et al., 2004). In this synaptic arrangement, dopamine depletion within the striatum not only removes tonic dopamine inhibitory control over corticostriatal glutamatergic drive, but also induces an imbalance between the "direct" and the "indirect" pathways (Fig. 1). In particular, this deficit produces an overactivity of the GABAergic projections from the striatum to the external part of the globus pallidus, leading to an excessive inhibition of thalamocortical and brainstem motor systems. From a pathological point of view, the hyperactivity of striatopallidal GABAergic neurons is considered one of the anomaly responsible for generation of motor parkinsonian symptoms. Pharmacological interventions

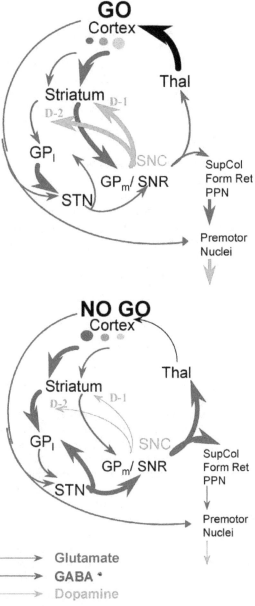

Fig. 1. The changes in the activity of basal ganglia circuits in normal state ('GO') vs Parkinson's Disease ('NO GO') are indicated. Heavy arrows, high activity; thin arrows, low activity. Abbreviations used: GP$_l$, globus pallidus, lateral; GP$_m$, globus pallidus, medial; SNC, Substantia nigra, zona compacta; SNR,Substantia nigra, zona reticulata; SupCol, Superior colliculus; Form Ret, formatio retucularis; PPN, Pedunculo pontine nucleus (from Tanganelli et al., 2004).

that can compensate for loss of dopamine and suppress the expression of motor symptoms in the pre-motor stages of Parkinson's disease are represented by the reduction of: *i)* the excitatory corticostriatal inputs that excite striatal output neurons of the "indirect pathway" or *ii)* the overactivity of striato-pallidal GABAergic neurons. The use of selective D_2 receptor agonist, A_{2A} adenosine receptor antagonism, blockade of GABA receptors in the external part of the globus pallidus or reduction of the excitatory NMDA receptor-mediated corticostriatal inputs, impinging upon striatal output neurons of the "indirect pathway", can be helpful for slowing progression of Parkinson's disease symptoms.

3. Neurotensin and its receptors

Neuropeptides represent undoubtedly one of the most common signaling molecules in the central nervous system. Accumulating evidence have implicated a vast number of neuropeptides and their receptors in the control of a wide range of physiological functions and pathological events, including neurodegenerative disorders.

Like all neuropeptides, neurotensin, an endogenous 13 amino acid peptide (Figure 2), is synthesized as part of a larger inactive precursor (Proneurotensin/neuromedin N).

Neurotensin tridecapeptide

pGlu-Leu-Tyr-Glu-Asn-Lys-Pro-Arg-Arg-Pro-Tyr-Ile-Leu-OH

Fig. 2. Sequence of neurotensin (modified from Ferraro et al., 2009).

The precursor molecule, a highly conserved polypeptide of 169-170 amino acid, contains one copy each of neurotensin and neuromedin N near the C-terminus and undergoes a differential tissue-specific cleavage at its four dibasic sites by proprotein convertases. Pro-neurotensin/neuromedin N may therefore be processed to generate different sets of peptides. Four biologically active products of Pro-neurotensin/neuromedin N processing have been described: neurotensin, neuromedin N, large neurotensin and large neuromedin N (Kitabgi, 2010). In the brain, Pro-neurotensin/neuromedin N processing mainly depends on proprotein convertase 2 activity and leads to high amounts of neurotensin and neuromedin N and small quantities of large neurotensin and large neuromedin N (Kitabgi, 2010). Using radioimmunoassay techniques, it has been demonstrated that the regional distribution of neurotensin and neuromedin N in brain tissues is, generally, the same. However, marked differences in the ratio of neurotensin over neuromedin N have been observed in different brain areas, being neurotensin generally more abundant in dopaminergic region such as substantia nigra pars compacta and ventral tegmental area.

Once processed as an active peptide in neurons, neurotensin is stored in dense core vesicles. The physiological inactivation of neurotensin is operated by endopeptidases belonging to the family of metallopeptidases, which act on primary cleavage sites in the peptide sequence: Arg8-Arg9, Pro10-Tyr11 and Tyr11-Ile12 bonds. Another mechanism that produces an inactivation of neurotensin transmission is the process of neurotensin internalization.

Neurotensin is widely expressed in nerve cells, fibers and terminals (Uhl, 1982; Emson et al., 1985) and exhibits diverse biological actions in the regulation of central nervous system functions of mammals, including man. The peptide is also highly expressed in the periphery, where it mainly acts as a modulator of the gastrointestinal and cardiovascular systems (Wang and Evers, 1999). Neurotensin was originally isolated and sequenced from bovine hypothalamus (Carraway and Leeman, 1973). Subsequent anatomical and functional studies have provided evidence that, in the brain, neurotensin behaves as neurotransmitter and/or neuromodulator (Nemeroff and Cain, 1985; Mendez et al., 1997). Neurotensin is released by neurons through sodium and calcium-dependent mechanisms. Once released, neurotensin produces its biological effects by interacting with three different receptor subtypes (NTS_1, NTS_2 and NTS_3/sortilin). The large distribution in the central nervous system of this family of membrane receptors explains the wide range of physiologic and pathologic effects mediated by the neuropeptide (Barroso et al., 2000). NTS_1 and NTS_2 receptors belong to the family of G-protein-coupled receptors with seven transmembrane domains, which share 60% homology. The NTS_1 receptor displays a high affinity for neurotensin, while NTS_2 receptor has a substantially lower affinity for the peptide and a high affinity to levocabastine, a histamine H_1 receptor antagonist (Chalon et al., 1996; Vincent et al., 1999). NTS_3/sortilin receptor is a single transmembrane protein located in intracellular vesicles of neurons and glia and appears involved in cell sorting and in tropism in cancer cells (Nouel et al., 1999; Mazella et al., 1998). NTS_1 receptor is coupled to a variety of signaling cascades, including production of inositol phosphates through activation of phospholipase C, formation of cAMP and cGMP, and induction of mitogen-activated protein kinase phosphorylation. Autoradiographic ligand binding, in situ hybridization, and immunohistochemical studies have yielded abundant information on the distribution of NTS_1 receptors in mammalian brain. NTS_1 receptors are markedly expressed in brain regions rich in dopamine cell bodies, such as the substantia nigra pars reticulata and pars compacta, the ventral tegmental area, and in projection areas of both nigrostriatal and mesocorticolimbic dopaminergic pathways, such as striatum, nucleus accumbens and frontal cortex (Palacios and Kuhar, 1981; Goulet et al., 1999; Boudin et al., 1998; Binder et al., 2001). In the striatum and nucleus accumbens, NTS_1 receptors are co-localized at post-synaptic level with dopamine D_2 receptors and, although in low density, at the pre-synaptic levels too (Pickel et al., 2001; Delle Donne et al., 2004). This receptor co-distribution together with the demonstration that neurotensin is localized within the nigrostriatal and mesolimbic dopamine neurons explain the role that the neuropeptide plays in the modulation of dopamine neurotransmission (Jennes et al., 1982). It is worth noting that in the striatum, NTS_1 receptors are significantly located on cortical glutamatergic terminals as well as on the striatopallidal GABA neurons (Boudin et al., 1996; Alexander and Leeman, 1998; Tanji et al., 1999). Finally, in the globus pallidus, neurotensin receptors (NTS_1 and NTS_2) exist in different neurons and are located both pre-synaptically and post-synaptically (Fassio et al., 2000; Sarret et al., 2003) thus regulating (mainly NTS_1 receptors), both pallidal glutamatergic and GABAergic transmission (Chen et al., 2004; 2006). Such distribution of NTS_1 receptors justifies the modulation that neurotensin exerts on the mesolimbic, mesocortical and nigrostriatal dopamine neurons, as well as on glutamatergic and GABAergic neurones (Deutch and Zahm, 1992; Fuxe et al., 1992 a,b; Rostene et al., 1992; Binder et al., 2001; Dobner et al., 2003; Petrie et al., 2005). Most of the central and peripheral functions controlled by NTS_1 receptors have been elucidated by the use of the non-peptide neurotensin antagonist SR48692, which preferentially binds NTS_1 receptors (Gully et al., 1993; Rostene et al., 1997).

4. Neurotensin levels, neurotensin binding sites and Parkinson's disease

The high concentrations of neurotensin in brain regions associated with dopaminergic cell bodies and projections, such as the striatum, substantia nigra, ventral tegmental area and globus pallidus (for a review, see Binder et al., 2001) indicate that neurotensin and dopamine are closely linked. In particular, the influence of neurotensin on nigrostriatal and mesocorticolimbic dopaminergic systems suggests that neurotensin may play a relevant role in dopamine-associated pathologies, such as some neurodegenerative disorders and neuropsychiatric diseases (Rostene et al., 1992; Lambert et al., 1995; St-Gelais et al., 2006).

In the following part of this section, data obtained from human and animal studies providing the existence of relationships between neurotensin and neurodegenerative disorders, will be shortly summarized.

Numerous studies have tried to determine whether, in humans, changes in the neurotensinergic system could be associated to Parkinson's disease. In an early study, high levels of neurotensin-like immunoreactivity were detected in lumbar cerebrospinal fluid from Parkinson's disease patients, whilst no significant changes in neurotensin content were observed (Emson et al., 1985). Successively, Fernandez et al. (1995, 1996) found that in post-mortem samples from basal ganglia of Parkinson's disease patients there were changes in the levels of different neuropeptides. In particular, substantia nigra neurotensin levels were two-fold higher in Parkinson's disease patients than in healthy subjects. It is worth noting that in incidental Lewy body disease, which is considered as a pre-symptomatic phase of Parkinson's disease, neurotensin levels tended to increase as in parkinsonian patients, even if this increase was not statistically significant (Fearnley and Lees, 1991). Similarly, in 6-hydroxydopamine-lesioned rats or in 1-methyl-4-phenyl-1,2,3,6-tetrahydropyridine-treated monkeys, two well-characterized animal models of Parkinson's disease, an increase in striatal and globus pallidus neurotensin levels was found, and such an enhancement was not modified by L-dopa treatment. In view of the above results, the authors suggested that changes in neurotensin levels and other neuropeptides may be considered as an early component of an integral part of the pathology rather than a secondary biochemical alteration resulting from loss of the nigrostriatal pathway or a drug-induced event. However, in contrast to the above results, in a previous study, Taylor et al. (1992) showed that substantia nigra neurotensin levels were unchanged following 6-hydroxydopamine lesion, but increased by a prolonged treatment with L-dopa. The authors concluded that changes in neurotensin levels appear to be only a secondary event, due to dopamine neuron loss in combination with protracted drug therapy. Despite these contrasting results, the hypothesis that an enhancement of neurotensin levels, associated to an activation of NTS_1 receptor located on the nigral dopamine neurons, contributes to the degeneration of these dopamine cells in Parkinson's disease, is supported by other animals studies. In particular, these findings indicate that a neurotensin-induced increase in both striatal and cortical endogenous glutamate release, is significantly coupled to an enhancement of neuronal excitotoxicity, which can contribute to nigral dopamine cell loss. In addition, it has been demonstrated that the neuropeptide increases the energy demands due to an increased firing rate in the dopamine cells. These enhancements are, at least in part, caused by a reduction of the D_2 autoreceptor signaling via an antagonistic NTS_1/D_2 receptor interaction (Fuxe et al., 1992a). These neurochemical and morphological results will be carefully described in the subsequent sections (5 and 6).

Besides the changes in neurotensin levels, biochemical and histological investigations in post-mortem brain tissues of parkinsonian patients have shown a significant reduction of neurotensin-binding sites in several specific brain areas of the basal ganglia as respect to healthy subjects (Chinaglia et al. 1990; Fernandez et al., 1994). In particular, Chinaglia et al. (1990), using a receptor autoradiography technique, compared the distribution of neurotensin receptors in post-mortem brain tissues from parkinsonian patients, with that found in patients affected by progressive supranuclear palsy and-in age-matched controls. Significant decreases in neurotensin receptor density were found in the substantia nigra, caudate nucleus, putamen and globus pallidus of both groups of patients in comparison to healthy subjects. In addition, a significant decrement of neurotensin receptor density was found in the ventral tegmental area, nucleus accumbens and dorsal part of caudate in patients with Parkinson's disease as regards to patients with progressive supranuclear palsy, indicating differential involvement of neurotensin receptor alterations in these two neurological disorders. Interestingly, in this cohort of Parkinson's disease patients, the reduction of striatal neurotensin binding sites was lower than the decrease of dopamine content in this nucleus, suggesting only a partial localization of neurotensin receptors on nigrostriatal dopaminergic projections. Using in situ hybridization, it has been possible to more specifically illustrate that NTS₁ receptor mRNA levels were decreased in the substantia nigra of patients with parkinsonism (Yamada and Richelson, 1995). These human results were confirmed in 1-methyl-4-phenyl-1,2,3,6-tetrahydropyridine-treated monkeys, where a decrease in the number of neurotensin-binding sites in the striatum and substantia nigra was found (Goulet et al., 1999; Tanji et al., 1999). The reduction of NTS₁ receptors in the substantia nigra of parkinsonian patients might be related to the loss of the nigrostriatal dopaminergic neurons. In contrast, the interpretation of the decrease in neurotensin-binding sites observed in the striatum of Parkinson's disease patients is certainly more difficult since, at present, the results concerning the pre-synaptic or the post-synaptic localization of striatal neurotensin receptors are still contradictory (Quirion et al., 1985; Cadet, 1991). However, it may be suggested that the decrease in striatal neurotensin-binding sites may reflect the loss of neurotensin receptors not only on dopaminergic nigrostriatal terminals but also on striatal GABAergic medium spiny neurons.

Taken together, the above mentioned studies from Parkinson's disease patients suggest a significant relationship between the alteration of neurotensinergic system and Parkinson's disease. On the basis of these findings, Schimpff et al. (2001) evaluated whether plasma neurotensin concentrations in parkinsonian patients could be considered as a marker in diagnosis and severity of this motor disorder. The results emerging from this study showed that the plasma neurotensin concentrations were significantly higher in Parkinson's disease patients than in healthy controls. Accordingly, neurotensin concentration in the plasma of untreated patients was higher than that observed in treated patients. It is worth noting that these findings were compatible with the enhancement of neurotensin levels detected in post-mortem brain tissues from parkinsonian patients and data obtained from animal studies. Thus, the authors concluded that in addition to the diagnostic criteria for Parkinson's disease "*measurement of extracted plasma neurotensin concentrations in patients with Parkinson may prove useful as an index in diagnosis*".

In summary, it can be concluded that the increase in striatal and nigral neurotensin tissue concentrations, as well as in cerebrospinal fluid and plasma levels may be due either to a loss of dopamine neurons and/or to a dysregulation of neurotensin transmission on striatal output, favoring the striatopallidal GABAergic pathway. Further work is needed to better understand the role of neurotensin in the pathophysiology of Parkinson's disease.

5. Striatal neurotensin and Parkinson's disease: neurochemical animal studies

5.1 Neurotensin modulation of pre- and post-synaptic D_2 receptors. Relevance for the control of striatopallidal GABAergic projections

As stated above, the motor deficits that characterize Parkinson's disease are associated to an imbalance on the functional activity of the "direct"–"indirect" circuits in favor of the "indirect pathway", *i.e.* reduced activity in the "direct pathway" and/or increased activity in the "indirect pathway" (Obeso et al., 2000; 2008). Several lines of evidence indicate that neurotensin is co-localized and co-distributed with dopamine neurons of the basal ganglia, including the somatodendritic complex and axon terminals of various neuronal elements in the substantia nigra and striatum. This close anatomical relationship, reinforces functional findings demonstrating the existence of reciprocal modulations between neurotensinergic and dopaminergic systems in these brain areas (Hökfelt et al., 1984; Nemeroff and Cain, 1985; Blaha et al., 1990; Castel et al., 1994; Tanganelli et al., 1994; Rostène et al., 1997; Werkman et al., 2000). Intensive animal studies have well documented that neurotensin, in addition to its direct excitatory effects on dopamine neurons, significantly modulates D_2 auto- and hetero-receptors functions through the activation of its high-affinity NTS_1 receptor (Kalivas and Duffy, 1990; Werkman et al., 2000; Binder et al., 2001). The regulation of dopaminergic transmission, especially at the level of nigrostriatal and mesocorticolimbic dopamine pathways, by neurotensin (Kitabgy et al., 1989; Deutch and Zahm, 1992) is mainly due to an antagonistic action of the activated NTS_1 receptor on D_2 receptor recognition and signaling. In the striatum, neurotensin has been shown to reduce the affinity of D_2 agonist binding sites and their transduction signals through a receptor-receptor interaction at both pre- and post-synaptic levels (Agnati et al., 1983; von Euler and Fuxe 1987; Shibata et al., 1987; Da-Silva et al., 1989; Fuxe et al., 1992 a,b). In particular, neurotensin by increasing the Kd value of D_2 receptor agonist binding, significantly decreases the affinity of D_2 receptors for endogenous dopamine and dopamine receptor agonists. The neurotensin-induced reduction of D_2 receptor agonist affinity has been demonstrated both in sections and in membrane preparations. The presence at the cellular level of NTS_1 and D_2 receptors in the same axon terminals and dendrites (Delle Donne et al., 2004), together with the demonstrated antagonistic intramembrane NTS_1/D_2 receptor–receptor interactions using biochemical radioligand binding analysis in striatal membranes (Agnati et al., 1983; von Euler and Fuxe 1987; Tanganelli et al., 1989; Fuxe et al., 1992b; Li et al., 1995; Diaz-Cabiale et al., 2002; Antonelli et al., 2007), give indirect evidence for the existence of NTS_1/D_2 receptor heteromerization. By using intrastriatal monoprobe microdialysis and measuring dopamine release from striatal terminals, in vivo evidence has been obtained that the neurotensin/D_2 antagonistic receptor–receptor interaction exists at the pre-junctional level in striatal dopamine transmission. This study demonstrate that, as expected, intrastriatal perfusion with the preferential dopamine D_2 receptor agonist pergolide decreased local dopamine outflow, an effect which reflects a stimulation of terminal D_2 auto-receptors causing the inhibition of striatal dopamine outflow. Interestingly, when neurotensin was co-perfused at a low nanomolar threshold concentration, together with pergolide, the inhibitory effect of the preferential dopamine D_2 receptor agonist on dopamine release is fully abolished as measured in the striatum of awake unrestrained rats. This provides a functional in vivo correlate to the binding results indicating the existence of antagonistic neurotensin/D_2 receptor–receptor interactions previously shown in neostriatal membranes and sections. A possible direct interaction between D_2 and NTS_1 receptors with the formation of heteromers has also been considered by Jomphe et al. (2006) as one of the possible, but not the exclusive, mechanisms underlying the functional control of striatal dopamine D_2-mediated transmission by neurotensin.

Biochemical and functional evidence suggests the existence of an antagonistic NTS_1/D_2 receptor-receptor interaction in rat neostriatum also at the post-synaptic level (Fuxe et al., 1992a; Ferraro et al., 1997). Post-synaptic D_2 receptors in the neostriatum exist predominantly on medium sized GABAergic neurons of the "indirect pathway", which project to the globus pallidus and exert an inhibitory influence on striopallidal GABA transmission (Reid et al., 1990; Ferre' et al., 1993). Converging evidence suggests that the behavioural catalepsy associated with blockade of striatal D_2 receptors is mediated by increased striopallidal GABA transmission, which leads to a decrease in thalamocortical motor drive (Drew et al., 1990; Osborne et al., 1994). Neurochemical findings, obtained employing in vivo dual-probe microdialysis technique, whereby one probe was implanted into the striatum and the other into the ipsilateral globus pallidus, demonstrated that intrastriatal perfusion with D_2 agonists inhibits striopallidal GABA release (Reid et al., 1990; Ferre' et al., 1993). On the contrary, D_2 receptor antagonists enhance striopallidal GABA release (Drew et al., 1990). Interestingly, intrastriatal co-perfusion of neurotensin, at a concentration by itself ineffective on pallidal extracellular GABA levels, in combination with pergolide, fully antagonizes the inhibitory effects of the preferential D_2 agonist on pallidal GABA release. The presence in the perfusate medium of the selective neurotensin receptor antagonist SR48692 removes the antagonistic effect of neurotensin, thus restoring the pergolide-induced inhibition of pallidal GABA levels. It is worth noting that higher concentrations of neurotensin, via a direct activation of NTS_1 receptor subtypes, significantly increase pallidal GABA outflow. SR48692 fully counteracts the facilitatory effects of neurotensin, indicating the involvement of NTS_1 receptors located on striopallidal GABAergic neurons in this effect. In view of the evidence showing that behavioural catalepsy in rodents and akinesia in humans are mediated by an increased striopallidal GABA transmission (Scheel-Kruger, 1986; Drew et al., 1990; Osborne et al., 1994), these findings suggest that the cataleptic profile of neurotensin (Shibata et al., 1987; Da-Silva et al., 1989) may be explained by its ability to influence neurotransmission in the "indirect pathway". In particular, the cataleptic action of neurotensin may be in part related to an enhancement of endogenous neurotensin signalling and in part to a reduction of post-synaptic D_2 receptors affinity. The existence of this intramembrane antagonistic neurotensin/D_2 receptor interaction is also supported by the finding that haloperidol-induced catalepsy is associated with an increase in pallidal GABA release (Drew et al., 1990; Osborne et al., 1994). Briefly, neurotensin-induced increase of pallidal GABA release and the consequent activation of striopallidal GABA transmission, may represent the neurochemical substrate to explain the behavioural data indicating that the activation of striatal NTS_1 receptors reduces motor activity (Poncelet et al., 1994).

5.2 Neurotensin modulation of striatal pre- and post-synaptic D_2 receptors. Functional consequences on the activity of the "indirect pathway"

As previously reported, in the "indirect pathway" the striatopallidal GABAergic projection corresponds to the first neuron of the trisynaptic connection that projects to the substantia nigra pars reticulata. The GABAergic projection from the globus pallidus to the subthalamic nucleus represents the second neuron whereas the subthalamic nucleus glutamatergic cells projecting terminals to the substantia nigra pars reticulata and collaterals to the internal part of the globus pallidus, the third one. Thus, changes in the activation of striatopallidal GABA neurons lead to modifications of the activity of subthalamic nucleus glutamate neurons and consequent variations in substantia nigra pars reticulata and pallidal glutamate release. In view of the above data and to analyze the functional relevance of striatal NTS$_1$ receptor activation on the activity of the "indirect pathway", a dual-probe microdialysis analysis was planed. One probe was implanted into the striatum and the other one in the ipsilateral globus pallidus of the awake rat; the effects of neurotensin on striatal and pallidal glutamate levels were then measured. In this part of the present section the results coming from these microdialysis studies, will be summarized.

5.2.1 Effects of striatal NTS$_1$ receptor activation on pallidal glutamate levels

Extracellular pallidal glutamate levels are mainly derived from the collaterals of the subthalamic nucleus-substantia nigra pars reticulata neurons (*see* above). Intrastriatal infusion with a high concentration of neurotensin increases striatal and pallidal glutamate as well as pallidal GABA levels (*see* also the above section). All these effects are counteracted by the local perfusion with the NTS$_1$ receptor antagonist SR48692. Thus, the intrastriatal neurotensin-induced increase of pallidal glutamate levels may be related to a direct activation of somatodendritic NTS$_1$ receptors located on the striatopallidal GABA neurons or to the antagonistic NTS$_1$/D$_2$ receptor-receptor interaction. The demonstration that the striatal neurotensin-induced increase in pallidal glutamate levels is counteracted by the intrapallidal perfusion of the GABA$_A$ receptor antagonist (-)-bicuculline, suggests that this effect is mediated via the activation of striatopallidal neurons. In fact, it seems likely that the stimulation of striatal NTS$_1$ receptors, by increasing striatopallidal GABA release, reduces the activity of GABAergic neurons projecting from the globus pallidus to the subthalamic nucleus, thus increasing pallidal glutamatergic transmission. In other words, this sequence of GABA-mediated inhibitory modulations induces a disinhibition of the excitatory glutamatergic subthalamic nucleus-substantia nigra pars reticulata efferents which send axon collaterals to the globus pallidus (Alexander and Crutcher, 1990). The intrapallidal (-)-bicuculline perfusion was employed since previous studies demonstrated the role of GABA$_A$ receptor activation in regulating the pallidal output system toward the subthalamic nucleus (Kita, 1992; Amalric et al., 1994). Accordingly, an electrophysiological study (Soltis et al., 1994) demonstrated that the infusion of bicuculline into subthalamic nucleus increased the firing rate of pallidal neurons.

5.2.2 Effects of NTS1 receptor activation on striatal glutamate levels

Extracellular striatal glutamate levels are derived in part, from the terminals of cortical and thalamic afferents (Sirinathsinghji and Heavens, 1989; Parent and Hazrati, 1995). As previously stated, intrastriatal perfusion with neurotensin at a high concentration increases striatal glutamate levels and this effect is fully counteracted by SR48692. Immunohistochemical studies have shown that in the striatum and nucleus accumbens, NTS$_1$ receptors and dopamine D$_2$ receptors are expressed on axon terminals, including the glutamatergic ones (Delle Donne et al., 2004). In this context, it seems possible that at least two mechanisms might underlay the neurotensin-mediated enhancement of striatal glutamate release. The first one may be related to a direct activation of local NTS$_1$ receptors expressed on striatal glutamate terminals. The second mechanism implies that the formation

Neurotensin as Modulator of Basal Ganglia- Thalamocortical Motor Circuit – Emerging Evidence for Neurotensin
NTS$_1$ Receptor as a Potential Target in Parkinson's Disease

165

of a NTS$_1$/D$_2$ heteromeric receptor complex mainly located on the plasma membrane of striatal glutamate terminals, antagonizes the inhibitory D$_2$ receptor mediated signaling (*see* above) on the glutamate terminals, leading to an increase of glutamate release. The presence of a functional antagonistic pre-synaptic NTS$_1$/D$_2$ interaction on glutamatergic striatal terminals has been demonstrated since a threshold concentration of neurotensin counteracts the D$_2$ agonist quinpirole-induced inhibition of K$^+$-evoked striatal glutamate levels.

5.3 Neurochemical studies: concluding remarks

The analysis of all the above microdialysis results suggests that the over-activity of striatopallidal GABA pathway is under the control of NTS$_1$ receptors located both on medium size spiny striatal GABAergic neurons and on striatal glutamatergic terminals. The mechanisms involved in this control are mainly associated to a direct activation of NTS$_1$ receptor homomer or to an antagonistic NTS$_1$/D$_2$ receptor-receptor interaction (Figure 3). Based on these molecular mechanisms, it might be suggested that the activation of NTS$_1$ receptors suppresses the inhibitory control mediated by nigrostriatal dopaminergic neurons on striatopallidal GABAergic neurons and enhances the excitatory cortico-striatal glutamatergic signaling. The final consequence of these combined opposite modulations is the hyperactivity of the striatopallidal GABAergic neurons of the "indirect pathway" which is considered one of the anomaly responsible for generation of motor parkinsonian symptoms (*see* section 2). Thus, neurotensin receptor antagonists, by counteracting the neurotensin-induced hyperactivity of striatopallidal GABAergic neurons, could be useful to reduce motor symptoms in Parkinson's disease patients.

6. Neurotensin and Parkinson's disease: biochemical and morphological analyses in neuronal cell cultures

The substantial elevation in extracellular glutamate accompanied by an excessive activation of excitatory amino acid receptors generates neuronal cell death (Sonsalla et al., 1998). Glutamate has been one of the major focus of research into the excitotoxic basis of neurodegenerative diseases (Choi, 1988; Meldrum and Garthwaite, 1990). In vivo and in vitro studies have shown that neurotensin significantly increases endogenous glutamate outflow in discrete rat brain regions, such as the striatum, globus pallidus, frontal cortex, substantia nigra and parabrachial nucleus-ventrobasal thalamus (Sanz et al., 1993; Saleh, 1997; Ferraro et al., 1998, 2000, 2001). These findings suggest that neurotensin may play a relevant role in reinforcing the effects exerted by glutamate on a variety of central nervous system functions. In particular, the observations that neurotensin amplifies glutamate levels and antagonizes the dopamine D$_2$ receptor-mediated inhibition of dopamine transmission in the basal ganglia (Fuxe et al., 1992 a,b), indicate that neurotensin may contribute to enhance the firing rate and energy demands in the nerve cells. In this context, as illustrated in section 4, a putative role of neurotensin in the development of Parkinson's disease, has been suggested (Fernandez et al., 1995, 1996; Tanji et al., 1999; Schimpff et al., 2001).

In this paragraph, the effects of neurotensin in modulating the glutamate-induced neurodegenerative effects in cultured rat mesencephalic dopaminergic (Antonelli et al., 2002) and cortical (Antonelli et al., 2004) neurons will be shortly summarized.

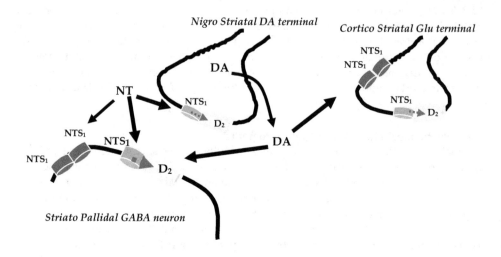

Fig. 3. Schematic representation of the pre-and postjunctional neurotensin (NT) receptor (NTS₁) and dopamine (DA) D₂ receptor interactions in the striatum taking place in NTS₁/D₂ heteromers in balance with excitatory NT receptor homomers (Modified from Ferraro et al., 2008).

6.1 Effects of neurotensin on glutamate-induced excitotoxicity in primary cultures of mesencephalic neurons

Biochemical and morphological approaches (Antonelli et al., 2002), provided evidence that the neurotoxic effects of glutamate on primary cultures of mesencephalic neurons are exacerbated by neurotensin.

Mesencephalic cell cultures, which contain dopaminergic neurons, express glutamate receptors (Meltzer et al., 1997; Yung, 1998; Mateu et al., 2000) as well as functional neurotensin receptors (Nalivaiko et al., 1998; Nouel et al., 1999). Thus, this in vitro preparation represents a suitable model for testing the influence of neurotensin on glutamate-induced neurotoxicity. Measurement of [³H]dopamine uptake in mesencephalic cell cultures has been proved a reliable parameter with which to evaluate the metabolic and structural integrity of the dopaminergic neurons in culture (Mount et al., 1989; Antonelli et al., 2002). In particular, in mesencephalic cell cultures intoxicated with glutamate, a reduction of [³H]dopamine uptake, is observed. The exposure of cells to neurotensin exacerbates the glutamate-induced neurotoxicity, causing a further reduction of [³H]dopamine uptake. Similar results were also obtained by evaluating the vulnerability of the mesencephalic cells to glutamate using tyrosine hydroxylase immunoreactivity. The tyrosine hydroxylase-immunoreactive cell count allows to quantify dopamine cell survival or loss of phenotype (Bowenkamp et al., 1996). As shown in Figure 4, the enhancing action of neurotensin on glutamate-induced toxicity in dopaminergic neurons has also been demonstrated by the increased disappearance of tyrosine hydroxylase-immunoreactive neurons pretreated with glutamate and neurotensin in combination. The selective neurotensin receptor antagonist SR48692 counteractes the above-mentioned effects of neurotensin, indicating that NTS₁ receptor was mainly involved in the neurotensin-induced

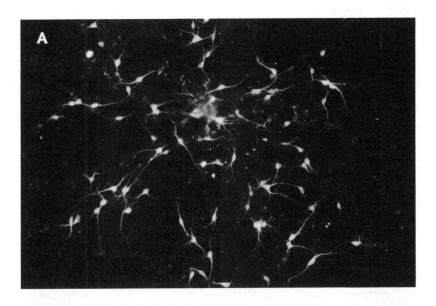

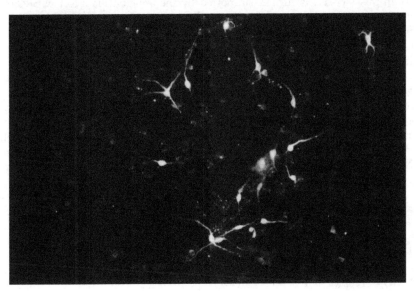

Fig. 4. Representative photomicrographs of tyrosine hydroxylase-immunoreactive mesencephalic cells in culture. **A** (control) shows a typical culture of tyrosine hydroxylase-immunoreactive neurons, with long processes and network. **B** shows a field of tyrosine hydroxylase-immunoreactive neurons exposed to 100 μM glutamate for 10 min, in which there is an evident neuronal loss (from Antonelli et al., 2002).

enhancement of glutamate injury. Since NTS_1 receptors are coupled to phospholipase C (Cathala and Paupardin-Tritsch, 1997; Trudeau, 2000), the effect of the combination of neurotensin with glutamate on [^{3}H]dopamine uptake was also evaluated in the presence of the specific protein kinase C inhibitor calphostin C (Kobayashi et al., 1989). The neurotensin-induced enhancement of glutamate neurotoxicity is completely prevented by calphostin C. Thus, it seems possible that the nigral NTS_1 receptors located on dopamine cells (Nalivaiko et al., 1998) enhance glutamate receptor subtype signaling through a protein kinase C activation. This finding suggests that neurotensin-mediated rise of glutamate excitotoxicity could be mediated by phosphorylation(s) of receptor-associated protein(s) involved in receptor signaling and/or trafficking.

6.2 Effects of neurotensin in modulating the neuronal activity of NMDA receptor in primary cortical cell cultures of rat

Evidence has been accumulated that the excessive activation of glutamate receptors, particularly NMDA receptors, may contribute to the neuronal cell death associated with chronic neurodegenerative disorders including Parkinson's disease and Alzheimer's disease. In this paragraph, the evidence for a functional role of NTS_1 receptors in modulating the neuronal activity of NMDA receptor in cortical glutamatergic nerve cells, will be discussed.

Accordingly to the above in vivo and in vitro experiments, neurotensin increases basal endogenous glutamate release from rat cortical cell cultures. The involvement of NTS_1 receptors in this increase is further supported by the antagonistic effect of SR48692. The exposure of cortical cell cultures to NMDA induces a concentration-dependent increase in endogenous extracellular glutamate levels, an increase that is enhanced in the presence of a sub-threshold concentration of neurotensin. These results indicate that NTS_1 receptor activation enhances the NMDA-receptor signaling and suggest the existence of facilitatory NTS_1/NMDA interactions at the membrane level. The lack of a neurotensin-mediated enhancement of glutamate outflow in the presence of NMDA receptor blockade further supports the hypothesis that neurotensin is a modulator of NMDA receptor function. Morphological analysis strengths the above hypothesis since neurotensin, in threshold concentration, enhances the glutamate-induced increase in the number of the apoptotic cells and such an effect is counteracted by SR48692 (Antonelli et al., 2004). A direct facilitatory NTS_1/NMDA interaction may therefore produce plastic changes in glutamate transmission and, if excessive, produce increases in glutamate-induced excitotoxicity. Under physiological conditions such a postulated NTS_1/NMDA heteromeric complex may modulate metaplasticity which is another main mode of homeostatic plasticity (*see* Perez-Otano and Ehlers, 2005), which serves to establish that receptor plasticity may exist in a proper working range, avoiding *e.g.* a dramatic NMDA receptor internalization and downregulation.

At the present, several mechanisms possibly underlying the demonstrated synergistic NTS_1/NMDA receptor interactions can be hypothesized: *i)* both receptors are known to produce an increase in intracellular Ca^{++} levels and their co-activation may therefore lead to a rapid and robust rise of intracellular Ca^{++} levels; *ii)* synergistic NTS_1/NMDA effect may involve a protein kinase C mediated phosphorylation of the NMDA receptors. It is worth noting that the inhibition of the protein kinase C by calphostin C suppresses the NTS_1-mediated enhancement of NMDA-induced increases of extracellular glutamate levels. (Antonelli et al., 2004). This finding assumes a particular relevance in view of the

Neurotensin as Modulator of Basal Ganglia- Thalamocortical Motor Circuit – Emerging Evidence for Neurotensin
NTS₁ Receptor as a Potential Target in Parkinson's Disease
169

demonstration that protein kinase C is likely to be an important regulator of neuronal NMDA receptors in vivo. The activation of protein kinase C increases NMDA channel opening rate and a rapid delivery of functional NMDA receptors to the cell surface. Thus, regulation of neuronal NMDA receptors by protein kinases plays a critical role in synaptic transmission and synaptic plasticity of NMDA receptors. Since phospholipase C–protein kinase C–inositol triphosphate pathway is the major signal transduction of NTS_1 receptors, it may be suggested that the existence of a neurotensin-mediated potentiation of NMDA receptors involves the activation of protein kinase C. Similarly to the above hypothesis, it has been demonstrated that mGluR1 activation potentiates NMDA receptors by an activation of protein kinase C (Skeberdis et al., 2001; Matsuyama et al., 2002); *iii)* it also seems possible that NTS_1 receptor by forming a receptor heteromer with the NMDA receptor (NTS_1/NMDA heteromer) may contribute to enhance NMDA receptor signalling and its surface expression; *iv)* a recent paper reported that neurotensin receptor agonists robustly increased extracellular concentrations of glycine in the rat prefrontal cortex (Li et al., 2010). It is well known that normal NMDA receptor function depends on not only the binding of glutamate to the receptor but also the binding of glycine to an allosteric site on this receptor. Thus, it could be suggested that neurotensin modulates NMDA receptor functions by modulating allosteric glycine activity.

Taken together, the results obtained in mesencephalic and cortical cell cultures suggest that neurotensin receptor antagonists, by counteracting the neurotensin-induced amplification of glutamate excitotoxicity could display neuroprotective properties.

7. Neurotensin receptor blockade in an animal model of Parkinson's disease

The postulated neuroprotective properties of neurotensin receptor antagonists are also supported by experiments (Ferraro et al., 2008) carried out in a rat model of Parkinson's disease [unilateral nigral 6-hydroxydopamine induced lesion of the nigrostriatal DA pathway, hemiparkinson model]. In this study, behavioural and biochemical experiments have been performed in control animals and in 6-hydroxydopamine unilaterally lesioned rats chronically treated with saline or with the NTS_1 receptor antagonist SR48692 from one-week before until one-week after the lesion. A conventional behavioural assessment using apomorphine-induced rotation was performed to quantify the unilateral nigrostriatal lesion-induced motor asymmetry after ipsilateral 6-hydroxydopamine injection. As expected, in 6-hydroxydopamine-lesioned rats, but not in control rats, the apomorphine injection produced a controlateral turning behaviour that significantly and progressively increased from week 1 to the 3rd week following the lesion. However, interestingly, in the SR48692-treated group, but not in the vehicle-treated group, the apomorphine-induced rotational behaviour is significantly reduced at each time of evaluation (day 7, 14 and 21 post lesion). Moreover, whereas the treatment stopped 2 weeks before, the effect of the compound remains significant. This finding suggests that systemic administration of NTS_1 antagonist decreased the functional consequence of a partial dopaminergic lesion induced by intranigral application of the neurotoxin 6-hydroxydopamine in the rat.

In view of the above behavioural findings, neurochemical experiments have been carried out in control animals and in rats chronically treated with SR48692 or its vehicle from one-week before until one week after the 6-hydroxydopamine injection. In particular, the responsivity to a challenge with NMDA has been assessed. The results obtained from this study demonstrate that in 6-hydroxydopamine-lesioned control and vehicle-treated rats, intrastriatal perfusion with NMDA induced a slight increase in glutamate extracellular levels that was significantly lower than that observed in sham-operated animals. Interestingly, in 6-hydroxydopamine-lesioned rats chronically treated with SR48692, the effect of intrastriatal perfusion of NMDA induced an increase in glutamate extracellular levels that was significantly higher with respect to that obtained in the group of 6-hydroxydopamine lesioned rats but still lower to that observed in control rats.

These neurochemical results are in line with previous microdialysis data indicating that dopamine denervation is associated with a reduction of the enhancement of striatal glutamate transmission induced by a high micromolar NMDA concentration. Since it has been demonstrated that endogenous dopamine in the striatum facilitates strong excitatory inputs, the reduction of NMDA-stimulated glutamate levels in lesioned-animals could imply a loss of facilitatory dopamine receptor mediated signals. In this view, the observation that in rats chronically treated with SR48692 the excitatory response to a NMDA stimulus on the striatal glutamatergic transmission is partially restored may support a protective action of the NTS1 antagonist against 6-hydroxydopamine-induced dopamine neuron degeneration.

8. Conclusion

Parkinson's disease is associated to a progressive loss of nigrostriatal dopaminergic neurons. The decrease of dopamine levels in the striatum of parkinsonian patients is responsible for the main motor disturbances characteristic of the disease such as akinesia, muscular rigidity and tremor. The strict interactions between the tridecapeptide neurotensin and the dopaminergic systems lead to hypothesize that the peptide could be involved in some aspects of Parkinson's disease. In this context, the present chapter discusses the putative role of neurotensin in the development and symptoms of Parkinson's disease.

Human studies provide evidence that in the basal ganglia of Parkinson's disease patients there is an increase in neurotensin levels. These changes might be an integral part of the pathology rather than a consequence of the dopamine neuron degeneration. In addition, neurotensin receptor binding sites, especially in the nigrostriatal dopamine system, are reduced in brains of Parkinson's disease patients and in the basal ganglia of hemiparkinsonian rats. This is probably a result of the ongoing degeneration of nigral dopamine cells in which the peptide actively participates.

Based on neurochemical and morphological animals studies, the hypothesis is now introduced that the activation of NTS_1 receptors by enhancing glutamate release and by amplifying the NMDA-mediated glutamate signalling contributes to the degeneration of dopaminergic neurons in Parkinson's disease. In addition, the reduction of the D_2 autoreceptor signaling due to the antagonistic NTS_1/D_2 receptor-receptor interaction, by enhancing the firing rate of dopamine neurons and energy demand may further contribute to this degeneration.

The neurochemical studies have also clearly demonstrated that increased striatal neurotensin levels, by leading to an over-activity to the "indirect pathway" in the basal ganglia, could also play a role in motor Parkinson's disease symptoms.

In closing, in view of the presented results, it could be suggested that NTS_1 antagonists, in combination with conventional drug treatments, may provide a possible novel therapeutic approach for the treatment of neurodegenerative pathologies, especially Parkinson's disease. This hypothesis is supported by studies demonstrating the putative neuroprotective effects of the neurotensin receptor antagonist SR48692 (systemically administered) in an in vivo animal model of Parkinson's disease. However, Mesnage et al. (2004) in an exploratory study reported that SR48692 could not improve parkinsonian motor disability. However, in this paper the authors reported that the lack of efficacy of NTS₁ receptor antagonists could be attributed to the low dose used, as demonstrated by the absence of adverse events observed in any of the patients tested. In fact, it was concluded that further studies with higher doses of neurotensin receptor antagonists are needed.

Taken together, the reported findings prompt to continue these preclinical studies in order to better understand the role of neurotensin in Parkinson's disease development and symptoms.

9. Acknowledgement

This work has been supported by grants from Sanofi-Aventis and University of Ferrara (Fondo di Ateneo per la Ricerca Scientifica).
The authors thank Dr. Jacqueline Fournier (Sanofi-Aventis) for her excellent scientific support during the research development.

10. References

Agnati, LF.; Fuxe, K.; Benfenati, F. & Battistini, N. (1983). Neurotensin in vitro markedly reduces the affinity in subcortical limbic [3H]N-propylnorapomorphine binding sites. *Acta Physiol. Scan.* 119, (December 1983), pp. 459-461, ISSN 0001-6772.

Alexander, GE. & Crutcher, M. (1990). Functional architecture of basal ganglia circuits: neuronal substrates of parallel processing. *Trends Neurosci.* 13, (July 1990), pp. 266-271, ISSN 0166-2236.

Alexander, MJ. & Leeman, SE. (1998). Widespread expression in adult rat forebrain of mRNA encoding high-affinity neurotensin receptor. *J. Comp. Neurol.* 402, (December 1998), pp. 475-500, ISSN 0021-9967.

Amalric, M.; Farin, D.; Dormont, JF. & Schmied, A. (1994). GABA-receptor activation in the globus pallidus and entopeduncular nucleus: opposite effects on reaction time performance in the cat. *Exp. Brain Res.* 102, pp.244-258, ISSN 0014-4819.

Antonelli, T.; Tomasini, MC.; Finetti, S.; Giardino, L.; Calzà, L.; Fuxe, K.; Soubriè, P.; Tanganelli, S. & Ferraro, L. (2002). Neurotensin enhances Glutamate excitotoxicity in mesencephalic neurons. *J. Neurosci. Res.* 70, (December 2002), pp. 766-773, ISSN 0360-4012.

Antonelli, T., Ferraro, L.; Fuxe, K.; Finetti, S.; Fournier, J.; Tanganelli, S.; De Mattei, M. & Tomasini, M. C. (2004). Neurotensin enhances endogenous extracellular glutamate levels in primariy cultures of rat cortical neurons. Involment of neurotensin receptor in NMDA induced excitotoxicity. *Cerebral Cortex* 1, (April 2004), pp. 466-473, ISSN 1047-3211.

Antonelli, T.; Tomasini, MC.; Fuxe, K.; Agnati, LF.; Tanganelli, S. & Ferraro, L. (2007) Receptor-receptor interactions as studied with microdialysis. Focus on NTR/D2 interactions in the basal ganglia. *J. Neural Transm.* 114, (January 2007), pp. 105-13. ISSN 0300-9564.

Bamford, NS.; Robinson, S.; Palmiter, RD.; Joyce, JA.; Moore, C. & Meshul, CK. (2004) Dopamine modulates release from corticostriatal terminals. *J. Neurosci.* 24, (October 2004), pp. 9541-9552, ISSN 0270-6474.

Barroso, S.; Richard, F.; Nicolas-Etheve, D.; Reversat, JL.; Bernassau, JM.; Kitabgi, P. & Labbè-Julliè, C. (2000). Identification of residues involved in neurotensin binding and modelling of the agonist binding site in neurotensin receptor 1. *J. Biol. Chem.* 275, (January 2000), pp. 328-336, ISSN 0021-9258.

Binder, EB.; Kinkead, B.; Owens, MJ. & Nemeroff, CB. (2001). Neurotensin and dopamine interactions. *Pharmacol. Rev.* 53, (December 2001), pp. 453-486, ISSN 0031-6997.

Blaha, CD.; Coury, A.; Fibiger, HC. & Phillips, AG. (1990). Effects of neurotensin on DA release and metabolism in the rat striatum and nucleus accumbens: cross-validation using in vivo voltammetry and microdialysis. *Neuroscience* 34, pp. 699-705, ISSN 0306-4522.

Boudin, H.; Pélaprat, D.; Rostène, W. & Beaudet, A. (1996). Cellular distribution of neurotensin receptors in rat brain: immunohistochemical study using an antipeptide antibody against the cloned high affinity receptor, *J. Comp. Neurol.* 373, (September 1996), pp. 76–89, ISSN 0021-9967.

Boudin, H.; Pelaprat, D.; Rostène, W.; Pickel, VM. & Beaudet, A. (1998). Correlative ultrastructural distribution of neurotensin receptor proteins and binding sites in the rat substantia nigra. *J. Neurosci.* 18, (October 1998), pp.8473-8484, ISSN 0270-6474.

Bowenkamp, KE.; David, D.; Lapchak, PL.; Henry, MA.; Granholm, AC.; Hoffer, BJ. & Mahalik, TJ. (1996). 6-hydroxydopamine induces the loss of the dopaminergic phenotype in substantia nigra neurons of the rat. A possible mechanism for restoration of the nigrostriatal circuit mediated by glial cell line-derived neurotrophic factor. *Exp. Brain Res.* 111, (September 1996), pp.1-7, ISSN 0014-4819.

Cadet, JL.; Kujirai, K. & Przedborski, S. (1991). Bilateral modulation of [3H]neurotensin binding by unilateral intrastriatal 6-hydroxydopamine injections: evidence from a receptor autoradiographic study. *Brain Res.* 564, (November 1991), pp. 37-44, ISSN 0006-8993.

Carraway, R. & Leeman, SE. (1973). The isolation of a new hypotensive peptide, neurotensin, from bovine hypothalami. *J. Biol. Chem.* 248, (October 1973), pp.6854-6861, ISSN 0021-9258.

Castel, MN.; Morino, P.; Nylander, I.; Terenius, L. & HöKfelt, T. (1994) Differential dopaminergic regulation of the neurotensin striatonigral and striatopallidal pathways in the rat. *Eur. J. Pharmacol.* 262, (September 1994), pp.1-10, ISSN 0014-2999.

Cathala, L. & Paupardin-Tritsch, D. (1997). Neurotensin inhibition of the hyperpolarization-activated cation current (Ih) in the rat substantia nigra pars compacta implicates the protein kinase C pathway. *J. Physiol.* 503, (August 1997), pp.87-97, ISSN 0022-3751.

Chalon, P.; Vita, N.; Kaghad, M.; Guillemot, M.; Bonnin, J. & Delpech, B. (1996). Molecular cloning of a levocabastine-sensitive neurotensin binding site. *FEBS Lett.* 386, (May 1996), pp. 91–94, ISSN 0014-5793.

Neurotensin as Modulator of Basal Ganglia- Thalamocortical Motor Circuit – Emerging Evidence for Neurotensin
NTS, Receptor as a Potential Target in Parkinson's Disease

173

Chen, L.; Yung, KK. & Yung, WH. (2004). Neurotensin depolarizes globus pallidus neurons in rats via neurotensin type-1 receptor. *Neuroscience* 125, pp.853-859, ISSN 0306-4522.

Chen, L.; Yung, KK. & Yung, WH. (2006). Neurotensin selectively facilitates glutamatergic transmission in globus pallidus. *Neuroscience* 141, (September 2006), pp.1871-1878, ISSN 0306-4522 .

Chinaglia, G.; Probst, A. & Palacios, JM. (1990). Neurotensin receptors in Parkinson's disease and progressive supranuclear palsy: an autoradiographic study in basal ganglia. *Neuroscience* 39, pp.351-360, 0306-4522.

Choi, DW. (1988). Glutamate neurotoxicity and diseases of the nervous system. *Neuron* 1, (October 1988), pp.623-34. ISSN 0896-6273.

Da-Silva, SL.; Brandão, ML. & Tomaz, C. (1989) Behavioral effects of neurotensin applied to periventricular structures of rats. *Braz. J. Med. Biol. Res.* 22, pp.711-715, ISSN 0100-879X.

Delle Donne, KT.; Chan , J.; Boudin, H.; Pélaprat, D.; Rostène, W. & Pickel, VM. (2004). Electron microscopic dual labeling of high-affinity neurotensin and dopamine D2 receptors in the rat nucleus accumbens shell. *Synapse.* 52, (June 2004), pp.176-187, ISSN 0887-4476.

Dobner, PR.; Deutch, AY. & Fadel, J. (2003). Neurotensin: dual roles in psychostimulant and antipsychotic drug responses. *Life Sci.* 73,(June 2003), pp.801-811. Rev, ISSN 0024-3205.

Deutch, AY. & Zahm, DS. (1992). The current status of neurotensin-dopamine interactions: issues and speculations. *Ann. N.Y. Acad. Sci.* 668, pp.232-252, ISSN 0077-8923.

Diaz-Cabiale, Z., Fuxe, K.; Narvaez, JA.; Finetti, S.; Antonelli, T.; Tanganelli, S. & Ferraro, L. (2002). Neurotensin-induced modulation of dopamine D2 receptors and their function in rat striatum: Counteraction by NTR1-lik receptor antagonist. *Neuroreport* 13, (May 2002), pp.763-766, ISSN 0959-4965.

Drew, KL.; O'Connor, WT.; Kehr, J. & Ungerstedt, U. (1990). Regional specific effects of clozapine and haloperidol on GABA and dopamine release in rat basal ganglia. *Eur. J. Pharm.* 187, (October 1990), pp. 385–397, ISSN 0014-2999

Emson, PC.; Horsfield, PM.; Goedert, M.; Rossor, MN. & Hawkes, CH. (1985). Neurotensin in human brain: regional distribution and effects of neurological illness. *Brain Res.* 347, (November 1985), pp.239-244 ISSN 0006-8993.

Fassio, A.; Evans, G.; Grisshammer, R.; Bolam, JP.; Mimmack, M. & Emson, PC. (2000). Distribution of the neurotensin receptor NTS1 in the rat CNS studied using an amino-terminal directed antibody. *Neuropharmacology* 39, (June 2000), pp. 1430–1442, ISSN 0028-3908.

Fearnley, JM. & Lees, AJ. (1991). Ageing and Parkinson's disease: substantia nigra regional selectivity. *Brain* 114, (October 1991), pp. 2283-2301, ISSN 0006-8950.

Fernandez, A.; De Ceballos, ML. & Jenner, P. (1994). Neurotensin, substance P, delta and mu opioid receptors are decreased in basal ganglia of Parkinson's disease patients. *Neuroscience* 61, (July 1994), pp.73-79, ISSN 0306-4522.

Fernandez, A.; Jenner, P.; Marsden, CD. & De Ceballos, ML. (1995). Characterization of neurotensin-like immunoreactivity in human basal ganglia: increased neurotensin levels in substantia nigra in Parkinson's disease. *Peptides.* 16, pp.339-346, ISSN 0196-9781.

Fernandez, A.; De Ceballos, ML.; Rose, S.; Jenner, P. & Marsden, CD. (1996) Alterations in peptide levels in Parkinson's disease and incidental Lewy body disease. *Brain* 119 (Pt 3), (June 1996), pp.823-830, ISSN 0006-8950.

Ferraro. L.; O'Connor, WT.; Antonelli, T.; Fuxe, K. & Tanganelli, S. (1997). Differential effects of intrastriatal neurotensin(1–13) and neurotensin(8–13) on striatal dopamine and pallidal GABA release. A dual-probe microdialysis study in the awake rat. *Eur. J. Neurosci.* 9, (September 1997), pp.1838-1846, ISSN 0953-816X.

Ferraro, L.; Tomasini, MC.; Siniscalchi, A.; Fuxe, K.; Tanganelli, S. & Antonelli, T. (2000). Neurotensin increases endogenous glutamate release in rat cortical slices. *Life Sci.* 66, pp.927-936, ISSN 0024-3205.

Ferraro, L.; Tomasini, MC.; Fernandez, M.; Bebe, BW.; O'Connor, WT.; Fuxe, K.; Glennon, JC.; Tanganelli, S & Antonelli, T. (2001). Nigral neurotensin receptor regulation of nigral glutamate and nigroventral thalamic GABA transmission: a dual-probe microdialysis study in intact conscious rat brain. *Neuroscience* 102, pp.113-120, ISSN 0306-4522.

Ferraro, L.; Tomasini, MC.; Mazza, R.; Fuxe, K.; Fournier, J.; Tanganelli, S. & Antonelli, T. (2008). Neurotensin receptors as modulators of glutamatergic transmission. *Brain Res. Rev.* 58 (August 2008) pp.365-373, ISSN 0165-0173.

Ferraro L, Tomasini MC, Beggiato S, Guerrini R, Salvadori S, Fuxe K, Calzà L, Tanganelli S, Antonelli T. Emerging evidence for neurotensin receptor 1 antagonists as novel pharmaceutics in neurodegenerative disorders. *Mini Rev Med Chem.* 9 (October 2009), pp. 1429-1438, ISSN: 1389-5575 (Print).

Ferrè, S.; O'Connor, WT.; Fuxe, K. & Ungerstedt, U. (1993). The striopallidal neuron: a main locus for adenosine-dopamine interactions in the brain. *J. Neurosci.* 13, (December 1993) pp.5402–5406, ISSN 0270-6474.

Fuxe, K.; von Euler, G.; Agnati, LF.; Merlo Pich, E.; O'Connor, WT.; Tanganelli, S.; Li, XM.; Tinner, B.; Cintra, A.; Carani, C. & Benfenati, F. (1992a). Intramembrane interactions between neurotensin receptors and dopamine D2 receptors as a major mechanism for the neuroleptic-like action of neurotensin. *Ann. N.Y. Acad. Sci.* 668, pp.186-204, ISSN 0077-8923.

Fuxe, K.; O'Connor, WT.; Antonelli, T.; Osborne, PG.; Tanganelli, S.; Agnati, LF. & Ungerstedt, U. (1992b). Evidence for a substrate of neuronal plasticity based on pre- and postsynaptic neurotensin-dopamine receptor interactions in the neostriatum. *Proc. Natl. Acad. Sci.* 89, (June 1992), pp.5591-5595, ISSN 0027-8424.

Galvan, A. & Wichmann T. (2008). Phatophisiology of Parkinsonism. *Clinical Neurophysiol.* 119, (July 2008), pp.1459-1474. Rew, ISSN 1388-2457.

Gerfen, CR. (1992). The neostriatal mosaic: multiple levels of compartmental organization in the basal ganglia. *Ann. Rev. Neurosci.* 15, pp.285-320, ISSN 0147-006X.

Gerfen, CR. (2003). D1 dopamine receptor supersensitivity in the dopamine-depleted striatum animal model of Parkinson's disease. *Neuroscientist* 9, (December 2003), pp.455-62, ISSN 1073-8584.

Neurotensin as Modulator of Basal Ganglia- Thalamocortical Motor Circuit – Emerging Evidence for Neurotensin
NTS₁ Receptor as a Potential Target in Parkinson's Disease

175

Goulet, M.; Morissette, M. & Grondin, R. (1999). Neurotensin receptors and dopamine transporters: effects of MPTP lesioning and chronic dopaminergic treatments in monkeys. *Synapse* 32, (June 1999), pp.153-64, ISSN 0887-4476.

Gully, D.; Canton, M.; Boidegrain, R.; Jeanjean, F.; Molimard, JC.; Poncelet, M.; Gueudet, C.; Heaulme, M.; Leyris, A.; Brouard, A.; Pelaprat, D.; Labbe-Jullie, C.; Mazella, J.; Soubrie, P.; Maffrand, JP.; Rostene, W.; Kitbagi, P. & Le Fur, G. (1993) Biochemical and pharmacological profile of a potent and selective nonpeptide antagonist of the neurotensin receptor. *Proc. Natl. Acad. Sci.* 90, (January 1993), pp.65–69, ISSN 0027-8424.

Kalivas, PW. & Duffy, P. (1990). Effect of acute and daily neurotensin and enkephalin treatments on extracellular dopamine in the nucleus accumbens. *J. Neurosci.* 10, (September 1990), pp.2940-2949, ISSN 0270-6474.

Kita, H. (1992). Responses of globus pallidus neurons to cortical stimulation: intracellular study in the rat. *Brain Res.* 589, (August 1992), pp.84-90, ISSN 0006-8993.

Kitbagi, P.; Herve, D.; Studler, JM.; Tramu, G.; Rostene, W. & Tassin, JP. (1989). Neurotensin/dopamine interactions. *Encephale* 15, (January-February 1989), pp.91–94, ISSN 0013-7006.

Kitbagi, P. (2010). Neurotensin and neuromedin N are differentially processed from a common precursor by prohormone convertases in tissues and cell lines. *Results Probl. Cell Differ.* 50, pp.50:85-96.

Kobayashi, E.; Nakano, H.; Morimoto, M. & Tamaoki, T. (1989). Calphostin C (UCN-1028C), a novel microbial compound, is a highly potent and specific inhibitor of protein kinase C. *Biochem. Biophys. Res. Commun.* 159, (March 1989), pp.548-553, ISSN 0006-291X.

Hökfelt, T.; Everitt, BJ.; Theodorsson-Norheim, E. & Goldstein, M. (1984). Occurrence of neurotensinlike immunoreactivity in subpopulations of hypothalamic, mesencephalic, and medullary catecholamine neurons. *J. Comp. Neurol.* 222, (February 1984), pp.543-59, ISSN 0021-9967.

Jennes, L.; Stumpf, WE. & Kalivas, PW. (1982). Neurotensin: Topographical distribution in rat brain by immunohistochemistry. *J. Comp. Neurol.* 210, (September 1982), pp.211-224, ISSN 0021-9967.

Jomphe, C.; Lemelin, PL.; Okano, H. & Trudeau, LE. (2006). Bidirectional regulation of dopamine D2 and neurotensin NTS1 receptors in dopamine neurons. *Eur. J. Neurosci.* 24, (November 2006), pp.2789-2800, ISSN 0953-816X.

Lambert, PD.; Gross, R.; Nemeroff, CB. & Kilts, CD., (1995). Anatomy and mechanisms of neurotensin–dopamine interactions in the central nervous system. *Ann. N. Y. Acad. Sci.* 757, (May 1995), pp. 377–389, ISSN 0077-8923.

Li, X M.; Ferraro, L.; Tanganelli, S.; O'Connor, WT.; Hasselrot, U.; Ungerstedt, U. & Fuxe, K. (1995). Neurotensin peptides antagonistically regulate postsynaptic dopamine D2 receptor in rat nucleus accumbens: a receptor binding and microdialysis study. *J. Neural Transm. [Gen Sect]*, 102, pp.125-137, ISSN 0300-9564.

Li, Z.; Boules ,M.; Williams, K.; Peris, J. & Richelson, E. (2010) The novel neurotensin analog NT69L blocks phencyclidine (PCP)-induced increases in locomotor activity and

PCP-induced increases in monoamine and amino acids levels in the medial prefrontal cortex. *Brain Res.*, 1311, (January 2010), pp. 28-36, ISSN 0006-8993.

Mateu, G.; Privat, A.; Thibault. J. & Vignon, J. (2000). Modulation of glutamate neurotoxicity on mesencephalic dopaminergic neurons in primary cultures by the presence of striatal target cells. *Int. J. Dev. Neurosci.* 18, (October 2000), pp.607–613, ISSN 0736-5748.

Matsuyama, S.; Higashi, H.; Maeda, H.; Greengard, P. & Nishi, A. (2002). Neurotensin regulates DARPP-32 thr34 phosphorylation in neostriatal neurons by activation of dopamine D1-type receptors. *J. Neurochem.* 81, (April 2002), pp.325-334, ISSN 0022-3042.

Mazella, J.; Zsurger, N.; Navarro, V.; Chabry, J.; Kaghad, M. & Caput, D. (1998) The 100-kDa neurotensin receptor is gp95/sortilin, a non-G-protein-coupled receptor, *J. Biol. Chem.* 273, (October 1998), pp.26273–26276, ISSN 0021-9258.

Meldrum, B. & Garthwaite, J. (1990). Excitatory amino acid neurotoxicity and neurodegenerative disease. *Trends Pharmacol. Sci.* 11, (September 1990) pp.379-387, ISSN 0165-6147.

Meltzer, LT.; Christoffersen, CL. & Serpa, KA. (1997). Modulation of dopamine neuronal activity by glutamate receptor subtypes. *Neurosci. Biobehav.* 21, (July 1997), pp.511–518. ISSN 0149-7634.

Mendez, M.; Souaze, F.; Nagano, M.; Kelly, PA.; Rostene, W. & Forgez, P. (1997). High affinity neurotensin receptor mRNA distribution in rat brain and peripheral tissues. Analysis by quantitative RT-PCR. *J. Mol. Neurosci.* 9, (October 1997), pp.93–102, ISSN 0895-8696.

Mesnage, V.; Houeto, JL.; Bonnet, AM.; Clavier, I.; Arnulf, I.; Cattelin, F.; Le Fur, G.; Damier, P.; Welter, ML. & Agid Y. (2004). Neurokinin B, neurotensin and Cannabinoid receptor antagonists and Parkinson disease. *Clin. Neuropharmacol.* 27, (May-June 2004), pp.108-110, ISSN 0362-5664.

Mount, H.; Welner, S.; Quirion, R. & Boksa, P. (1989). Glutamate stimulation of3H]dopamine release from dissociated cell cultures of rat ventral mesencephalon. *J Neurochem* 52, (april 1989) pp.1300–1310, ISSN 0022-3042.

Nalivaiko, E.; Michaud, JC.; Soubrié, P. & Le Fur, G. (1998). Electrophysiological evidence for putative subtypes of neurotensin receptors in guinea-pig mesencephalic dopaminergic neurons. *Neuroscience* 86, (October 1998), pp.799-811, ISSN 0306-4522.

Nemeroff, CB. & Cain, ST. (1985). Neurotensin-dopamine interactions in the CNS. *Trends Pharmacol. Sci.* 6, pp.201-205. ISSN 0165-6147.

Nouel, D.; Sarret, P.; Vincent, JP.; Mazella, J. & Beaudet, A. (1999). Pharmacological, molecular and functional characterization of glial neurotensin receptors. *Neuroscience* 94, pp.1189-1197, ISSN 0306-4522.

Obeso, JA.; Linazasoro, G.; Guridi, J.; Ramos, E. & Rodriguez-Oroz, MC. (2000). High frequency stimulation of the subthalamic nucleus and levodopa induced dyskinesias in Parkinson's disease. *J. Neurol. Neurosurg. Psychiatry* 68, (January 2000), pp.122-3, ISSN 0022-3050.

Obeso, JA.; Marin, C.; Rodriguez-Oroz, C.; Blesa, J.; Benitez-Temiño, B.; Mena-Segovia. J.;
    Rodríguez, M. & Olanow. CW. (2008). The basal ganglia in Parkinson's disease:
    current concepts and unexplained observations. *Ann Neurol.* 64 Suppl2, (December
    2008), S30-46, ISSN 0364-5134.

Osborne, PG.; O'Connor, WT.; Beck, O. & Ungerstedt, U. (1994). Acute vs chronic
    haloperidol; Relationship between tolerance to catalepsy and caudate and
    accumbens DA, GABA and Acetylcholine release. *Brain Res.* 643, (January 1994),
    pp.20–30, ISSN 0006-8993.

Palacios, JM. & Kuhar, MJ. (1981).Neurotensin receptors are located on dopamine-
    containing neurones in rat midbrain. *Nature.* 294, (December 1981), pp.587-589,
    ISSN 0028-0836.

Parent, A. & Hazrati, LN. (1995). Functional anatomy of the basal ganglia. I. The cortico-
    basal ganglia-thalamo-cortical loop. *Brain Res Brain Res Rev* 20, (January 1995),
    pp.91–127, ISSN 0165-0173.

Perez-Otano, I. & Ehlers, M.D. (2005). Homeostatic plasticity and NMDA receptor
    trafficking. *Trends Neurosci.* 28, (May 2005), pp. 229-238, ISSN 0165-6147.

Petrie, Ak.; Schmidt, D.; Busber, M.; Fadel, J.; Carraway, RE. & Deutch, A. (2005)
    Neurotensin activates GABAergic interneurons in the prefrontal cortex. *J. Neurosci.*
    25, (February 2005), pp.1629-1636, ISSN 0270-6474.

Poncelet, M.; Gueudet, C.; Gully, D.; Soubriè, P. & Le Fur, G. (1994) Turning behavior
    induced by intrastriatal injection of neurotensin in mice: sensitivity to non-peptide
    neurotensin antagonists. *Naunyn Schmiedeberg's Arch. Pharmacol.* 349, (January
    1994), pp.57-60, ISSN 0028-1298.

Pickel, VM.; Chan, J.; Delle Donne, KT.; Boudin, H.; Pélaprat, D. & Rosténe, W. (2001). High-
    affinity neurotensin receptors in the rat nucleus accumbens: subcellular targeting
    and relation to endogenous ligand. *J. Comp. Neurol.* 435, (June 2001), pp.142-155,
    ISSN 0021-9967.

Quirion, R.; Chiueh, CC.; Everist, HD. & Pert, A. (1985). Comparative localization of
    neurotensin receptors on nigrostriatal and mesolimbic dopaminergic terminals,
    Brain Res. 327, (February 1985), pp.385–389, ISSN 0006-8993.

Reid, MS.; O'Connor, WT.; Herrera-Marschitz, M. & Ungerstedt, U. (1990). The effect of
    intranigral GABA and dynorphin A injections on striatal dopamine and GABA
    release: evidence that dopamine provides inhibitory regulation of striatal GABA
    neurons via D2 type receptors. *Brain Res.* 519, (June 1990), pp.255–260, ISSN 0006-
    8993.

Rostene, W.; Brouard, A.; Dana, C.; Masuo, Y.; Agid, F.; Vial, M.; Lhiaubet, AM. Rostene, W.
    & Pelaprat, D. (1992). Interaction between neurotensin and dopamine in the brain.
    Morphofunctional and clinical evidence. *Ann. N.Y. Acad. of Sci.* 668, pp. 217–231,
    ISSN 0077-8923.

Rostene, W.; Azzi, M.; Boudin, H.; Lepee, I.; Souaze, F.; Mendez-Ubach, M.; Betancur, C. &
    Gully, D. (1997). Use of nonpeptide antagonists to explore the physiological roles of
    neurotensin. Focus on brain neurotensin/dopamine interactions. *Ann. N.Y. Acad.
    Sci.* 814,(April 1997), pp.125-141, ISSN 0077-8923.

Saleh, TM.; Kombian, SB.; Zidichouski, JA. & Pittman, QJ. (1997). Cholecystokinin and neurotensin inversely modulate excitatory synaptic transmission in the parabrachial nucleus in vitro. *Neuroscience* 77, (March 1997), pp. 23-35, ISSN 0306-4522.

Sanz, B.; Exposito, I. & Mora, F. (1993). Effects of neurotensin on the release of glutamic acid in the prefrontal cortex and striatum of the rat. *Neuroreport* 4, (September 1993), pp.1194-1196, ISSN 0959-4965.

Sarret, P.; Perron, A.; Stroh, T. & Beaudet, A. (2003). Immunohistochemical distribution of NTS2 neurotensin receptors in the rat central nervous system. *J. Comp. Neurol.* 461, (July 2003), pp.520–538, ISSN 0021-9967 .

Scheel-Krüger, J. (1986). Dopamine-GABA interactions: evidence that GABA transmits, modulates and mediates dopaminergic functions in the basal ganglia and the limbic system. *Acta Neurol. Scand. Suppl.* 107, pp.1-54, ISSN 0065-1427.

Shibata, K.; Yamada, K. & Furukawa, T. (1987). Possible neuronal mechanisms involved in neurotensin-induced catalepsy in mice. *Psychopharmacology (Berl).* 91, pp.288-292, ISSN 0033-3158.

Schimpff , RM.; Avard, C.; Fénelon, G.; Lhiaubet, AM.; Tennezé, L.; Vidailhet, M. & Rostène, W. (2001). Increased plasma neurotensin concentrations in patients with Parkinson's disease .*J Neurol Neurosurg. Psychiatry* 70, (June 2001), pp.784–786, ISSN 0022-3050.

Silkis, I. (2001). The cortico-basal ganglia-thalamocortical circuit with synaptic plasticity. II. Mechanism of synergistic modulation of thalamic activity via the direct and indirect pathways through the basal ganglia. *Biosystems.* 59, (January 2001), pp.7-14, ISSN 0303-2647.

Sirinathsinghji, DJS. & Heavens, RP. (1989). Stimulation of GABA release from the rat neostriatum and globus pallidus in vivo by corticotropinreleasing factor. *Neurosci. Lett.* 100, (May 1989), pp. 203–209, ISSN 0304-3940.

Skeberdis, VA.; Lan, J.; Opitz, T.; Zheng, X.; Bennett, MV. & Zukin, RS. (2001). mGluR1-mediated potentiation of NMDA receptors involves a rise in intracellular calcium and activation of protein kinase C. *Neuropharmacology* 40, (June 2001), pp.856-865, ISSN 0028-3908.

Smith, Y. & Villalba, R. (2008). Striatal and extrastriatal dopamine in the basal ganglia: an overview of its anatomical organization in normal and Parkinsonian brains. *Mov Disord.* 23 Suppl (3), S534-547, ISSN 0885-3185.

Soltis, RP.; Anderson, LA.; Walters, JR. & Kelland, MD. (1994). A role for non-NMDA excitatory amino acid receptors in regulating the basal activity of rat globus pallidus neurons and their activation by the subthalamic nucleus. *Brain Res.* 666, (December 1994), pp.21-30, ISSN 0006-8993.

Sonsalla, PK.; Albers, DS. & Zeevalk, GD. (1998). Role of glutamate in neurodegeneration of dopamine neurons in several animal models of parkinsonism. *Amino Acids.* 14, pp.69-74, ISSN 0939-4451.

St-Gelais, F.; Jomphe, C. & Trudeau, LE. (2006). The role of neurotensin in central nervous system pathophysiology: what is the evidence? *J. Psychiatry Neurosci.* 31, (July 2006), pp. 229-245, ISSN 1180-4882.

Neurotensin as Modulator of Basal Ganglia- Thalamocortical Motor Circuit – Emerging Evidence for Neurotensin
NTS, Receptor as a Potential Target in Parkinson's Disease

179

Tanganelli, S.; von Euler, G.; Fuxe, K.; Agnati, LF. & Ungerstedt, U. (1989). Neurotensin counteracts apomorphine-induced inhibition of dopamine release as studied by microdialysis in rat neostriatum. *Brain Res.* 502, (November 1989), pp.319-324, ISSN 0006-8993.

Tanganelli, S.; O'Connor, WT.; Ferraro, L.; Bianchi, C.; Beani, L.; Ungerstedt, U. & Fuxe, K. (1994). Facilitation of GABA release by neurotensin is associated with a reduction of dopamine release in rat nucleus accumbens. *Neuroscience* 60, (June 1994), pp.649-657, ISSN 0306-4522.

Tanganelli, S.; Sandager Nielsen, K.; Ferraro, L.; Antonelli, T.; Kehr, J.; Franco, R.; Ferré, S.; Agnati, LF.; Fuxe, K. & Scheel-Krüger, J. (2004). Striatal plasticity at the network level. Focus on adenosine A2A and D2 interactions in models of Parkinson's Disease. *Parkinsonism Relat. Disord.* 10, (July 2004), pp.273-80, ISSN 1353-8020.

Tanji, H.; Araki, T.; Fujihara, K. (1999). Alteration of neurotensin receptors in MPTP-treated mice. *Peptides* 20, pp.803-807, ISSN 0196-9781.

Taylor, MD.; De Ceballos, ML.; Rose, S.; Jenner, P. & Marsden, CD. (1992). Effects of a unilateral 6-hydroxydopamine lesion and prolonged L-3,4-dihydroxyphenylalanine treatment on peptidergic systems in rat basal ganglia. *Eur. J. Pharmacol.* 219, (August 1992), pp.183-192, ISSN 0014-2999 .

Trudeau, LE. (2000). Neurotensin regulates intracellular calcium in ventral tegmental area astrocytes: evidence for the involvement of multiple receptors. *Neuroscience* 97, pp.293-302, ISSN 0306-4522.

Uhl, GR. (1982). Distribution of neurotensin and its receptor in the central nervous system. *Ann. N. Y. Acad. Sci.* 400, pp.132-49, ISSN 0077-8923.

Vincent, J.P.; Mazella, J. & Kitabgi, P. (1999). Neurotensin and neurotensin receptors. *Trends Pharmacol. Sci.* 20, (July 1999) pp.302-309, ISSN 0165-6147.

Von Euler, G. & Fuxe, K. (1987). Neurotensin reduces the affinity of D2 receptors in rat striatal membranes. *Acta Physiol. Scand.* 131, (December 1987), pp.625-626, ISSN 0001-6772.

Wang, Z.; Kai, L.; Day, M.; Ronesi, J.; Yin, HH. & Ding, J. (2006). Dopaminergic control of corticostriatal long-term synaptic depression in medium spiny neurons is mediated by cholinergic interneurons. *Neuron* 50, (May 2006), pp.443–452, ISSN 0896-6273.

Wang, XM. & Evers, BM. (1999). Characterization of early developmental pattern of expression of neurotensin/neuromedin N gene in foregut and midgut. *Dig. Dis. Sci.* 44, (January 1999), pp.33-40, ISSN 0163-2116.

Werkman, TR.; Kruse, CG.; Nievelstein, H., Long, SK. & Wadman, WJ. (2000). Neurotensin attenuates the quinpirole-induced inhibition of the firing rate of dopamine neurons in the rat substantia nigra pars compacta and the ventral tegmental area. *Neuroscience* 95, pp.417-423, ISSN 0306-4522.

Yamada, M. & Richelson, E. (1995). Heterogeneity of melanized neurons expressing neurotensin receptor messenger RNA in the substantia nigra and the nucleus paranigralis of control and Parkinson's disease brain. *Neuroscience* 64, (January 1995), pp.405-417, ISSN 0306-4522.

Yung, KK. (1998). Localization of ionotropic and metabotropic glutamate receptors in distinct neuronal elements of the rat substantia nigra. *Neurochem. Int.* 33, (December 1998), pp.313–326, ISSN 0197-0186.

9

Role of ^{123}I-Metaiodobenzylguanidine Myocardial Scintigraphy in Parkinsonian Disorders

Masahiko Suzuki

Department of Neurology, The Jikei University School of Medicine, Aoto Hospital, Tokyo,
Japan

1. Introduction

Parkinson's disease (PD) is a relatively common neurological disorder in the elderly. However, only 76% of patients considered clinically to have PD are confirmed to have PD after postmortem examination (Hughes et al., 1993). The most common atypical form of parkinsonism is multiple system atrophy (MSA) (Hughes et al., 1994). MSA is clinically characterized by a combination of parkinsonian, autonomic, pyramidal and/or cerebellar symptoms and signs. The differential diagnosis of disorders with parkinsonism is very important because prognosis and treatment options differ substantially (Wenning et al., 1997). However, although the diagnoses of PD and MSA are based on current clinical criteria (Gelb et al., 1999; Gilman et al., 1999), they continue to lack sufficient specificity (Hughes et al., 1992; Litvan et al., 1997), particularly early in the disease course (Osaki et al., 2002).

Extrapyramidal signs in dementia with Lewy bodies (DLB) resemble those seen in PD, although less rest tremor and left/right asymmetry, but more severe rigidity, favors a diagnosis of DLB. The subtle differences in the nature of extrapyramidal signs between DLB and PD may be of limited help in clinically differentiating the two disorders. This is particularly true in the early disease stages because the sensitivity of the clinical diagnosis of DLB based on the consensus criteria of the DLB International Workshop was 0.22 compared with 0.83 based on a neuropathological diagnosis (McKeith et al., 1996).

The clinical features of PD and autosomal recessive juvenile parkinsonism (AR-JP) are also similar. Thus, it may be difficult to differentiate these two disorders. Neuropathological studies in AR-JP have revealed selective degeneration with gliosis of the pigmented neurons of the substantia nigra and locus ceruleus, but generally no Lewy bodies (Takahashi et al., 1994; Mori et al., 1998; Paviour et al., 2004), suggesting that the pathological findings and disease process of AR-JP differ from those of PD.

Metaiodobenzylguanidine (MIBG) is a physiological analogue of noradrenaline (norepinephrine) (Wieland et al., 1981) and ^{123}I-MIBG myocardial scintigraphy has been used to evaluate postganglionic cardiac sympathetic innervation in parkinsonian disorders (Braune et al., 1999; Orimo et al., 1999; Druschky et al., 2000; Taki et al., 2000; Suzuki et al., 2005). ^{123}I-MIBG myocardial scintigraphy can be performed safely and is clinically used to estimate local myocardial sympathetic nerve damage in PD (Braune et al., 1998; Orimo et al., 1999; Takatsu et al., 2000a). Myocardial innervation imaging using ^{123}I-MIBG has also emerged as a useful method to confirm or exclude the presence of PD (Jost et al., 2010). Thus, ^{123}I-MIBG scintigraphy is the only method that can distinguish with a high degree of sensitivity and specificity between parkinsonian disorders and PD.

In the present study, we evaluated ^{123}I-MIBG myocardial scintigraphy in patients with PD, DLB, AR-JP, and MSA in order to enhance the differentiation of PD from these other neurological diseases that mimic PD.

2. Material and methods

2.1 Patients

A total of 74 subjects were enrolled prospectively based on the criteria outlined below for PD (n = 36), DLB (n = 6), MSA (n = 14), AR-JP (n = 2), and normal control groups (NC; n = 16). There was no significant difference in age between patients with parkinsonism and NC (P = 0.25), and none of the enrolled subjects had clinical evidence of diabetes mellitus or cardiovascular disease. Cases were excluded if no relevant clinical information was provided. In addition, none of the participating subjects were taking drugs that might interfere with ^{123}I-MIBG uptake (Solanki et al., 1992; Wafelman et al., 1994; Braune et al., 2001).

The diagnosis of probable DLB was made based on the criteria of DLB adopted by the International National Workshop on DLB (McKeith et al., 1996). Six patients with DLB had early recurrent visual hallucinations and delusions unrelated to therapy, marked fluctuations in alertness, progressive cognitive decline, and spontaneous motor features of parkinsonism. These psychiatric symptoms became worse with administration of anticholinergic agents and dopamine agonists.

Thirty-six patients with idiopathic PD (Hoehn and Yahr (HY) stage 1, 8 patients; HY 2, 22 patients; HY 3, 6 patients) showed two or more of the following cardinal features of PD: rest tremor, bradykinesia, muscular rigidity, loss of postural reflexes, and unilateral symptoms; thus fulfilling standard diagnostic criteria 6. All PD patients had a good or excellent initial response to levodopa treatment.

Fourteen patients presented with probable MSA according to the criteria reported by Gilman and colleagues (Gilman et al., 1999); all showed extrapyramidal symptoms and corticospinal dysfunction, sporadic adult-onset, and rapid disease progression without dementia. These patients tended to be unresponsive to levodopa or dopamine agonist therapy.

The study included two patients with AR-JP. Both had consanguineous parents and were only first generation. Their clinical features included early-onset (in the 20s) and levodopa-responsive parkinsonism, diurnal fluctuation, and slow progression of the disease. The disease presented initially with dystonic posture of the legs followed by a gradual development of parkinsonism. Their parkinsonian symptoms were responsive to levodopa, although a gradual decline in the efficacy was noted. The parkinsonian triad was mild, and the tremor was usually fine and postural. The levodopa efficacy was sufficient and the clinical course was benign; however, both showed a clear wearing-off phenomenon.

2.2 ^{123}I-MIBG myocardial scintigraphy

^{123}I-MIBG myocardial scintigraphy was performed in all subjects using an intravenous injection of 111 MBq ^{123}I-MIBG (Daiichi Radioisotope Laboratories Co, Tokyo, Japan). Single positron emission computed tomographic and planar images of the chest were obtained after 30 minutes for early images and after 4 hours for delayed images, using a triple-headed

gamma camera (MULTI SPECT III, Siemens, IL, USA) equipped with low-energy and high-resolution collimators. The photopeak of ¹²³I was centered at 159 keV with a 20% energy window. For the anterior planar image, the data was acquired for 4 minutes with a 256 x 256 matrix for image acquisition. The organ uptake of ¹²³I-MIBG was determined by setting the region of interest (ROI) on the anterior view. An ROI was drawn in the left ventricle of the heart and an angular ROI was also set in the upper mediastinum in early imaging, with the same also used for the delayed imaging. The heart to mediastinum ratio (H/M ratio) represented the average counts per pixel in the heart (H) and mediastinum (M).

2.3 Statistical analysis

All data are expressed as mean ± standard deviations. Differences in continuous variables were examined for statistical significance using Student's t-test. A P value less than 0.01 was considered to denote a significant difference. All tests were performed with the STATA 8.0 software program (STATA Corporation, College Station, TX). The AR-JP group was excluded from the analysis because of the small number of subjects.

3. Results

The normal mean values of the H/M ratio in 16 NC were 2.04 (SD 0.18) (range; 1.86-2.55) in the early phase and 2.12 (0.15) (1.91-2.43) in the delayed phase (Table 1). The mean H/M ratio in the early/delayed phase was 1.25 (0.11) (1.11-1.37)/1.18 (0.12) (1.01-1.39) in patients with DLB, 1.45 (0.19) (1.13-1.79)/1.36 (0.22) (1.03-1.99) in those with PD, and 1.88 (0.27) (1.46-2.34)/1.88 (0.40) (1.33-2.47) in those with MSA, respectively. In patients with DLB, the H/M ratio in the early/delayed phases was significantly lower than in MSA and NC groups. In patients with PD, the H/M ratio in the early/delayed phases was also significantly lower than that in MSA and NC groups. In the early phase, the mean value of H/M ratio in patients with DLB was significantly lower than that in patients with PD. However, the H/M ratio in the delayed phase for patients with DLB was lower than that in PD patients, although the difference was not significant (P = 0.015) (Table 1). Overall, there was no significant difference in the early/delayed H/M ratio between the MSA and NC groups (P = 0.077, P = 0.054, respectively). In the two patients with AR-JP, the H/M ratios in the early/delayed phases were preserved within the same range (1.99/2.13, 2.00/2.10, respectively) as the mean value of H/M ratio in NC (Figure 1).

| Diagnosis | n (M/F) | Age (years) | H/M ratio | | WR (%) |
			Early image	Delayed image	
DLB	6 (5/1)	68 ± 8	1.3 ± 0.1*†¶	1.2 ± 0.1*†	39 ± 5
PD	36 (24/12)	64 ± 9	1.5 ± 0.2*†	1.4 ± 0.2*†	42 ± 6
MSA	14 (8/6)	63 ± 8	1.9 ± 0.3 ns	1.9 ± 0.4 ns	35 ± 7 ns
NC	16 (11/5)	64 ± 9	2.0 ± 0.2	2.1 ± 0.2	35 ± 4

Data are mean±SD. *P < 0.001, compared with normal control subjects; ns, not significant, compared with normal control subjects; †P < 0.001, compared with MSA; ¶P < 0.004, compared with PD. DLB, dementia with Lewy bodies; PD, Parkinson's disease; MSA, multiple system atrophy; NC, normal control subjects; M, male; F, female; H/M ratio, heart to mediastinum ratio.

Table 1. Subjects' background and data summary

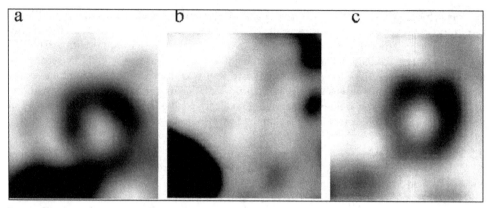

Fig. 1. Short-axis views of ^{123}I-MIBG myocardial scintigraphy

Short-axis views in the early phase of single-photon emission computed tomography of iodine-123–labeled metaiodobenzylguanidine (^{123}I-MIBG) myocardial scintigraphy in a 62-year-old man with autosomal recessive juvenile parkinsonism (a), a 58-year-old man with idiopathic Parkinson's disease (Hoehn and Yahr Stage II, b), and a healthy 62-year-old man (c).

4. Discussion

The major findings of the present study were that 1) ^{123}I-MIBG uptake of the myocardium was significantly lower in patients with Lewy body disease (LBD) including PD and DLB than in controls, 2) the mean values of both the early and delayed H/M ratios in patients with DLB were significantly lower than those in patients with PD, and 3) the mean values of H/M ratios in the early and delayed phases in patients with MSA and AR-JP were well within the range of healthy control subjects.

Decreased cardiac uptake of ^{123}I-IMIBG has been reported in LBD (Yoshita et al., 2001; Watanabe et al., 2001; Nagayama et al., 2005; Suzuki et al., 2006; Suzuki et al., 2007), and a role for postganglionic cardiac sympathetic nerves in PD was demonstrated (Orimo et al., 2001). Thus, reduced uptake of ^{123}I-MIBG is considered to reflect lesions in postganglionic cardiac sympathetic neurons in PD. Lower amounts of cardiac ^{123}I-MIBG uptake were also reported in DLB, even in the early disease stage (Watanabe et al., 2001; Yoshita et al., 2001; Suzuki et al., 2006). These studies suggested that uptake of ^{123}I-MIBG reflects myocardial sympathetic nerve function and that lowered myocardial ^{123}I-MIBG uptake could reflect a disturbance of the postganglionic cardiac sympathetic nerves. In this context, the present study indicated marked reduction of ^{123}I-MIBG uptake in DLB, indicating impairment of the cardiac sympathetic nervous system in this disorder and possible lesions in the postganglionic cardiac sympathetic neurons in DLB, as in PD (Suzuki et al., 2006). These observations might indeed reflect actual cardiac sympathetic denervation, which precedes the neuronal loss in the sympathetic ganglia (Orimo et al., 2005). Cardiac uptake of 6-^{18}F fluorodopamine on positron emission tomography, which can also assess cardiac sympathetic innervation, was decreased in patients with PD (Goldstein et al., 1997; Goldstein et al., 2000), supporting that cardiac sympathetic denervation occurs in LBD.

Decreased cardiac uptake of MIBG has been reported even in the early stages of PD, which suggests early involvement of the cardiac sympathetic nerves. To investigate this proposal,

Orimo et al. (2007) immunohistochemically examined heart tissues, the sympathetic ganglia, and the medulla oblongata at the level of the dorsal vagal nucleus in 20 patients with incidental Lewy body disease (ILBD), which is thought to represent a presymptomatic stage of PD, and 10 control subjects, using antibodies against TH and NF. TH- and NF-immunoreactive nerve fibers of fascicles in the epicardium were well preserved in 10 of the 20 patients with ILBD and in all control subjects. In contrast, TH-immunoreactive nerve fibers had almost entirely disappeared in 6 patients and were moderately decreased in 4 of the 20 patients with ILBD. In addition, none of these ILBD patients showed neuronal loss in the dorsal vagal nucleus or sympathetic ganglia (Orimo et al., 2007). These findings suggested that degeneration of the cardiac sympathetic nerve begins even in the presymptomatic stage of PD, when neuronal loss in the dorsal vagal nucleus is not yet evident.

The present study also revealed relatively preserved cardiac ¹²³I-MIBG uptake in MSA, consistent with previous studies (Yoshita et al., 1998; Nagayama et al., 2005). Taki et al. (2004) previously reported preserved ¹²³I-MIBG uptake in MSA, suggesting that central and preganglionic neurons are predominantly affected, while postganglionic sympathetic neurons are usually spared. Thus, cardiac ¹²³I-MIBG uptake could be unimpaired, indicating the significance of ¹²³I-MIBG imaging as a discriminator between PD and MSA (Yoshita et al., 1998; Braune et al., 1999; Orimo et al., 1999; Druschky et al., 2000; Takatsu et al.; 2000a, 2000b). Postmortem studies demonstrated that postganglionic cardiac sympathetic nerve fibers are markedly decreased in all PD patients, but not necessarily in those with MSA, providing substantial evidence of discrepant ¹²³I-MIBG uptake between PD and MSA (Orimo et al., 2001, 2002). Recent myocardial innervation imaging with ¹²³I-MIBG scintigraphy also demonstrated a high sensitivity for PD detection and adequate specificity for discriminating between PD and MSA (Köllensperger et al., 2007; Chung et al., 2009; Fröhlich et al., 2010). However, Nagayama et al. (2010) recently suggested that MSA cannot consistently be distinguished from PD based on ¹²³I-MIBG myocardial scintigraphy. Their study clearly showed that cardiac MIBG uptake is not always preserved in patients with MSA and that approximately 30% of patients with MSA showed decreased MIBG uptake without any correlation to disease duration or severity. The precise mechanisms underlying low cardiac MIBG uptake in MSA patients remain unclear. The same authors also reported an autopsied patient with MSA showing low cardiac MIBG uptake with an incidental LB pathology in addition to a typical MSA pathology (Nagayama et al, 2008). Therefore, the presence of LB pathology may be a suitable explanation for the low myocardial MIBG uptake observed in patients with MSA. The second consensus statement on the diagnosis of MSA gave no advice about the usefulness and reliability of MIBG scintigraphy scanning in the workup of suspected patients with MSA (Gilman et al., 2008), while the Quality Standards Subcommittee of the American Academy of Neurology found insufficient evidence to recommend MIBG cardiac imaging for differentiating PD from MSA (Suchowersky et al., 2006).

In contrast, myocardial uptake of ¹²³I-MIBG in AR-JP was normal in our study (Suzuki et al., 2005). The H/M ratios in the early and delayed phases in two patients were well within the range for healthy control subjects. These findings might explain the tendency for cardiac sympathetic function to be normal in patients with AR-JP. The pathological background of PD is a systemic distribution of Lewy bodies and Lewy neuritis, spreading to the peripheral autonomic nervous system, including the cardiac plexus (Wakabayashi et al., 1997; Iwanaga et al., 1999). Thus, although the present study included only two patients with AR-JP, it indicated that cardiac sympathetic nerve denervation occurs in PD, and thus accounted for the decrease in cardiac uptake of ^{123}I-MIBG in PD patients and not in those with AR-JP. In this regard, quantification of cardiac ^{123}I-MIBG uptake is considered a valuable tool to identify patients with PD and to distinguish them from patients with other parkinsonian syndromes, including AR-JP (Braune et al., 1999; Orimo et al., 1999; Druschky et al., 2000; Taki et al., 2000). However, a recent study of PD patients showed a low myocardial ^{123}I-MIBG uptake in one patient with PARK2 mutation and autonomic dysfunction, while early-phase MIBG uptake was normal in all other patients free of autonomic dysfunction (Yoritaka et al., 2011). Similar to the above study, a low uptake of ^{123}I-MIBG was reported in 1 of 4 patients with PARK2 mutations, with disease duration of 12 years and ill-defined autonomic dysfunction (Quattrone et al., 2008). In addition, 3 patients in the above study who had low ^{123}I-MIBG uptake were slightly older than the other patients. Incidentally, Estorch et al. (1995) reported that the uptake of ^{123}I-MIBG decreases with age, suggesting that aging could affect patients with PARK2 mutations. Decreased myocardial uptake of ^{123}I-MIBG is also considered to indicate the presence of α-synuclein aggregates in the axons of PD patients (Orimo et al., 2008), while the H/M ratio of patients with PARK2 mutations was reported to be within the range of the normal controls (Suzuki et al., 2005). Moreover, postmortem examination of patients with PARK2 mutations showed well preserved tyrosine hydroxylase immunoreactive nerve fibers in the epicardium (Orimo et al., 2005), suggesting normal functioning myocardial sympathetic nerve terminals in patients with PARK2 mutations. MIBG scintigraphy might be a marker for α-synuclein in patients with PARK2 mutations; however, there are no pathological reports on the presence of Lewy bodies in patients with PARK2 mutations with low MIBG uptake (Yoritaka et al., 2011).

5. Conclusion

The results of the present study indicated that inclusion of ^{123}I-MIBG myocardial scintigraphy in the clinical assessment can potentially increase the chance of correctly distinguishing LBD from the other parkinsonian syndromes. Our study also indicated a difficulty in the differential diagnosis of PD from DLB by ^{123}I-MIBG findings alone. In comparison with PD, mild degeneration of the cardiac sympathetic nervous system may occur in patients with MSA. Finally, abnormalities of ^{123}I-MIBG uptake in genetically identified cases of AR-JP are rare and inconsistent findings. Together, our findings support the conclusions of previous studies that ^{123}I-MIBG myocardial scintigraphy is a potentially useful tool for the differential diagnosis of LBD based on the decreased ^{123}I-MIBG uptake in cardiac postganglionic sympathetic nerve fibers.

6. References

Braune, S., Reinhardt, M. & Bathmann, J. (1998). Impaired cardiac uptake of meta-123I iodobenzylguanidine in Parkinson's disease with autonomic failure. *Acta Neurologica Scandinavia* Vol. 97, pp. 307-314, ISSN 0001-6314

Braune, S., Reinhardt, M. & Schnitzer, R. (1999). Cardiac uptake of ^{123}I-MIBG separates Parkinson's disease from multiple system atrophy. *Neurology* Vol. 53, pp. 1020-1025, ISSN 0028-3878

Braune, S. (2001). The role of cardiac metaiodobenzylguanidine uptake in the differential diagnosis of parkinsonian syndromes. *Clinical Autonomic Research* Vol. 11, pp. 351-355, ISSN 0959-9851

Chung, E.J., Lee, W.Y. & Yoon, W.T. (2009). MIBG scintigraphy for differentiating Parkinson's disease with autonomic dysfunction from Parkinsonism-predominant multiple system atrophy. *Movement Disorders* Vol. 24, pp. 1650-1655, ISSN 1531-8257

Druschky, A., Hilz, M.J. & Platsch, G. (2000). Differentiation of Parkinson's disease and multiple system atrophy in early disease stages by means of I-123-MIBG-spect. *Journal of Neurological Sciences* Vol. 175, pp. 3-12, ISSN 0022-510X

Estorch, M., Carrio, I. & Berna, L. (1995). Myocardial iodine-labeled metaiodobenzylguanidine 123 uptake relates to age. *Journal of Nuclear Cardiology* Vol. 2, pp. 126-132, ISSN 1071-3581

Fröhlich, I., Pilloy, W. & Vaillant, M. (2010). Myocardial MIBG scintigraphy: a useful clinical tool? : A retrospective study in 50 parkinsonian patients. *Neurological Sciences* Vol. 31, pp. 403-406, ISSN 1590-3478

Gelb, D.J., Oliver, E. & Gilman, S. (1999). Diagnostic criteria for Parkinson disease. *Archives of Neurol* Vol. 56, pp. 33-39, ISSN 0003-9942

Gilman, S., Low, P.A. & Quinn, N. (1999). Consensus statement on the diagnosis of multiple system atrophy. *Journal of Neurological Sciences*, Vol. 163, pp. 94-98, ISSN 0022-510X

Gilman, S., Wenning, G.K. & Low, P.A. (2008). Second consensus statement on the diagnosis of multiple system atrophy. *Neurology*, Vol. 71, pp. 670-676, ISSN 1526-632X

Goldstein, D.S., Holmes, C. & Cannon, R.O. III. (1997). Sympathetic cardioneuropathy in dysautonomias. *New England Journal of Medicine*, Vol.336, pp. 696-702, ISSN 0028-4793

Goldstein, D.S., Holmes, C. & Li, S-T. (2000). Cardiac sympathetic denervation in Parkinson disease. *Annals of Internal Medicine*, Vol.133, pp. 338-347, ISSN 0003-4819

Hughes, A.J., Daniel, S.E. & Kilford, L. (1992). Accuracy of clinical diagnosis of idiopathic Parkinson's disease: A clinico-pathological study of 100 cases. *Journal of Neurology, Neurosurgery, and Psychiatry*, Vol. 55, pp. 181-184, ISSN 0022-3050

Hughes, A.J., Daniel, S.E. & Blankson, S. (1993). A clinicopathologic study of 100 cases of Parkinson's disease. *Archives of Neurology*, Vol.50, pp. 140-148, ISSN 0003-9942

Iwanaga, K., Wakabayashi, K. & Yoshimoto, M. (1999). Lewy body-type degeneration in cardiac plexus in Parkinson's and incidental Lewy body diseases, *Neurology*, Vol. 52, pp. 1269-1271, ISSN 0028-3878

Jost, W.H., Del Tredici, K., & Landvogt, C. (2010). Importance of ¹²³I-metaiodobenzylguanidine scintigraphy/single photon emission computed tomography for diagnosis and differential diagnostics of Parkinson syndromes. *Neurodegenerative Diseases* Vol. 7, pp. 341-347, ISSN 1660-2862

Köllensperger, M., Seppi, K. & Liener, C. (2007). Diffusion weighted imaging best discriminates PD from MSA-P: A comparison with tilt table testing and heart MIBG scintigraphy. *Movement Disorders*, Vol. 22, pp. 1771-1776, ISSN 0885-3185

Litvan, I., Goetz, C.G. & Jankovic, J. (1997). What is the accuracy of the clinical diagnosis of multiple system atrophy? A clinicopathologic study. *Archives of Neurology*, Vol. 54, pp. 937-944, ISSN 0003-9942

McKeith, I.G., Galasko, D. & Kosaka, K. (1996). Consensus guidelines for the clinical and pathologic diagnosis of dementia with Lewy bodies (DLB): Report of the consortium on DLB international workshop. *Neurology,* Vol. 47, pp. 1113-1124, ISSN 0028-3878

Mori, H., Kondo, T., & Yokochi, M. (1998). Pathologic and biochemical studies of juvenile parkinsonism linked to chromosome 6q. *Neurology,* Vol. 51, pp. 890-892, ISSN 0028-3878

Nagayama, H., Hamamoto, M. & Ueda, M. (2005). Reliability of MIBG myocardial scintigraphy in the diagnosis of Parkinson's disease. *Journal of Neurology, Neurosurgery and Psychiatry,* Vol. 76, pp. 249-251, ISSN 0022-3050

Nagayama, H., Yamazaki, M. & Ueda, M. (2008). Low myocardial MIBG uptake in multiple system atrophy with incidental Lewy body pathology: an autopsy case report. *Movement Disorders,* Vol. 23, pp. 1055–1057, ISSN 1531-8257

Nagayama, H., Ueda, M. & Yamazaki, M. (2010). Abnormal cardiac ^{123}I-meta-iodobenzylguanidine uptake in multiple system atrophy. *Movement Disorders,* Vol. 25, pp. 1744-1747, ISSN 1531-8257

Orimo, S., Ozawa, E. & Oka, T. (2001). Different histopathology accounting for a decrease in myocardial MIBG uptake in PD and MSA. *Neurology,* Vol. 57, pp. 1140-1141, ISSN 0028-3878

Orimo, S., Ozawa, E. & Nakade, S. (1999). ^{123}I-metaiodobenzylguanidine myocardial scintigraphy in Parkinson's disease. *Journal of Neurology, Neurosurgery, and Psychiatry,* Vol. 67, pp. 189-194, ISSN 0022-3050

Orimo, S., Oka, T. & Miura, H. (2002). Sympathetic cardiac denervation in Parkinson's disease and pure autonomic failure but not in multiple system atrophy. *Journal of Neurology, Neurosurgery, and Psychiatry,* Vol. 73, pp. 776-777, ISSN 0022-3050

Orimo, S., Amino, T. & Itoh, Y. (2005). Cardiac sympathetic denervation precedes neuronal loss in the sympathetic ganglia in Lewy body disease. *Acta Neuropathologica (Berlin)* Vol. 109, pp. 583-588, ISSN 0001-6322

Orimo, S., Takahashi, A, & Uchihara, T. (2007). Degeneration of cardiac sympathetic nerve begins in the early disease process of Parkinson's disease. *Brain Pathology,* Vol. 17, pp. 24-30, ISSN 1015-6305

Orimo, S,. Uchihara, T. & Nakamura, A. (2008). Axonal α-synuclein aggregates herald centripetal degeneration of cardiac sympathetic nerve in Parkinson's disease. *Brain,* Vol. 131, pp. 642-650, ISSN 1460-2156

Osaki, Y., Wenning, G.K. & Daniel, S.E. (2002). Do published criteria improve clinical diagnostic accuracy in multiple system atrophy? *Neurology,* Vol. 59, pp. 1486-1491, ISSN 0028-3878

Paviour, D.C., Surtees, R.A. & Lees, A.J. (2004). Diagnostic considerations in juvenile parkinsonism. *Movement Disorders,* Vol. 19, pp. 123-135, ISSN 0885-3185

Quattrone, A., Bagnato, A. & Annesi, G. (2008). Myocardial [123]metaiodobenzylguanidine uptake in genetic Parkinson's disease. *Movement Disorders* Vol. 23, pp. 21-27, ISSN 1531-8257

Solanki, K.K., Bomanji, J. & Moyes, J. (1992). A pharmacological guide to medicines which interfere with the biodistribution of radiolabelled meta-iodobenzylguanidine (MIBG). *Nuclear Medicine Communications,* Vol.13, pp. 513-521, ISSN 0143-3636

Suchowersky, O., Reich, S. & Perlmutter, J. (2006). Practice parameter: diagnosis and prognosis of new onset Parkinson disease (an evidence-based review): report of the Quality Standards Subcommittee of the American Academy of Neurology. *Neurology*, Vol. 66, pp. 968-975, ISSN 1526-632X

Suzuki, M., Hattori, N. & Orimo, S. (2005). Preserved myocardial ¹²³I-metaiodobenzylguanidine uptake in autosomal recessive juvenile parkinsonism: First case report. *Movement Disorders*, Vol.20, pp. 634-636, ISSN 0885-3185

Suzuki, M., Kurita, A. & Hashimoto, M. (2006). Impaired myocardial ¹²³I-metaiodobenzylguanidine uptake in Lewy body disease: Comparison between dementia with Lewy bodies and Parkinson's disease. *Journal of Neurological Sciences*, Vol. 240, pp. 15-19, ISSN 0022-510X

Suzuki, M., Urashima, M. & Oka., H. (2007). Cardiac sympathetic denervation in bradykinesia-dominant Parkinson's disease. *Neuroreport*, Vol.18, pp. 1867-1870, ISSN 0959-4965

Takahashi, H., Ohama, E. & Suzuki, S. (1994). Familial juvenile parkinsonism: Clinical and pathologic study in a family. *Neurology*, Vol. 44, pp. 437-441, ISSN 0028-3878

Takatsu, H., Nishida, H. & Matsuo, H. (2000a). Cardiac sympathetic denervation from the early stage of Parkinson's disease: Clinical and experimental studies with radiolabeled MIBG. *Journal of Nuclear Medicine*, Vol. 41, pp. 71-77, ISSN 0161-5505

Takatsu, H., Nagashima, K. & Murase, M. (2000b). Differentiating Parkinson disease from multiple-system atrophy by measuring cardiac iodine-123 metaiodobenzylguanidine accumulation. *Journal of the American Medical Association*, Vol. 284, pp. 44-45, ISSN 0098-7484

Taki, J., Nakajima, K. & Hwang, E.H. (2000). Peripheral sympathetic dysfunction in patients with Parkinson's disease without autonomic failure is heart selective and disease specific. *European Journal of Nuclear Medicine*, Vol. 27, pp. 566-573, ISSN 0340-6997

Taki, J., Yoshita, M. & Yamada, M. (2004). Significance of ¹²³I-MIBG scintigraphy as a pathophysiological indicator in the assessment of Parkinson's disease and related disorders: It can be a specific marker for Lewy body disease. *Annals of Nuclear Medicine*, Vol. 18, pp. 453-461, ISSN 0914-7187

Wafelman, A.R., Hoefnagel, C.A. & Maes, R.A. (1994). Radioiodinated metaiodobenzylguanidine: A review of its biodistribution and pharmacokinetics, drug interactions, cytotoxicity and dosimetry. *European Journal of Nuclear Medicine*, Vol. 21, pp. 545-559, ISSN 0340-6997

Wakabayashi, K. & Takahashi, H. (1997). Neuropathology of autonomic nervous system in Parkinson's disease. *European Neurology*, Vol. 38, Suppl 2:2-7, ISSN 0014-3022

Watanabe, H., Ieda, T. & Katayama, T. (2001). Cardiac ¹²³I-meta-iodobenzylguanidine (MIBG) uptake in dementia with Lewy bodies: Comparison with Alzheimer's disease. *Journal of Neurology, Neurosurgery, and Psychiatry*, Vol. 70, pp.781-783, ISSN 0022-3050

Wenning, G.K., Tison, F. & Ben Shlomo, Y. (1997). Multiple system atrophy: A review of 203 pathologically proven cases. *Movement Disorders*, Vol. 12, pp. 133-147, ISSN 0885-3185

Wieland, D.M., Brown, L.E. & Rogers, W.L. (1981). Myocardial imaging with a radioiodinated norepinephrine storage analog. *Journal of Nuclear Medicine*, Vol. 22, pp. 22-31, ISSN 0161-5505

Yoshita, M. (1998). Differentiation of idiopathic Parkinson's disease from striatonigral degeneration and progressive supranuclear palsy using iodine-123 meta-iodobenzylguanidine myocardial scintigraphy. *Journal of Neurological Sciences,* Vol. 155, pp. 60-67, ISSN 0022-510X

Yoritaka, A., Shimo, Y. & Shimo, Y. (2011). Nonmotor symptoms in patients with PARK2 mutations. *Parkinson's Disease,* Vol. 2011, pp. 1-5, ISSN 2042-0080

Yoshita, M., Taki, J. & Yamada, M. (2001). A clinical role for ^{123}I-MIBG myocardial scintigraphy in the distinction between dementia of the Alzheimer's-type and dementia with Lewy bodies. *Journal of Neurology, Neurosurgery, and Psychiatry,* Vol. 71, pp. 583-588, ISSN 0022-3050

Permissions

The contributors of this book come from diverse backgrounds, making this book a truly international effort. This book will bring forth new frontiers with its revolutionizing research information and detailed analysis of the nascent developments around the world.

We would like to thank Dr. Juliana Dushanova, for lending her expertise to make the book truly unique. She has played a crucial role in the development of this book. Without her invaluable contribution this book wouldn't have been possible. She has made vital efforts to compile up to date information on the varied aspects of this subject to make this book a valuable addition to the collection of many professionals and students.

This book was conceptualized with the vision of imparting up-to-date information and advanced data in this field. To ensure the same, a matchless editorial board was set up. Every individual on the board went through rigorous rounds of assessment to prove their worth. After which they invested a large part of their time researching and compiling the most relevant data for our readers. Conferences and sessions were held from time to time between the editorial board and the contributing authors to present the data in the most comprehensible form. The editorial team has worked tirelessly to provide valuable and valid information to help people across the globe.

Every chapter published in this book has been scrutinized by our experts. Their significance has been extensively debated. The topics covered herein carry significant findings which will fuel the growth of the discipline. They may even be implemented as practical applications or may be referred to as a beginning point for another development. Chapters in this book were first published by InTech; hereby published with permission under the Creative Commons Attribution License or equivalent.

The editorial board has been involved in producing this book since its inception. They have spent rigorous hours researching and exploring the diverse topics which have resulted in the successful publishing of this book. They have passed on their knowledge of decades through this book. To expedite this challenging task, the publisher supported the team at every step. A small team of assistant editors was also appointed to further simplify the editing procedure and attain best results for the readers.

Our editorial team has been hand-picked from every corner of the world. Their multi-ethnicity adds dynamic inputs to the discussions which result in innovative outcomes. These outcomes are then further discussed with the researchers and contributors who give their valuable feedback and opinion regarding the same. The feedback is then collaborated with the researches and they are edited in a comprehensive manner to aid the understanding of the subject.

Apart from the editorial board, the designing team has also invested a significant amount of their time in understanding the subject and creating the most relevant covers. They scrutinized every image to scout for the most suitable representation of the subject and create an appropriate cover for the book.

The publishing team has been involved in this book since its early stages. They were actively engaged in every process, be it collecting the data, connecting with the contributors or procuring relevant information. The team has been an ardent support to the editorial, designing and production team. Their endless efforts to recruit the best for this project, has resulted in the accomplishment of this book. They are a veteran in the field of academics and their pool of knowledge is as vast as their experience in printing. Their expertise and guidance has proved useful at every step. Their uncompromising quality standards have made this book an exceptional effort. Their encouragement from time to time has been an inspiration for everyone.

The publisher and the editorial board hope that this book will prove to be a valuable piece of knowledge for researchers, students, practitioners and scholars across the globe.

List of Contributors

Jorge Diaz
INSERM UMR-894, Psychiatry and Neurosciences Center, Paris, France
Paris Descartes University, Faculty of Pharmacy / Laboratory of Neurobiology and Molecular Pharmacology (UMRs894 INSERM), Paris, France

Renaud Massart
INSERM UMR-894, Psychiatry and Neurosciences Center, Paris, France

Pierre Sokoloff
Pierre Fabre Research Institute, Neurology and Psychiatry Department, Castres, France

Louise M. Collins, André Toulouse and Yvonne M. Nolan
Department of Anatomy and Neuroscience, University College Cork, Ireland

Marlene Jimenez-Del-Rio and Carlos Velez-Pardo
School of Medicine, Medical Research Institute, Neuroscience Research Group, University of Antioquia, Medellin, Colombia

Hassan Niknejad
Nano medicine and Tissue Engineering Research Center, Shahid Beheshti University of Medical Sciences, Tehran, Iran

Emma Thornton and Robert Vink
University of Adelaide, Australia

Shigeru Takasaki
Toyo University, Izumino 1-1-1, Ora-gun Itakuracho, Gunma, Japan

Amal Alachkar
University of Aleppo, Syria

Luca Ferraro, Tiziana Antonelli, Sarah Beggiato, Maria Cristina Tomasini, Antonio Steardo and Sergio Tanganelli
Department of Clinical and Experimental Medicine, Section of Pharmacology, University of Ferrara, Italy and IRET Foundation, Ozzano Emilia, Bologna, Italy

Kjell Fuxe
Department of Neuroscience, Karolinska Institute, Stockholm, Sweden

Masahiko Suzuki
Department of Neurology, the Jikei University School of Medicine, Aoto Hospital, Tokyo, Japan